A Miracle
and
A Privilege

RECOUNTING A HALF CENTURY
OF SURGICAL ADVANCE

Francis D. Moore, M.D.

JOSEPH HENRY PRESS
Washington, D.C.   1995

JOSEPH HENRY PRESS • 2101 Constitution Avenue, N.W. • Washington, D.C. 20418

The Joseph Henry Press, an imprint of the National Academy Press, was created with the goal of making books on science, technology, and health more widely available to professionals and the public. Joseph Henry was one of the founders of the National Academy of Sciences and a leader of early American science.

Library of Congress Cataloging-in-Publication Data

Moore, Francis D. (Francis Daniels), 1913-
    A miracle and a privilege : recounting a half century of surgical advance / Francis Daniels Moore.
        p.   cm.
    Includes bibliographical references and index.
    ISBN 0-309-05188-6(alk. paper)
    1. Moore, Francis D. (Francis Daniels), 1913- . 2. Surgeons—
United States—Biography. I. Title.
    [DNLM: 1. Moore, Francis D. (Francis Daniels), 1913-
2. Surgery—personal narratives. WZ 100 <8185 1995]
RD27.35.M6496A3   1995
617′.092—dc20
[B]
DNLM/DLC
for Library of Congress   95-1645
                                                                                CIP

Cover photo: FDM assisting Robin Goodfellow at an operation in 1974. Goodfellow was the first woman appointed Chief Resident Surgeon at the Brigham and one of the first women to occupy such a position at any of the Harvard teaching hospitals.

Printed in the United States of America

To Laura and Katharyn

Be not slow to visit the sick.
Ecclesiasticus 7:35

Contents

Preface

My surgical experience as a child was confined to appendicitis at age 12 and a fractured knee at 14. After the appendix operation, my rowdy friends came to call, and we got to laughing. It hurt. Surgery. As for the knee, maybe that carried some sort of an academic message, because Frederick Christopher, a surgeon of Winnetka, thought my fractured knee was unusual (as I was certain, of course, that it was). It was depicted in his *Textbook of Minor Surgery*. Impressive. I still have the volume as a memorial to my adolescent trauma.

In 1933 as a sophomore in college, I decided to apply for admission to medical school. As a third-year medical student in 1937 I resolved to try for a surgical internship and started out as a fledgling surgeon on July 1, 1939. Just halfway between those two decisions, in June 1935, Laura Bartlett and I were married.

My decisions to enter medicine as a profession and the field of surgery as a calling had at least some basis in my childhood experiences. Although there were no physicians on either side of my family as far back as we could trace, I enjoyed science and especially biological science. As a child I had the privilege of being the patient of several remarkable doctors, two of them surgeons. Surgery was probably the inevitable choice, as I enjoyed a certain degree of manual dexterity, whether it be playing the piano or tinkering in the tool shop. Being by nature more a participant than an observer, I favored the interventionist mode as an approach to human illness. With regard to the decision for marriage, Laurie and I had attended school together. As college graduation approached, our mutual chemistry of attraction naturally led to marriage. In those days that was the only acceptable way to consummate our desire.

This is the story of a privileged childhood, of wonderful years at school and college, of working as a surgeon for more than half of this century, and of living with a remarkable family for four-fifths of it. For me as a surgeon in a university and its teaching hospitals, and later as professor and department head, teaching and research have always been a prominent part of my life. During these years there has been a massive increase in the scope and effectiveness of biomedical science and of surgery. Our research played a role in that growth. The central theme of this book is surgery in an era of change.

Now entering my ninth decade and approaching the end of both this century and this life, I look back on a satisfying career and a spate of extraordinary happenings. I have enjoyed writing these stories, both of my own experiences and of a revolution in the science of human biology and the art of surgery. For many readers born before 1950, these matters may have a familiar timbre. For others—especially those of a younger generation—these tales may be mere bits of ancient life, or history retold.

This account would be incomplete without telling of individual patients, whose stories are strong threads woven into the fabric of a surgeon's life. Many of these stories are of patients (often under fictitious names) who lived despite severe challenge. A surgeon sees much of life. Wonderful, joyous, human life. And hopes to ensure a few more good years for many people.

There are also stories here of death. A surgeon caring for the seriously ill or injured, for cancer, sees much of death. A man who lost his wife after 53 years of wonderful marriage cannot help but consider the meaning of death. And now, there is an urgent need to ease the end along for some who are facing painful and hopeless illness.

All these tales are of medical, surgical, and scientific friends, leaders, stars; and of the family that decorated my life.

F.D.M.
Boston, Massachusetts
April, 1995

Acknowledgments

I am deeply indebted to friends and family who have stuck with me faithfully through the conception and gestation of this book. Laurie went over some of the earlier stories with me, and Katharyn has been over the whole book in its later stages, offering much helpful advice.

Four faithful readers have helped mold and organize the book in detail. I am grateful to Fisher Howe III, former Foreign Service Officer, currently consultant on funding for nonprofit organizations; Henry Saltonstall, surgeon of Exeter, New Hampshire; Leroy D. Vandam, Professor Emeritus of Anaesthesia at Harvard, our staff anesthetist for 26 years; and Charles F. Haas, classmate and Hollywood author producer. All are familiar with many of the happenings, stories, and people of this book.

I am also indebted to colleagues at the Brigham, Harvard, and other institutions who have made contributions and detailed suggestions. These include Marcia Angell, Clyde Barker, Robert Bartlett, Saul Benison, Donald Brief, E. Langdon Burwell, Sir Roy Calne, Andrea Chambers, John Collins, James Dalen, Robert Demling, Lewis Dexter, Ben Eiseman, Dwight Harken, John Howard, Richard Lower, John Mannick, Robert Mayer, Anthony Monaco, Joseph Murray, John Najarian, Israel Penn, Lucie Prinz, Steven Rosenberg, Jay Sanford, Richard Shemin, Thomas Starzl, Judith Swazey, Richard Warren, Douglas Wilmore, and Lawrence Zaroff. Richard Wolfe, Curator of Rare Books and Manuscripts at the

Countway Library, opened his collection generously for reference and illustrations. John Dusseau, formerly editor at WB Saunders, who assisted with two of my previous books, has generously given advice on this one.

For retrieval of archival pictures from the medical school and the hospital, I am indebted to Madeleine Mullin and Susan Berg; for photographic reproduction of slides and illustrations, to Ken Bates; and for aerial photography of the hospital and the medical school, to Joseph Melanson of Wareham, Massachusetts.

Scott Lubeck, Director, and Stephen Mautner, Executive Editor, and their staff at the Joseph Henry Press have been responsive and helpful throughout the production of a finshed book from the original manuscript.

Dr. Oglesby Paul, author of several medical biographies, gave me experienced help. To Diane Q. Forti, medical editor extraordinaire, I am indebted for her detailed suggestions throughout the book. Susan Lang Cramer contributed her skills abundantly as both editor and typist through the long period of preparation and revision of this manuscript. To all, I am most grateful.

A Miracle
and
A Privilege

BOOK ONE

Student of Man

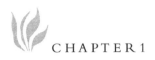

CHAPTER 1

Medical Student

(1935-1939)

Getting acquainted with the human body is the first task of the medical student. As it was 60 years ago, so it is (or should be) today. Learning how this awe-inspiring and remarkably intricate piece of machinery is assembled—how it works, its control and communication systems, and its central programming—occupied the full attention of the 120 young men (my classmates) as we dissected our first cadavers in the marble quadrangle of the Harvard Medical School. We had begun our journey toward a medical career. It was September 1935.

For any medical student, that first close-up view of a dead person is shocking, startling, and sometimes upsetting. But even when you have become accustomed to that inglorious, lifeless carcass as a suitable object for close examination, any sense of beauty or worship requires a bit of imagination, of sublimation. The object of our anatomical researches bore little resemblance to the real beauty of a living being. Brown, dried out, smelling strongly of formaldehyde, this cold, stiff flesh retained little that could be recognized as the fabric of man.

For me and many of my colleagues, this task of dissecting a human body also served as our introduction to surgery. Taking in our unskilled hands the ancient tools of sharp scalpel and grasping forceps we gently, at first gingerly, at times clumsily, exposed the inner workings to our view, with as much excitement as did those first Paduan anatomists

3

400 years before. These inner workings were to be the focus of our attention, one way or another, for about 50 years, the expectable career of most doctors. As we began to learn more, the beauty and efficiency of the body's exquisite structure and organization would impress us and the impact of that knowledge would never leave us.

In those first few months we also studied physiology and biochemistry, the function of the human body. In the laboratory these functions were reduced to chemical assays, such as salts in the blood, protein in the plasma, urea in the urine. The minutiae of scientific reductionism. As we had with the cadaver, we carried out these analyses with our own two hands, breaking a lot of glassware as we went along. We tangled up or snapped the connections of elaborate and expensive devices used to analyze gases such as oxygen, carbon dioxide, nitrogen, and hydrogen in the blood. These baffling apparati were named after their inventors, Van Slyke or Haldane. Until we had mastered the procedures and ultimately recognized the genius of those inventive scientists, we daily cursed the devilish intricacy of their inventions. To understand the meaning of these measurements demanded a bit of imagination, lofty conceptualization, and, again, sublimation. In time we learned to appreciate these matters as examples of the magnificently sensitive chemical and physiological adjustments of lung, brain, heart, gut, liver, and kidney—the organs that keep us alive.

Dr. Robert Green, our Professor of Anatomy, was an obstetrician by trade, a classical scholar in his spare time, and an orator-actor at heart. Great stuff for a teacher of anatomy. Affectionately known as Bobby Green, he encouraged us to learn enough so we could add to the Roman platitude, "Nihil humanum mihi alienum est" ("Nothing human is foreign to me"), an additional assertion: " .. et nihil anatomicum." Thus we should strive always to improve our knowledge of anatomy through the decades ahead.

Huddled in groups of four around this dead bit of humankind, we dissected, made drawings, learned names and terms, and tried to reconcile what we saw with what was depicted in the textbook propped up on the bench nearby. John Adams, Guy Hayes, and Charlie Mixter were my dissection team-mates. Guy Hayes was to become a director of the international division of the Rockefeller Foundation and accomplish great works, particularly the foundation of the medical school in Cali, Colombia. The rest of us were destined to become surgeons. Charlie Mixter and I would remain in Boston while John Adams became Professor of Neurological Surgery at the University of California, San Francisco.

The work was demanding and the hours as long as we wanted to make them. When we finished our anatomy course in January of 1936, we had in our minds at least a précis of human anatomy, that interwoven collection of structures that Andreas Vesalius had termed the "Fabrick of Man" in 1543. Although large gaps in our knowledge of anatomy remained, we retained at least a few details until the final examination and even a bit thereafter. We had spent four solid months in this concentrated effort.

How did he die, that person to whose remains we devoted so much attention? How did he live? Intuitively we did not consider the answers to those questions. The cadaver attended by our laboratory neighbors had a bullet lodged in the heart. But we found no such clues. A certain amount of austere impersonality and disconnectedness is probably best in this initial attempt to understand the fabric before we try to treat its tears or patch its holes.

Bobby Green had reworded another platitude. He taught us not to say, "I am a body, I have a soul," rather, "I am a soul, I live in a body." This put human anatomy where it belongs, as the structure that serves as a dwelling place. Injury and disease can so destroy that warm dwelling place that it is no longer habitable, and the dweller—energy, mind, and soul—had best be permitted to depart.

We learned, as does every novice looking for the first time at the organization of the human brain, that the brain, despite its structural difference from all other organs and its additional complexity, is also but a dwelling place. This ultimate computer houses the thinking, cognitive mind. We know the mind is there because it communicates with us. Without its dwelling place or when its machinery ceases, when it ceases to convert energy into thought and ceases to communicate, the mind ceases its function and, as with the rest of the resident, no longer lives there.

Some consider the soul a religious concept, others a literary metaphor. However you define it, the soul is a transcendental entity tethered more to the mind than to the brain. Without embracing any concepts of immortality, I have always interpreted the soul as an epiphenomenon of the mind that requires an observer, a "third party," for its validation and to achieve reality. Just as the mind is an expansion of the brain, so also the soul is an extension, an expression, of the mind. This became part of our emerging picture of that former person and, by extension, the thousands of patients we would care for over the five decades ahead. Our job would be to keep their dwelling places suitable for habitation.

So here we were in the very first weeks of our courses, just setting out on our study of anatomy, physiology, and biochemistry, already beginning to think about the mind–body dualism. This might seem presumptuous for rank neophytes, a matter that has challenged the most profound philosophers for centuries and most advanced neurochemists for decades.

That's just how it was. These concerns are inescapable in your first encounter with the basic human via the body and its workings. As beginning students of human biology we could not avoid considering (though often privately, personally) these issues of body, mind, and soul. We found ourselves thinking about them right from the start. If you plan to help maintain that dwelling place intact by treating injured or threatened people, these concerns become very important and practical. One question that would engage us many years later was, Could we, by treatment, keep the dwelling place warm and alive too long?

Maybe it seems a long transit from the dross of a preserved carcass to these transcendent musings. But it was exhilarating to be starting out on this pathway. What a prospect lay ahead!

Sometimes we found it hard to philosophize very much on those waning afternoons, as the New England twilight turned to darkness in the late fall, the leaves gone by. We would put down our instruments, take off our lab coats, and don our jackets. I, for one, wanted to get away from that smelly place and back to the apartment to see my bride, Laurie. Maybe the next day was a Saturday and we could get a ticket to the game. Or we might "spread it" and go out for supper in Chinatown.

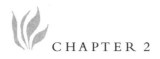

CHAPTER 2

Harvard Medical School in the 1930s

The Harvard Medical School of 1935 was uncluttered and straight-forward: proud, even splendid, in its simplicity. It had been pursuing a straight-line development in the teaching of college graduates to become physicians, a clear continuity of concept and curriculum dating back to its origin as the Medical Faculty of Harvard College in 1782. It had emerged from its miserable nineteenth century trough of mediocrity as a diploma factory, rescued by President Charles W. Eliot when, about 1870, he introduced entrance examinations and a final measure of achievement leading to the M.D. degree.

In 1935 the Harvard Medical School was still a simple graduate school. There was neither government nor corporate funding to speak of. Tuition was $400 per annum. The science was solid but not static, challenging but not arcane. Patients were looked after in a two-tiered system with charity wards for the care of the poor and for the teaching of students, interns, and residents, while the fancier private wings offered a more elegant version of hospital care with lots of amenities, private nurses, fancy accommodations, the operative hand (and fees) of senior staff only, and flowers on the breakfast tray.

In 1935 such matters as understanding human disease in terms of molecular mechanisms, looking for the responsible gene or its absence, still lay far in the future. Massive federal financing of research was not even a dream. And at the same time, such nightmares as a plague of malpractice suits, open-ended government payment systems leading to excessive billing, paperwork by the forestful, insurance companies telling physicians what to do, were unheard of. Changes such as these were to start with a rush after World War II.

The tax-supported city and county hospitals were the charity hospitals of the time. The Boston City Hospital was a prime example. The university hospitals, particularly those of the middle west, were coming into their own as unique institutions where the state owned both medical school and hospital. While these institutions contained charity beds reserved for the care of residents of their own states, private patients were also cared for. The ancient, privately endowed, trustee-operated, university-affiliated hospitals of the eastern cities and a few to the west and south (Chicago, New Orleans, San Francisco) seemed to dominate the quest for excellence. They set the standard for care and creativity.

In private as well as university hospitals many patients were cared for as a charitable enterprise. Few physicians were paid to give medical care to charity patients, surely not the interns and residents, most of whom received meager salaries of up to $25 a month or nothing at all. Even in those days such a pittance scarcely covered carfare or cigarettes. Reward to interns and residents took the form not of cash, but rather of the prestige of appointment, the privilege of teaching, the opportunity for research, and above all, the eventual possibility of being appointed to the staff. The Harvard Medical School was affiliated with no fewer than seven major hospitals, most of them private and trustee-governed. The Boston City and the Boston Psychopathic were the only exceptions.

The Harvard Medical School was serene, even complacent, in its social view. At Harvard College there was a beginning stir about inequities in the medical care system. The Committee on Costs of Medical Care had first published its report in 1929 at the University of Chicago. Fifteen years before this the Flexner Report on the State of Medical Education, critical of many medical schools and hospitals as being little more than tuition-hungry factories churning out diplomas, had also criticized the Harvard teaching hospitals because of their seeming commitment to community service rather than the advancement of learning. In 1935 the Harvard Medical School and its faculty careened (or serened) along, brilliant professors leading the way, students' families scratching up pennies for tuition, the faculty secure in their practice and university work. Secure, but less than prosperous.

A Married Student

For Laurie and me, existence was idyllic. From our apartment on Longwood Avenue, only a block from the medical school, we looked out on a scene of a few low buildings and quite a few open lots. Now this vista is filled with hospital skyscrapers and research towers. Across from us, in an old wooden tenement, lived a dark-complected, mustachioed Italian who tended his garden and, with a special pride, harvested his tomatoes in August. He gave us some. Our automobile could be parked at the curb 24 hours a day. Because we had bought our first car on our Wyoming honeymoon, it bore a Wyoming license plate that began with the number 3. This showed it was from Sheridan County. So, periodically, people would come up the stairs knocking at our door looking for "the people from Sheridan," and we would talk about mutual friends.

I probably thought I was working pretty hard. Each student was given a box of bones to take home so he could study some hard-core anatomy. One evening as I took the box out from under the bed and started to pore over these bones, Laurie, rarely querulous or skeptical, said, "Alright, Moorie, let's take the bones back to the morgue."

At Harvard College our class consisted of about 1,000 young men, largely drawn from the eastern part of the country. Our class was a moderate, middle-of-the road group of congenial students, many of whom became lifelong friends. Only later did we learn—and then rather inadvertently—that our college class was hardly a hand-picked group! We had been admitted in 1931 during the steep economic downswing after the 1929 crash that was to lead to the depths of the Depression. Applicants to Harvard College in those days were not very numerous. There were not as many scholarships as now and many families couldn't afford college. In 1931 every single applicant to Harvard College had been admitted. That was us.

Our Harvard Medical School class was filled with brilliant people. Many would later become leaders at medical schools all over the country or research scientists or both. We were a small but interesting group, intentionally drawn from all parts of this country and a few foreign countries. Only a few of us came from monied or privileged families. We represented all economic groups, large towns, small towns, large colleges, small colleges. A stimulating mix. But there were no women. Harvard Medical School did not inaugurate coeducation until about 10 years later, admitting its first women in the class that entered in 1945.

Science for Beginners

The medical school curriculum is totally new to most incoming students. All have taken some chemistry at college and even some courses in the chemistry of living organisms (organic chemistry and biological chemistry). The rest is new. The underlying chemical reactions of disease, medical biochemistry, are new to every student. Many have studied some sort of physiology, especially in their biology and zoology courses at college, and have some idea of how the heart works, the structure of muscles, the function of endocrine glands. They may have dissected a frog, a dogfish, or even worked up to the pinnacle complexity of a cat. But the detailed study of human anatomy, of microbiology (the study of bacteria and viruses), and above all, of pathology is totally new to these young minds fresh from college. It is fascinating to watch bright young people with inquisitive minds as they grapple with scientific concepts with which they have had no prior experience.

The most spectacular of the preclinical sciences, and the newest to us, was human pathology, the science of understanding human disease. It is largely descriptive. Phenomenology. Pathology examines how disease has changed cells, tissues, organs, and how those changes came about. Pathology is the science that underlies every detail of clinical medicine, surgery, and pediatrics. It has always been taught by the examination of diseased tissues as seen by the unaided eye or through the microscope. In our time this subject occupied the entire second year of medical school.

Of major importance in the development of this knowledge, and in teaching pathology, is the examination of the recently deceased by the autopsy. For the medical student, the first autopsy can be an emotional experience (like that first cadaver) as well as a scientific milestone. We

10

were required to attend several autopsies. There were many euphemisms or hospital double-talk for patients who had died. Some were referred to as having been "transferred to Ward X" or "sent to Allen Street," that being the street behind the Massachusetts General Hospital where the hearses came to call. When an autopsy was imminent, such lingo was used to post the event on a bulletin board at the medical school. My first autopsy, that of a patient I had tried to help a few days before, proved to be more of a wrench than the first cadaver in the anatomy course. Again, it became essential for us as proto-physicians to remain disconnected.

Exposure to these new fields of human thought may be exciting, stimulating, and exhausting, but for some it can also be frightening, overwhelming, and discouraging. Happily, I found myself in the first group. I loved it, was thrilled by it all, considered each new field as a possible and attractive career, and was not overwhelmed, overburdened, or assaulted by this mass of learning.

Visiting the Sick

Ecclesiasticus advises us, "Be not slow to visit the sick." We began to follow this biblical admonition in our second and third years. I remember the first patient I saw in outpatient medicine, a third-year course we took at the Beth Israel Hospital. Three of us met together to talk with her and carry out a physical examination under the watchful eye of our instructor, Dr. Benjamin Banks. Her name was Mrs. Szintax. The three of us, a bit nervous, stood out in the hall with the instructor, while the nurse tended to the proper accoutrement of the patient: the usual immodest hospital johnny with a little extra covering. The nurse was slow. A bit nervous herself. Dr. Banks becoming restless (looking at his watch), opened the curtain a bit and said, "Are you ready, Mrs. Szintax?"

He used the tone usually reserved for a frightened child at Halloween, about to be assaulted by a team of hobgoblins. "Are you ready, Mrs. Szintax?" became a sort of jocular greeting that we used for years, remembering that very sober moment with our first patient, and Dr. Banks trying to put her at ease.

I remember Mrs. Szintax clearly because she later became my patient. I saw her periodically, operated on her, and some years later she

11

sent her daughter to me as a patient. I am very proud of the confidence she placed in me as a mere beginner. It is with fondness and respect that I remember that first moment in the autumn of 1937. In a manner of speaking, Mrs. Szintax was my first patient.

American medical students meet patients very early in their education. That it is possible for immature students to meet patients is one of the miracles of modern American medical education. In many other countries, the medical schools are too big for this sort of instruction so early in the curriculum; the European tradition sees the beginning medical student as a rowdy tramp (often intoxicated) yet to be civilized, not a person for whom such doors are to be opened.

Sometime during the first year, and possibly even during the first month or first week, the American medical student, clad perhaps for the first time in a white coat, will confront a sick and often apprehensive patient. The patient is apt to assume that the examiner is a physician. We were leery of this and took pains to tell the patient frankly that we were nothing but medical students. Most patients examined by students or whose care is discussed with students welcome this, both in the hope that it may help them and in the assurance that it will help others. The student's humanity and human empathy are here given their first opportunity for display. Some students came to it naturally, others slowly, and still others, never. This relationship of patient with student was simple, straightforward. It was unquestioned. It gave us our first contact with sick people.

On District

In addition to those notable early visits with hospital patients, we were each required to deliver 12 babies "on District" (i.e., at the patient's home). Because of some happenstance, possibly the illness of an upperclassman, four of us were assigned to District at the end of our second year, rather than the third year. "District" was a term for a way of life for mothers, babies, and students in obstetrics, stretching back into the early nineteenth century, and within a few years to be swept away by Modern Medical Care. Medical students (externes) were assigned an area of Boston (a district) in which, under the watchful eye of first-year house officers (internes) from the obstetrical hospital (the Boston Lying-In), they were to deliver the babies of very poor women.

Here was the bottommost layer of two-tiered medicine, carried to its extreme. No anesthesia. Instruments sterilized by boiling on a gas stove (unless the gas company had turned it off). These settings did not always display the loftiest of home life. There might be a single dangling electric bulb (again, assuming bills paid). A husband sometimes drunk. I remember on one occasion where the sniffling, dirty, measly children were huddled bug-eyed on a bed in the only other room, sneaking a door-crack preview of the advent of a new brother or sister, the young mother, grunting, panting, sometimes crying out, cussing the children, telling them to shut the door. She had been there before. Between uterine contractions she often told the sweating young externe what to do next.

After the slippery but perfect little neophyte slides out in a sudden rush, "Now you tie the cord and cut it," the mother says. Then the placenta. Then clean up. Maybe glasses of Chianti all around from a straw-covered bottle. Another member added to a family already unable to enjoy the richness of their wonderful and rapidly growing brood because of the worry of caring for them.

In case of trouble during labor, our instructions were to give the husband a nickel. He was to go to a pay phone and call the interne, who would drive over to help us in his rickety jalopy, or maybe take the streetcar. Leisurely assistance.

I delivered the requisite 12 such babies. On two occasions I dispensed with the leisurely arrival of help and told the husband to call an ambulance to take his wife to the hospital immediately. One was a patient who had an epileptic convulsion while I was boiling up the kit on the stove. Not for a home delivery! The other patient looked sick when I first entered her room. Her ankles were swollen and her color a bit blue. Even to my second-year ear the telltale soft rumbling heart murmur of a narrowed mitral valve was detectable. Then she told me that she had been an outpatient at House of the Good Samaritan. This was a hospital devoted to the care—often terminal—of young people with rheumatic heart disease such as hers. I knew that there was a good chance this woman might die in labor. After her arrival at the hospital by ambulance she was delivered by cesarean. I felt exonerated for my caution. The senior obstetrician grumbled that I had done a good job and that the system—which should have identified such a high-risk mother—had failed.

In addition to the discouraging derelicts, we saw some joyous members of our civilization out there in the slums, on District. One woman I recall particularly. She lived on Gold Street, then the most squalid street in South Boston. But her little apartment was spotlessly clean. Her few sticks of furniture were carefully placed on a clean floor, tiny pictures were arranged on the wall, a rusty old third-hand refrigerator, neat and clean inside. She was well-spoken, of dark brunette Irish beauty. When I went to see her and the baby a few days later (as we were supposed to do), she thanked me and gave me a prized silver dollar. This was the first money I had ever earned from a patient, and it was a gift at that. I had it framed. Years later it still hung on the wall of my office and I often told its story to interested visitors. Then one night it disappeared. Someone, I do not know who, saw the dollar, broke the glass, and stole it. Of such petty greed is one thread woven into the fabric of man.

A Medical Faculty

The faculty of the Harvard Medical School included (then, as now) several figures of world renown. They were immensely impressive and inspiring to us. Walter Cannon elucidated the function of the autonomic nervous system. He showed by his experimental work that the mind and body work together, that fright, hunger, anger, produce bodily changes. Why are people still puzzled and amazed to find that mind and body work together? Why must we suffer the expensive rhetoric of Eastern cults and wealthy gurus to understand this? Walter Cannon taught us physiology. As a senior professor he met regularly with the most junior students and in small groups. A wonderfully human and inspiring figure.

Hans Zinsser was one of the great bacteriologists of his day, a dynamic ego, lecturer, and writer (*Rats, Lice and History*) and autobiographer (*As I Remember Him*). Zinsser was a showman, but he could show real accomplishment and we enjoyed his showy lectures. One of the young members of his department was John Enders, who was awarded the Nobel Prize 20 years later for discovering how to culture the poliomyelitis virus, making it possible for Salk and Sabin to develop vaccines. In so doing Enders helped to wipe out a major disease of mankind in his lifetime. John Enders sat with the other members of the department in the front row of each of Professor Zinsser's lectures. All the faculty in that department were assigned to this sometimes hard duty. In later years, I often wondered what John Enders thought when Zinsser voiced his doubt that a vaccine against poliomyelitis would ever be possible. Later on, through other circumstances, John Enders became a close friend of mine (though 15 years older), adviser, and role model.

A. Baird Hastings was a leading biochemist, who brought arcane chemical methods to bear on clinical medicine. Now, they are all commonplace. He had a strong impact on me, as I later tried to bring quantitative chemistry to the study of surgical convalescence and the care of surgical illness. A few years later, as a young surgical instructor, I was asked by Baird Hastings to give clinics for the whole first-year class in their biochemistry course, discussing some surgical problems (hemorrhage, shock, fracture, infection) to demonstrate how biochemical understanding underlies many aspects of surgical care and how prompt and skillful surgical operation can minimize complications and metabolic burdens during convalescence.

On the clinical side, our professors of medicine and surgery were also prominent not only in Boston, but over the world. During World War II the care of all the wounded American soldiers in the European theater was supervised by one of our professors of surgery, Elliott Cutler, later promoted to brigadier general. Military surgery in the Mediterranean theater was under the leadership of Edward D. Churchill, another professor of surgery, and later my boss at the Massachusetts General. It is not generally known that the care of our wounded in both the European and the Mediterranean theaters was guided by these two fellow professors of surgery from the Harvard Medical School. Cutler was our principal teacher at the Peter Bent Brigham, as was Churchill at the Massachusetts General. Both men were deeply imprinted on our class and contributed to its apparent bias toward surgery. To observe and assist such men as these while they were operating, to hear them think out loud, and to gather a little of their skill and their philosophy was an immense privilege.

In internal medicine few exceeded Fuller Albright and Soma

Weiss in their influence on our class. Albright was an endocrinologist, the prototypical clinical investigator, who showed the world about metabolic bone disease and hyperparathyroidism (in which the parathyroid glands are overactive). He showed us both the joy and the effectiveness of his researches in the care of the sick, translating their sometimes subtle message into everyday practical experience. Soma Weiss was the brilliant Hungarian clinician who led us through the intricate mysteries of diseases of the heart and blood vessels. He died at an early age. While on an airplane he had a sudden severe headache, recognized the ominous symptoms, made his own diagnosis of a brain hemorrhage, knew the prognosis, and died a few days later at the age of 42. I still quote his teachings. His widow remains a close friend.

College students also teach each other. They influence each other strongly. In medical school the influence is even stronger. The impact of each student on the thought and learning of fellow students is often more crucial than the knowledge imparted by learned professors. Not only is it group learning, it is group teaching. Physiology and biochemistry were often taught with students working in groups or teams. Students often saw patients together, one or two students interviewing or examining a patient (such as Mrs. Szintax) and talking to the patient's family. We carried out minor operations together in the outpatient department or stitched up cuts and lacerations. The influence we had on each other was so much a part of the educational process that now, in retrospect, it is almost impossible to distinguish it from the impact of the faculty.

Student Research

Research was a key component of our medical education because our teachers were deeply involved in the biomedical sciences. Many of them were guilty of talking too much about their research when they should have been talking about broader issues. But the research of these men was usually at the cutting edge of thought anyway, so it was not too distracting.

Participation in research is now a requirement at many medical schools. While this was not so in the 1930s, doors were opened and research was made possible. In our second and third years Bill Carleton and I carried out a research study that occupied Sundays and holidays for many months. We were studying the dramatic and abrupt fall in a certain pregnancy hormone that disappeared from the mother soon after delivery. The source of this hormone was unknown, but its absence a few days after delivery suggested that the hormone (present during pregnancy in huge amounts) arose either in the placenta or in the infant. We discovered that the infant's urine showed almost none of this hormone, ruling out the baby as its source. If the hormone came from the placenta, its secretory rate would fall to zero very rapidly when the placenta was expelled from the mother's body at the time of birth. We showed, by documenting the exact rate of the hormone's disappearance after delivery, that the placenta had to be the source. The hormone was all gone in about 2 hours. Such a finding had not been previously recorded.

Our wives had served as the subjects of this research at the time of the birth of our children, so we had lots of cooperation in collecting the urine samples! While our findings were original and conclusions correct, this research was never published. Based on too few cases. It taught us a lot of things about research, how mistakes could be made and how hard it is to do it right. It also showed that simple theories could be sound, and research was the way to elucidate them. Other students in our class carried out research that was more telling and soon published.

Another bit of my research was more historical than scientific. The Boylston Medical Society was an undergraduate group that required a member to give a talk at one of the meetings. It is said to be the oldest medical society in the western hemisphere (founded 1811). I had become interested in Civil War surgery. During spring vacation of our third year (1938), Laurie and I borrowed an old book of photos by Matthew Brady and took off to drive over some of the battlefields. We visited Chancellorsville, Fredericksburg, and the Wilderness, all within one area of Northern Virginia. We stood where Brady seemed to have had his camera, and we took pictures to show the same scenes 70 years later. The sunken road at Fredericksburg, the Inn at Chancellorsville. They bore a strong resemblance to Brady's gruesome scenes right after the battles. No more corpses. But even some of the small trees were recognizable. Bigger, now. Today those same scenes have weathered 130 years since their epic battles.

We visited Richmond where a classmate, Dan Ellis, showed us the Confederate Museum with its store of medical records and memorabilia. By a curious coincidence we were invited to a small dinner given for Douglas Southall Freeman, the author of Robert E. Lee's biography and *Lee's Lieutenants*. Freeman was a famous patriarch of the history of the War Between the States. It was a great privilege for Laurie and me to dine with him on our visit to the battlefields.

When we returned from Virginia, I presented my paper on Civil War surgery before the Boylston Medical Society. I asked two senior surgeons whose fathers had been surgeons in that war—Dr. John Homans and Dr. Thaddeus Stevens—to discuss my paper. I showed the pictures and told of the accounts of treating the wounded. It was quite an evening. For many years students looking over the records and seeing my title in the list came to see me for references and memoirs so they could enjoy that remarkable bit of surgical history: the care of the wounded in a huge military action with hundreds of thousands of casualties. It defined the state of surgery after the discovery of anesthesia (chloroform was used more than ether) but before the advent of surgical cleanliness (Lister's first paper on antisepsis was not published until 1867). Amputation was the most common major operation in that war. Open fractures were universally fatal unless the limb was amputated.

Our First Four Years

Married students were rare in those days. There was still a bias against marriage by medical students. In a class of 120 only two of us were married at the beginning (John Adams and I); a third, also a close friend (Henry Swan), was married the next summer. Clearly the fiscal realities of the Depression fed this bias. Few parents could undertake, as mine did, to support a medical student and his wife. The going theory was that this bias against marriage was supported if not instituted and promoted by Harvey Cushing, who was engaged to Kate Crowell for 6 or 8 years before taking the plunge. If he had waited so long, certainly others should! Considering that such a bias was almost universal in medical schools, I doubt we can blame it all on Cushing. The bias against medical student marriage rapidly diminished and was about gone by 1940,

18

even before Pearl Harbor, which ended it completely. After the war, medical schools were filled with men (and later women) who had already seen military service. They were older and many were already married.

Because Laurie and I did not live in the dormitory, I had less daily contact with fellow students than did my unmarried classmates. Laurie often cooked supper for our small group of students, and each supplied his share of steak, green peas, and beer. They came to love this petite, brilliant, hospitable, and unselfish lady I could proudly call my wife. During those Depression years, senior members of the Harvard College faculty gave evening extension courses. Laurie enrolled in them as an extension (i.e., night) student for a year or two, until our children occupied all her time. She thought it was great to take a course in Chinese history under John Fairbank. About 45 years later a small group of us visited China. The knowledge Laurie had gained as a young student made the trip more interesting for all of us.

Making It to Internship

Medical students enjoy raucous jokes and risque humor, and in those days we often drank too much. Prohibition had been repealed in 1934 while we were at college, and a widespread tendency to uproarious alcoholic parties was certainly notable in our medical school years. While these parties sometimes bothered the neighbors, they seemed to be a generally harmless way of blowing off steam and getting out from under the intense pressures of medical school. The biggest party of all came in the spring of our fourth year, when interns were appointed and we learned where each of us was going for that all-important next step.

Sometime during the second year of medical school or early in the third year, I had decided to go into surgery. This resolve was further strengthened by the fact that I did not enjoy my fourth-year courses in internal medicine. Too much talk and theory; not enough action. It was commonplace at that time for students to move around and take courses at other medical schools. I took courses in New York at the Columbia-Presbyterian Medical Center and at the University of Chicago (Billings Hospital), where I intended to return to practice. Whatever turned my resolve to surgery is unclear and probably unimportant. Possibly, my early encounters with three remarkably able and appealing surgeons in Winnetka and Chicago—Fred Christopher, Vernon David, and Dallas Phemister—two of whom (FC, VD) practiced their craft on me, and the third (DP), a close friend of my father, was a strong factor. George Dick was a friend of my mother. He was Professor and Head of the Department of Medicine at the University of Chicago. It was he who, on hearing I was going into surgery, said, "Surgery is the specialty of getting people well." Coming from a professor of internal medicine, that was an impressive endorsement!

While most of our class took internships in internal medicine (some heading toward pediatrics or psychiatry), we were a very surgical class with an unusually large number of internships in surgery. Eighteen professors of surgery emerged from those 120 men. The intern year was merely the first of 3 to 5 years of residency. The hospital of internship became the hospital for those crucial years of residency. Our 4 years at medical school had somehow produced weathered veterans of learning the medical sciences and arts, with little practical experience. Internship and residency supplied just that.

Education consists of a series of peaks scaled, followed by a fall to the bottom of the abyss before the next pinnacle looms ahead. This boom-and-bust phenomenon is nowhere more apparent than at the time when recent medical graduates first proudly flourish their medical degrees, realizing among other things that for the rest of their lives they will be addressed as "Doctor." A few short days or weeks later they reappear in a white suit as the lowly intern, the lowermost icon on the vast totem pole of medical practice in the United States.

We all expected this transition, this *sic transit gloria*. We were not the least worried about our change in status. Instead, we were terribly worried about where we would intern, since we wanted to intern at a hospital that would give us the best possible residency and a good start in our profession. Along with seven other fourth-year students I was appointed to the surgical internship at the Massachusetts General Hospital. I felt grateful and tremendously excited by this opportunity. I remember only the first hour or so of the party that followed these internship announcements. My long-suffering wife, who shared fully the joy of our joint triumph in this appointment, had dinner with all of us out on the town. Though small in stature, she was able to prop me up and get me home.

How did I come to this happy moment that marked the beginning of my surgical life? My decision to become a doctor was not grounded in any ambitions my parents had for me, nor was I one of those youngsters who always knew that medicine was going to be his life's work. Yet, when I think back on it, there were several influences that might have made more of an impression on me than I knew at the time.

I must have been a fairly bookish child, though I didn't think of myself in those terms. The public library was not far from our school. I avidly read books to feed my interest in the history of World War I, a subject on which I had become a self-taught expert. Then one of my teachers suggested that I read Valery-Radot's *Life of Pasteur*. While I enjoyed the book, I could not understand the chemistry described in it. It told the story of a research academic in biomedical science, the kind of career I was later to follow, but I cannot honestly claim that the book affected me deeply.

Still, I had developed an interest in science, which was encouraged by my mother who had a love of science in her soul. Among her circle of friends were several physicians, including Dr. Rollin Woodyatt, of the Presbyterian Hospital in Chicago, an early pioneer in the study of insulin and diabetic physiology; Dr. C. Anderson Aldrich, pediatrician and author of one of the leading texts in pediatrics; and Dr. David Danforth, a prominent obstetrician. Our family doctor was George Dick, alluded to above. The surgeons I mentioned previously, inspiring men, gave me a very attractive image of what it would be like to be a doctor, and I am certain that the many personal and friendly contacts I had with them played a role in my ultimate choice.

BOOK ❦ TWO

Middlewesterner: Born, Bred, Schooled, Wed

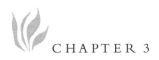

CHAPTER 3

Family Origins, Childhood in the Trenches

Born and bred a middlewesterner, I will always cherish that brand name, despite 60 years in Boston and my parents' New England origins. The deeply ingrained sense of regional superiority held by most New Englanders may or may not be justified, but it is well designed to grind down the home-grown pride of people from other, flatter, windier, and colder regions, especially that large flat place between the Rockies and the Appalachians. Bostonians may travel in Europe from earliest childhood, but they can't seem to get completely straight in their minds the difference between Ohio and Iowa: flat states with short names, mostly vowels. Their children may move to California. But not to Illinois. Most of them will have visited Cairo, Egypt, before they get to Cairo, Illinois. I must confess to some humility, since I too have been to the former twice and the latter only once. Even though a middlewesterner I have now come to feel at home and even a little sentimental about this beautiful northeast corner, where passes are notches and straits are holes.

Our family home was at 1621 Judson Avenue in Evanston, Illinois, about a block west of Lake Michigan. A block or two farther west—a short walk for father—was the C&NW Railroad (the Northwestern), whose tracks running north from Chicago (a mile or so from the lake) defined the line of affluent suburbs called the North Shore.

Mother's maiden name was Caroline Seymour Daniels. The

Seymour line had its origins in Connecticut, specifically the general region of New Haven and Hartford, and boasted a long line of Seymour ministers. Her mother, Harriet Burnham Seymour, came from Hartford. The Daniels ancestry traced back to Vermont on her father's side. Her father, my grandfather, Francis Barrett Daniels, after whom I was named, was born in 1848 in Grafton, Vermont, a village about 12 miles west of Bellows Falls. From vacations in such a beautiful little village as Grafton, it was easy to understand the regional pride of New Englanders. It is a storybook place nestled among the hills, with white church spires sticking up through the pine trees. In my childhood those open pastures with dairy herds, cow bells ringing as they grazed, were a joy. Now, the farms abandoned, dense pine and hardwood growth covers all the hills. Bare Hill is no longer bare and is usually mislabeled Bear Hill.

Starting out as a schoolboy from a one-room school in Grafton, Grandfather Daniels had attended Phillips Academy, Andover, Massachusetts, then Harvard College (class of 1871) and Columbia Law School. He started his law practice when he moved to Dubuque, Iowa, in 1876. There he married Harriet Seymour, the daughter of the Reverend Seymour of Hartford, who had founded Griswold, an Episcopal College (like his alma mater Trinity at Hartford) in Davenport, Iowa. It was because of this Iowa migration of the Seymours and one Daniels lawyer, and their marriage, that my mother was born in Dubuque. She attended The Baldwin School in Philadelphia, then Bryn Mawr College (class of 1901). In 1899, Francis Barrett Daniels, the young lawyer from Dubuque, was made corporation counsel for the Pullman Company. The family moved to Evanston.

My father's name was Philip Wyatt Moore. The Moore family had its origins in Quincy and Braintree, Massachusetts, and prior to that in the general region of Ellsworth, Maine. That is where two of the Maine Moores, the Wyatt Moores (père et fils), saw militia service in the French and Indian Wars, about 1750. Father's family later moved to Boston and his parents lived in Brookline. Grandfather Moore commuted to Boston where he was a clerk in one of the banks. He never attended college. His mother was of the Tompson family, a long line of Puritan, later Congregational, ministers in Quincy, Massachusetts. The first Harvard alumnus in the Tompson family graduated in the class of 1652. Father attended

Brookline High School ('97) and the Massachusetts Institute of Technology ('01). He wrote his senior thesis on the characteristics of an oil-fired internal combustion engine that relied on compression rather than electricity for ignition. He was studying what we now call a diesel, not yet used very much in 1901 or known by that name, though its invention by Herr Diesel is mentioned in the thesis.

Father graduated in 1901 with a degree in metallurgy and went to work with the Bethlehem Steel Company. There he got into an argument with his boss and left. He moved to Chicago, hooked up with an acquaintance, Fred Poor, and the two of them bought out a patent for a device known as a rail anchor, or anticreeper, and started a new company. His former boss, now a close friend, was a major investor. A rail anchor is a device placed on the rail that bears against the tie and keeps the rail from creeping along when the heavy train deforms it slightly and tends to push a ripple of metal ahead of the wheels.

Father and Mother met in Evanston and became members of a congenial set of unmarrieds. They took the big step in 1909. Over the next 4 years they had three children I was the youngest.

My early years coincided with the years of World War I, known then as The Great War. One of my earliest memories was of running outdoors whenever I heard the sound of an airplane overhead to look up and see a biplane flying low and maybe doing a loop-the-loop. Probably it was a JN4, or "Jenny," the standard training plane for aviators in WWI. There was an airfield just west of Evanston. I also remember going downtown to my father's office on the thirteenth floor of the Railway Exchange Building above Michigan Boulevard, where we stood on the balcony, looked down from that dizzying height, and watched the victory parade coming down Michigan Boulevard. This was not long after Armistice Day, November 11, 1918. I was five. I remember General Pershing on his horse and many squads of cavalry before the horse-drawn artillery came along, followed by the doughboys marching in a line eight abreast as far as you could see. Lots of horses but only a few noisy rumbling tanks.

That war was brought home to me in a more immediate form in our backyard. A couple of trenches had been excavated by my brother (4 years older than I) and his malevolent squad of buddies. Gas masks were commonplace during that war. We made ours from a brown paper grocery bag with two eyes cut out. I was given a stick as a proxy for a rifle and was told to get down in the trench, representing Kaiser Bill. Philip, my brother, and his warlike pals, then possibly 7 or 8 years old, rifles in hand, would charge toward crouching, huddling me (gas mask in place, rifle at the ready) with the announced object of bayonetting me, thus putting an end to both the hated Kaiser and the war. Psychiatrists might regard this as an early episode of terror, some form of sibling harrassment that left an indelible mark. Quite the reverse; I look back on it all with a good deal of pleasure. It is said that a Labrador dog would rather be beaten than ignored.

Winnetka and Hubbard Woods

As the war ended, we moved a few miles north from Evanston to Hubbard Woods. Hubbard Woods does not refer to some boreal hamlet in the subarctic, but instead to an affluent assortment of dwellings on the shore of Lake Michigan about 25 miles north of Chicago. Here my family had acquired a large home on a wooded lot on the edge of a ravine, and it is here that I greatly enjoyed growing up from ages 5 to 18, when I went away to college.

The name Hubbard Woods still fascinates people strange to the area. Some years later I was inducted into a student honor society at the Harvard Medical School. One of the professors, a balding Bostonian of high-grade provinciality (the type often referred to as a Boston Baked Bean) handed me my diploma, saying, "Well, Moore, you certainly have done well coming from such a remote place." I did not disillusion him about the average size of the dwellings in that remote hamlet, the average number of cars, the chauffeurs employed by the isolated and primitive inhabitants, their folk dances conducted to the music of drums and horns at clubs where they indulged in a quaint game of whacking little round white balls into holes in the ground, or the uniformity of the political clan to which they belonged.

Our family life was both serene and affluent. I certainly was spoiled. Plenty of help around the house. Summer vacations in New England or Wyoming. At Thanksgiving we went to Boston where we had a big Thanksgiving dinner either with my father's sister, Aunt Isabelle, or at 80 Commonwealth Avenue with my father's Uncle Warren. My Uncle Warren was Dr. Hayward Warren Cushing, a surgeon of Boston, a member of the faculty of Harvard Medical School. He carried out his practice and teaching at the Boston City Hospital, which at that time had a very strong Harvard Surgical Service under David Cheever, David Sears, and my uncle. He was no relation of Harvey Cushing, whom he scorned as an upstart, nor of the surgical Warrens of Boston, of whom more later.

Father never discussed his work with us kids, except to tell us what a rail anchor was. We were asked to visit his office from time to time. I always had the sense there of quiet industry, of people working hard and knowing exactly what they were doing. Father was a hard-working industrial executive. He took the 7:47 to town and came home late in the afternoon or in the early evening. His company, originally Poor and Moore, or the P&M Company, manufactured railroad track equipment and acquired a number of foundries to make these products. The company prospered.

If Father was the achiever, Mother was the intellectual of the family. She was well-read, enjoyed the classics in the original (both Latin and Greek), and was always willing to engage in discussion on intellectual topics, the sort of a discussion my father avoided completely. It is rather surprising that they had such a satisfactory marriage.

While differing in many ways, they were both gregarious with a wide group of close friends, played a great deal of bridge and golf, and frequently entertained at large dinner parties. Growing up with them I developed a severe distaste for bridge and never learned to play golf. Yet I enjoyed doing things with other people and developed my own brand of gregariousness. The combination of these parents produced some hard-working scholarly achievers. Both my brother and sister were brilliant students with fine academic records and high honors at Harvard and Bryn Mawr College.

Maybe one thing about being born a middlewesterner is that you are apt to travel a good deal. It is quite a few miles to get anywhere else. For the son and grandson of men in the railroad business, railroad travel was bound to become an integral part of my young life.

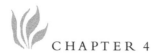

CHAPTER 4

Trains, Family Doings, and Travels

To a small boy brought up in Chicago, who spent his summer vacations on the east coast or in Wyoming, who had a father in the railway supply business and a grandfather as corporation counsel for the Pullman Company, trains were a way of life. Trains were wonderful. They went everywhere, and all that came to Chicago stopped and terminated there. In Chicago there were a great many terminals, or depots, as they were called.

On trains they served pancakes every day. You could have them any day of the week, not just on Sundays. Those dining cars were a joy, rattling along, the water jiggling and the ice tinkling in the glass but rarely spilling, while we watched the landscape go by. The large, black waiters wore spotless white uniforms and moved deftly with perfect control and grace in the lurching car. The whole place had an unforgettable smell of bacon and fresh coffee. Always clean, never sloppy.

Leaving the dining car, you would get a glimpse into the long, narrow kitchen, very hot, filled with busy men working in close quarters, laughing and yelling. How could they make hot mulligatawny soup there and still have the loganberry juice so cold?

And as for the sleeping cars, each was named. I cannot remember ever riding in the same one twice. The green drapes down at night, the ladders to the upper berth. Mother often took the drawing room at the end of the car that sometimes had an adjoining compartment, if there were lots of us. The little sink and toilet. When you flushed the toilet, you looked down on the tracks and the ties (and rail anchors) whizzing by. You suddenly heard the loud unmuffled clatter of railroad travel. There was a sign on the toilet seat: "Kindly do not flush the toilet while standing in the station." To a small boy, the English here was confusing. If you were standing in the station, how could you possibly flush the toilet? Why would you want to?

Spotless, clean sheets. Tawny yellow-brown blankets that had a freshly cleaned smell. Little green nets strung along the outer side of the berth to put kits or books in. Leave your shoes on the aisle floor at night, and they would be polished in the morning. To this small boy there were no finer people than Pullman porters. They were cheerful and delighted in telling stories to the kids. At the end of the trip even little boys were offered a brush-up as we closed in on the depot. You went to the noisy cold vestibule between the cars—or even on the station platform as people got out. The porter had an oversized whisk broom with which he brushed you thoroughly, front and back. It felt good. That was when you were supposed to give him his tip. Father gave us a silver dollar to tip the porter, who put a little stool below the lower step of the car to ease a small person's stepping down to the platform.

The roadway crossing whistle calling in the night seemed far away. As it passed, its pitch suddenly fell as the Doppler effect of approach led to a receding, longer wavelength of sound. The red shift at an Iowa road crossing. Then the distant warning wail of a train that seems way ahead, so rapidly followed by the sudden shocking rush of the passing train going the other way only a foot or two away. The clickety-clack of the rails. Father said that each rail was the same length. So if you counted the clicks and had a stopwatch, you could calculate the speed of the train. An easy bit of algebra but we often forgot to divide by 5,280 or multiply by 60, or something equally basic. He never worked out the problem for us. Just left us with it. Maybe that's one sign of a good teacher.

Because of Grandfather's work with the Pullman Company, at the time of his death we were given a private car for the family to accompany him to his burial on a hilltop in Grafton, the Vermont village where he had been born in 1848. All the members of the Daniels family are buried there. It was a sad time, but an unforgettable journey for a small boy. All that switching of the private car from one train to another. Big chugging steam engines emitting little short signals on the steam whistle to direct the switchmen, the way an ocean liner signals to the swarming tugboats as it comes in to dock.

A train trip to Wyoming—frequent in my life—took two nights and the better part of three days. I enjoyed seeing the flat land and the treeless plains and the sometimes surprising contrasts. There is a strip of northwestern Nebraska that runs on into Wyoming where the thick, dark-green pines of the Black Hills suddenly cease to grow. The CB&Q (Burlington Route) went right along that line for many miles. So, looking out the dining car to the north, you saw a dense pine forest; to the south were endless flat plains without a tree or distinguishing feature all the way to the horizon.

The trip back to Chicago on the cow train after the beef roundup (conducted early in the fall) took five nights and six days. It was slow because of a ruling of the Interstate Commerce Commission that cattle had to be released from their cars and given food and water once every 24 hours while on the way to slaughter (in Chicago).

Uncle Fred was a good deal older than his brother, my father. He, too, had attended MIT. He was keen on the theater and often took us to see plays in Chicago. I can remember going with him to see the Irish Players perform Sean O'Casey's *The Plough and the Stars* in about 1922. Grandmother Daniels looked after our musical education and took me to many concerts of the Chicago Symphony and an impressive array of soloists. As a little boy I had the privilege of hearing Kreisler play the violin; Paderewski, Rachmaninoff, and Horowitz the piano; and an orchestra under Frederick Stock that was especially strong in the works of Bach, Haydn, Handel, and Beethoven.

On one occasion Uncle Fred took me to visit his foundry in Hoopeston, Illinois, where they made rail anchors. It was a typically middlewestern scene, etched clearly in my mind: a small town of brick dwellings with a town square and white fences. It was early summer. Huge cornfields stretched in every direction as far as you could see. In the town was one set of brick buildings a bit taller than the rest of the town. It had a couple of smokestacks chugging out smoke. This was the foundry. The iron ore was melted down in open-hearth furnaces. Huge ladles of molten, white-hot iron poured their burden delicately into tiny sand molds to make rail anchors. These shapes were then annealed by slow heat treatment to make the iron malleable, so it would bend without breaking. The workers were sweaty, stripped to the waist, smiling at their young visitor. They looked like friends. Hoopeston is on the Vermillion River. This was the Vermillion Malleable Iron Co. at work.

Mother had several medical theories. As children we laughed at them behind her back. As we grew older and realized that she could be tolerant and often laughed at herself, we would kid her about these theories and the things she did. This was an era abounding in theories about various medical and health practices. Many of them were very different from today's fads. For instance, there was the idea that children should sleep outdoors at night. Many of the houses in Winnetka and along the North Shore had big sleeping porches. Ours had several so we could all sleep outdoors. In the absolute dead of winter with the temperature about 10 below, it was difficult to see what manner of health benefit was obtainable from sticking the tip of your nose out of a pile of blankets. I don't think it did us any harm. But we would sometimes retreat indoors.

One summer in the early 1920s there was a severe poliomyelitis epidemic. We were taking the train from Chicago to Bellows Falls, Vermont, for one of our many summer visits. Mother was suspicious of everything as the cause of this terrible disease. Especially filth. As it turned out, she was right. She got hold of some formaldehyde or formalin, possibly an ancestor of Lysol or Clorox or some similar antiseptic solution, and went over the entire sleeping car to get everything nice and clean. Needless to say, this was greeted with severe reprimands, if not angry objections, by the other passengers in the car. There were enough of us to fill up one end of the car and one of the drawing rooms. While there were many cases of polio in Vermont, and my cousin from Providence, Rhode Island, came down with severe paralytic polio (which affected her seriously throughout her life), none of our immediate family contracted the disease. Knowing what we now know about polio—and the fact that it is a filth disease spread in much the same manner as typhoid fever—Mother was certainly correct in trying to clean everything up. But at the time and for years afterward, it was just the source of a big laugh, telling the story about how she drove everyone else out of the Pullman car.

Our widely ranging summer vacations in New England or Wyoming were in part traceable to our parents' desire for us to see the world as youngsters. Our vacations at first were spent in Grandfather's farmhouse on the top of the hill at Grafton, Vermont. There we learned horseback riding, watched the farmhands milk the cows, chased the chickens, plucked out the feathers after the chickens were beheaded with an axe on a chopping block, swung on the swing attached to the high roof beams of the barn with the haylofts on each side smelling of wonderful fresh timothy hay. Then, when Father could not summer as a guest of in-laws anymore, we spent a summer on Cape Cod and another one near the Cape in a little place called Marion, Massachusetts, where I went at the age of 13, unaware that it would come to dominate much of our family life 20 years later.

In 1923, when I was 10, we took a long trip to Europe. When Mother took a trip, she took it in a big way. One or two maids or nurses came along to supervise the children. There were trunks and porters. A fair show of a royal progress. We spent about a month in London at a tiny hotel called the Garland House, not too far from Picadilly. There, Mother engaged the daughter of a member of Parliament to show us London and take care of us. She gave us all a marvelous time. Mother was always hospitable to her friends' children, and we brought along many schoolmates from Hubbard Woods and Winnetka. We spent a couple of weeks in Paris. I detested Paris. It was hot, dry, dirty, dusty, and totally uninteresting. Things improved when we went to see the World War I battlefields. We took a charabanc, an open bus, out to Château Thierry and Belleau Wood near Paris. These battles marked the high-water mark of the German advance in the spring of 1918 that almost overwhelmed the Allies. The American Army, though small in those months, played a role in turning back the advance. As we tramped through Belleau Wood only 5 years after the battle, there were still broken trees, helmets, and belt buckles (*Gott Mit Uns*) on the ground. We saw occasional bones. Now, that war is as remote in the past as was the Civil War when Laurie and I visited those battlefields of Virginia in 1938.

The fields along the road had little platforms on the side where unexploded shells were carefully placed. The farmers in their plowing often encountered these shells and placed them on those little plank benches. Then the army would come along and take the shells away. There must have been some lethal explosions from those encounters, though I do not remember hearing about them at the time.

We spent some time in a villa in southern France (Father rented it for a month). It was an ancient farm on Lac d'Annecy, a magical region of Haute Savoie. The villa was on the west side of the lake, about halfway down from the ancient castled town of Annecy, near a hamlet called St. Jorioz. We looked across the lake at the French Alps. The little sharp peaks immediately across the lake were Les Dents des Enfants. I was at an age when learning a language is easy, and I became reasonably adept at speaking French. We rented the villa from Dr. André Varay. He was a charming man, the leading surgeon of the area. While we were living at the Villa Varay, someone spilled a pot of tea on my right arm. Dr. Varay dressed this burn with picric acid, a rather painful procedure. He explained that this was the way he had treated *les poilus* at Verdun. My career in treating burns started out the right way—as a patient.

Many years later a French visitor, a Dr. Varay, came to visit our department of surgery. He was not a surgeon. We invited him to dinner. I did not make the connection at first. But then after a couple of martinis, he announced that he had come to see me not for any profound medical knowledge, but because I had been the 10-year-old boy who had taught him, then 7, how to play *le beisbol*. He was now a successful French practitioner, quite impressive in his double-breasted vest and spats. His office was on l'Avenue Foch, one of the streets that makes the points of the star of La Place de l'Etoile. Fashionable. Like Harley Street in London. What a reunion so many miles and years from that rustic villa in Haute Savoie!

Mother's classical scholarship gave her a special interest in the Roman ruins in the south of France. I remember her helping my brother Philip with his first Latin lesson in the Roman amphitheater in Avignon while we were all on a family trip to England and France. I did not yet understand the appropriateness of giving a Latin lesson in a Roman amphitheater.

My parents were a part of a small group who founded a new private day school in Winnetka called the North Shore Country Day School. They obtained the services as headmaster of an educator named Perry Dunlap Smith. It was at that school that I was educated from first through twelfth grade. I graduated from high school there, and then was off to college.

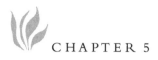

CHAPTER 5

A Great School

(1919-1931)

Back in the 1920s, I encountered people in the Mountain West who considered a private school to be a retreat for retarded children. The idea of sending children to a school where parents paid large tuitions seemed outrageous. Removing children from a comfortable bed and home-cooked food in exchange for a hard bed and bad food at great expense seemed a ridiculous waste of money.

Today private schools are found in every part of this country, but they are still a larger slice of the educational pie in the East and the Northeast than they are elsewhere. Some private boarding schools in New England have multi-million-dollar endowments and vast brick-colonial campuses, the envy of any freshwater college.

By those standards, the North Shore Country Day School was simplicity itself. It was dedicated to the proposition that most of its students should easily achieve admission to the colleges of the eastern seaboard with—in addition—a broad education based on a rich mixture of scholarship, athletics, music, and art.

Our school was situated in a community inhabited by people of affluence who were given to liberal views of education, such as those endorsed by Dewey in the last quarter of the nineteenth century, but who at the same time were prone to conservatism in politics, social intercourse, and business, and harbored their own full share of ethnic prejudice.

The school was rather small, graduating about 30 students a year.

It was coeducational, which was lucky for me, since the student body included Laura Bartlett. The school encouraged intellectual inquiry on any and all topics and was more liberal in its view of politics than was the surrounding community.

North Shore Country Day School nourished my interest in music. The headmaster played the bass fiddle in the school orchestra where I played clarinet. As a member of the orchestra, our authority figure was completely subject to the baton of the conductor. The headmaster had also been a famous athlete in his college days and an officer in World War I. He inspired not only by his philosophy, avoiding the zealotry of overenthusiasm, but also by his joy in achievement and by his quest for excellence. In addition, he could be found having a good time at school dances or enthusiastically singing with the students.

Despite my egregious shortcomings in athletics, I found it possible to struggle through with studies and exams and to enjoy proms, dances, Gilbert and Sullivan operas, and the other obsessive-compulsive disorders of private teenage education. My life certainly could not be described as hardscrabble. While I can remember walking those 2 miles to school and taking the trolley on many occasions, our children later insisted that I was regularly driven to school by a uniformed chauffeur. This disaster happened, but only rarely. When it did happen, I got out of the car a block or two from the school to avoid a pretentious arrival. The understanding chauffeur (friend and confidant) always laughed over this.

Courses in algebra, history, Latin, English, and psychology were my favorites. I made music with several members of the music department, with whom I performed two-piano recitals. One, Arthur Landers, later became music director at Phillips Exeter Academy in New Hampshire. I played *Rhapsody in Blue* at a graduation celebration, using Gershwin's own two-piano arrangement about 6 years after Gershwin first performed it. My partner on the other piano on that occasion was Eleanor Cheney, a classmate and far better pianist than I.

Our class did pretty well in fulfilling the college-entrance mission of North Shore Country Day School. Harvard, Yale, Princeton, and Williams welcomed a good many of the boys, while the girls were admitted to Vassar, Smith, Radcliffe, Bryn Mawr, and Wellesley. Our class picture shows the 28 boys and girls, standing awkwardly on the auditorium steps in the June sunlight. The year was 1931.

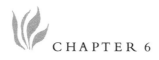

CHAPTER 6

Harvard College

(1931-1935)

F reshly sprung from 12 years at North Shore Country Day School, three of my classmates and I came to Harvard together. We were Fisher Howe, member of the State Department for many years, still one of my closest friends; Thomas Lynde Dammann, later to become a wide-ranging reporter for *The New York Times*; Charles Friedman Haas, later a film writer and director in Hollywood; and I.

We arrived in Cambridge, Massachusetts, in mid–September 1931. I came by train, straight from a glorious Wyoming summer pitching hay, punching cows, and concocting mint juleps for my father's houseguests. The four of us had pored over catalogues and selected our courses and rooms. Three of us were to room in Harvard Yard in the same room in Lionel Hall that my brother had occupied while finishing college the previous June. We were the first freshmen to live in the Yard, formerly occupied only by seniors.

Although I considered myself to have been privileged by family upbringing and private schooling, I was not prepared for the excitement, challenge, and mix of experiences that awaited me at college. I was far from home. Most members of our Harvard freshman class seemed to have dozens of close friends from prep school, whereas I knew only my three high school buddies. The locals (of whom there were a great many in those days) went home frequently for weekends. I had to make new friends and learn new social customs. Early on I learned that, when I responded "Hubbard Woods" to the question, "Where are you from?" the riposte would be, "Where's that?" Answering "Winnetka" helped, but not much. "Chicago" was the simplest reply to those many students (most of our class) whose families lived east of the Appalachians, the majority in New England and New York.

In spite of the advantages of having an achiever father, an intellectual mother, and a wonderful high school education, my academic career in college was somewhat less than spectacular. I concentrated in anthropology because I was interested primarily in human evolution: physical anthropology. The curriculum for anthropology included several premedical courses in its concentration list, so, when I decided to go to medical school in sophomore year, I found I could meet two requirements with one sign-up: concentration in anthropology, and the pre-med curriculum.

We were required to spread our course selections widely. Particularly prominent for me were philosophy and music. The most stimulating philosophy course I took was Philosophy 4b, taught by Professor Perry entitled "American Ideals and Standards with Special Reference to Puritanism and Democracy." Professor Perry enlightened us on the interaction of three cultural traits that make American society at least reasonably successful: a puritanical point of view (essential to stay the overweening greed of capitalism); capitalism (generally competent to organize commercial activity); and democracy, "one man, one vote" (providing the public with a means to restrain the excesses of the other two).

By far the best course I took in college was organic chemistry taught by Louis Fieser. Our textbook was written by James Bryant Conant, Professor of Organic Chemistry, who was appointed President of Harvard during 1933, our sophomore year. The course was beautifully organized and taught without frills or distractions. Professor Fieser gave all the lectures himself. It may be hard to believe that a course in chemistry can be a thing of beauty. It was.

Although I finally graduated cum laude in general studies, any academic achievement beyond that was impeded by several diversions. First among these was the fact that Laura Bartlett was attending Sarah Lawrence College in Bronxville, New York. Obviously, it was necessary to journey to Bronxville as often as possible. I did so with such frequency that I was accused of seeking my degree at Sarah Lawrence. This commuting was accomplished mostly by bumming rides (I did not have a car), taking the train, or occasionally taking the old N.Y. steamer, via the Cape Cod Canal. This packet was by far the cheapest way to get from Boston to New York (about $1.75 one way). Boarding at a broken-down old wooden wharf on the Boston waterfront at about 5:00 PM, we would transit the canal a few hours later and wake up (if possible) early enough to see the New York skyline and Statue of Liberty emerge from the morning mist. This skyline soon changed drastically because the Empire State Building was completed in 1933 and the Chrysler Building soon thereafter. Please recall that for some years the Woolworth Building was the highest building in New York (and the entire world), and the Wrigley Building, a monument to the invention of chewing gum, the tallest in Chicago.

In addition to New York trips to see Laurie, other diversions were traceable to various extracurricular activities. I enjoyed writing prose and poetry (supposedly humorous) and became a staffer of that famous magazine (also supposedly humorous), the *Harvard Lampoon*. At this time we stole the Sacred Codfish, a wooden icon that hung in the State House in Boston, and—a year later—the Yale bulldog. Much as I would like to claim credit for these brilliant literary coups as president of that magazine in my junior year, it was my buddies to whom all the credit was due. Fortunately, no one went to jail or was expelled from college. The bulldog (valuable according to the Elis) and the codfish (sacred according to the state senate) were returned in the same state of health and carving they had been in when purloined.

Music, Serious and Comic

I took some music courses at college. One was on composition, at which I fancied myself adept. I wrote a chorus for orchestra and male voices, set to Shelley's *Ozymandias*:

"... Round the decay
Of that colossal wreck, boundless and bare,
The lone and level sands stretch far away."

40

Open fifths. High strings. Octave voices. Terrific. When our turn arrived, my roommate, Warren Sturgis, and I performed this epic on two pianos for the professor and the assembled class. The professor remained curiously, remarkably, and unexpectedly unmoved. When our performance was over, the class offered us some polite applause, which quickly died down when the professor stalked up to my piano, pointed to one measure of the composition and said, "Francis, don't you realize, that F natural should be an F sharp? Next!"

The one bright spot in the music department was our visiting professor, Gustav Holst, the great English composer. He exemplified the eclectic view of music that has always appealed to me. If Duke Ellington was in town, Holst always went to that night club to hear him. The Holst *Dirge for Two Veterans* was part of our glee club repertoire at the time that I accompanied and later sang second bass. It is a tremendously moving piece for men's voices, on the burial of two veterans of the Civil War. Much more interesting than anything our stuffy old music professor had written.

Early in our sophomore year I was asked to join the Hasty Pudding Club, a college club dating back to 1770, whose main claim to fame rested on its theatricals. I wrote some music for the shows, the first was a jazzy tune called "Hot Stuff" for the Hasty Pudding show in the spring of 1933. It owed a debt to Gershwin and Tin Pan Alley, then at a peak of popularity. With a name like that how could you lose? I was then elected president of the Hasty Pudding Theatricals and wrote the show for 1934, which imagined the unthinkable: Harvard College as a coeducational institution (shades of North Shore Country Day). It was entitled "Hades! The Ladies!" This sitcom turned out to be prophetic. By the time of our 20th reunion the Harvard campus was full of students of the gentler gender. They were certainly more appealing aesthetically than all those acne-pocked teen-age males. This particular Hasty Pudding show enjoyed the collaboration of many of my classmates, including my high school buddy, Charles Haas. Our theatrical mentor was a young English student named Alistair Cooke. He was in the United States on a Commonwealth Fund International Fellowship studying the American language. He spent most of his fellowship year in Baltimore studying with H.L. Mencken. We had a great time with this noble adventure, and

41

Alistair later rose to eminence in the world of TV here and in Great Britain with his series "America" and Masterpiece Theatre.

We took "Hades! The Ladies!" on a road trip that included Washington, D.C., where dwelt many Harvard alumni, not a few of whom were brain-trusters in the first Roosevelt term. You could always count on Harvard alumni to purchase tickets to a Hasty Pudding show. This venue was particularly appropriate because our cast included Teddy Roosevelt III (grandson of the former president) and Mike Garfield (also grandson of a former president). Robert Hepburn (brother of Katherine Hepburn, then at her first of many peaks in popularity) was the third member of what we called the "publicity trio." We could count on the press to give us all sorts of advance publicity with lots of pictures. We did very well, at least in the newspapers.

This was in April 1934. President Franklin D. Roosevelt had been a member of the Hasty Pudding Club during his Harvard years (class of '04) and had been in the cast of the Pudding show in 1903. Franklin and Eleanor invited the cast to the White House for tea in the East Room. I played the piano while the cast sang our songs. We had looked up the show in which FDR was a chorus girl. So we sang some of his songs: a pleasant surprise for our hosts.

Depression Years

Our college years coincided with the Great Depression, known by that term even then. The Great Crash of '29 had occurred when we were sophomores in high school. During this period of economic anguish, the world also moved from post-war to pre-war. There was an ominous prescience based on strong clues: the sudden emergence of Hitler and Mussolini as "dictators" (then a new term), the inflation in post-Versailles Germany, and lingering hatreds and polarization resulting from a war that had not really ended 15 years before with the signing of the Armistice in 1918. I had studied Sidney Fay's *Origins of the World War*. It took no genius to realize that we were heading in that direction again. It was a time of dark forebodings: the Spanish Civil War, the occupation of the Saar.

Harvard tuition was $400 per year, $100 a course. I took five courses each year ($500). My father was very generous to stake me to this additional tuition. But many people couldn't afford such a large outlay. To put it in some perspective, $400 dollars was the cost of our first automobile—a Ford sedan—when Laura and I married. Nowadays a two-door Ford costs somewhere around $12,000, and tuition at a private college starts somewhere around $20,000.

From our earliest days at school we had been exposed to the concept that privilege imposes obligation, *noblesse oblige*. Many of our college classmates were active in helping the poor. The Phillips Brooks House at Harvard was devoted to social work. In recent decades earning a salary doing summertime jobs starting at about the age of 16 has become almost universal among American youth. All our children and grandchildren have undertaken such jobs. Many of them have worked during college in social welfare activities with sick, crippled, or underprivileged people. But in the 1930s altruism was not so common. In the summer of 1934 I studied German and went to Germany hoping among other things to perfect my spoken German. It was Hitler's first year in power, and Germany was already permeated with racist terror. Another summer, I worked in Chicago on a dialysis project for the treatment of kidney failure—prophetic of things to come. But mostly I just had a good time in the summertime with my friends, especially Laura, in Winnetka or Wyoming.

In the fall of our senior year quite a few members of our class were admitted to medical schools (mostly on the east coast). In January Laurie and I informed our families that we would like to be married. No one was very surprised.

My final term at Harvard College, the spring of 1935, was enjoyable and exciting beyond all belief, largely because we were engaged to be married. I returned from Cambridge to Winnetka in June 1935, a few days after graduation, to begin what was the greatest privilege of my life, that of being married to Laura, who became the steadfast guide of my life.

After graduation, as we clutched our diplomas and started to look for scarce jobs or apply to graduate school, we tried to forget about the Depression and the ominous pre-war tensions of Europe. We tried not to consider such matters as part of our own personal future. Laura and I set out on our honeymoon with excitement, love, joyousness, and nothing but the challenge of a medical career ahead and possibly, if we were lucky, a family.

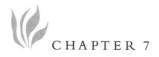

CHAPTER 7

Laura: Wife for Life

Laura Benton Bartlett and I had met when we were students at school. Meeting her certainly formed a great divide in my life, a little bit upstream of the age of 15.

Falling in love is not subject to close analysis. You can list all its aspects, ranging from the crudest sort of lustful eroticism to the most refined sense of joy in cherry pie, in conversation about Restoration drama, or the way she sits a horse. All treasure is surrounded by dragons. There was plenty of competition. Some of her boyfriends were actually friends of mine, and one was the brother of one of my closest friends. So maybe I shouldn't call them dragons. But anyway, there they were. Challengers. Competitors.

Laura

Laurie was an only child. Her father was a native of Peoria, Illinois, descended from a long line of New Hampshire Bartletts. He was a bond broker and securities underwriter in Chicago, a graduate of St. Paul's School in Concord, New Hampshire, and college at Yale. Her mother's origins were in Toledo and Granville, Ohio, and Sewickley, Pennsylvania. Like my parents, the Bartlett ancestors had moved west to find business opportunities in the decades prior to World War I. Mr.

Bartlett had been a machine-gun officer and instructor in the service. He went into the securities business right after the war.

The senior Bartletts were good friends of the Moores. They lived only about a mile away. On high school evenings I was often allowed to borrow the car to drive to the Bartlett home. After a couple of years of this, my father claimed that the car would go there automatically without anybody at the wheel.

When I was at Harvard, Laurie often came to Cambridge from Sarah Lawrence, and we attended various functions at Eliot House or at the Hasty Pudding Club. Everyone who saw her fell in love with her. I was worried that I might be exposing her to a variety of men more able, more attractive, taller, and better looking than I. Fortunately, she never wavered.

But there was an additional twist to this. In the course of the Boston debutante cotillions and other affairs of that stripe, held with big-name dance orchestras (Duke Ellington, Cab Calloway, Guy Lombardo) in major hotels, such as the Somerset, the Copley, the Ritz, or at The Country Club, I had met an interesting group of young Bostonian women. They were cordial but cautious when they first met Franny's girl from Winnetka. They quickly took a shine to her, and several of them became Laurie's closest friends for the next 50 years. What better dividend from four college years in Boston?

Wedding, and Some Electricity

Our wedding was on June 24th in 1935, at the Congregational Church in Winnetka. The reception was at the Bartlett home. Lots of our friends of both generations were there. We took off in a Model A Ford sedan Mother had given us, with tin cans attached to the back, and headed for Milwaukee for our wedding night. On the way there, something happened that in retrospect, 53 years later, turned out to have been foreboding and ominous, though at the time we did not appreciate anything except physical danger.

We were overtaken by one of those sudden, overpowering, frightening middlewestern electric storms (squalls and thunderstorms). Storms of such ferocity are rarely seen in the east except far out at sea, and then it is wind and rain and not so much electricity. We were about halfway to Milwaukee. There were some high-tension towers near us. The sky suddenly became very dark, like late evening. There were tremendous strokes of lightning all around us. Shattering crashes of thunder. We sort of tingled, not for love alone. Sparks flew from the electric power lines in the distance. The downpour was torrential. We pulled to the side of the road and watched this magnificent outpouring of nature's energy onto the flat, hot plains. I knew that in a car you were in the safest possible place because with tires as the only ground contact there was no electrical grounding. It was all over in minutes, to be followed by one of those spectacular and beautiful middlewestern sunsets. Fifty-three years later, in just such a storm, Laurie's and my life together would end.

Young Marrieds and a Growing Family

One October evening, 4 months after our wedding, was the kind of Saturday night we enjoyed relaxing a little bit. Neither of us consumed very much alcohol. I offered Laurie a rum old-fashioned. I don't know what ever possessed me to offer my beautiful bride such a dreadful drink. But she downed it with gusto, as I did mine. A few hours later she began to have severe abdominal pain. I called Bill Marlowe, the only internist I knew at that time in Boston. He diagnosed appendicitis and asked if I knew any surgeons. I didn't know many people because as a newly married couple we had just moved to Boston. The only surgeon I knew of was David Cheever, who presented the first-year clinics in anatomy. At that time I did not appreciate his eminence. He removed Laurie's appendix, and there began a friendly relation with the Cheever family over many years. Laurie never touched rum again.

About 3 months after this, Laurie became pregnant, and in October 1936, Nancy was born. First we named her Laura. But then we realized that if I was resting comfortably in my favorite chair, lounging robe in place (like Archie Bunker), and called "Laura," two people would respond. Unlikely. But that was the operative theory. So we changed her name from Laura Bartlett to Nancy Holmes, after her great-grandmother.

Over the next few years we moved to several small houses in the general vicinity of Boston and Brookline, and soon other children came along to keep Nancy company. Peter Bartlett Moore (1939) was given his grandfather Edmund's nickname, Peter. Sarah Sewall Moore, named after her great-great-great-grandmother, was born a couple of years later (1941), and then in 1944 came Caroline Daniels Moore, named after my mother. There was a gap of fully 6 years before FDM, Jr., was born. All are achievers, successful in what they do. Our five children are now the parents of our 17 grandchildren.

Nancy, like her mother, married a medical student (Lucius Hill) when she was only 19. They have four children. She is a consultant in learning disabilities in the schools of Portsmouth, New Hampshire. Luke is a senior surgeon of Exeter. Peter went to Yale and is now professor of chemistry there, and has taken his turn as head of the Department of Chemistry. Like his grandfather, he married a girl from Iowa, Margaret Murphy. They have two children. Sarah (Sally) is an artist and teacher in Grafton, Vermont. She married Richard Warren, the son of a surgeon, our close friend. They have three children. She has started a school for teachers in Vermont. Caroline is dean of admissions at The Day School in New York. To be original, she married a lawyer, James Tripp, also the son of friends in Brookline. Jim is now senior counsel for the Environmental Defense Fund. They have two children. Our youngest, FDM, Jr., "Chip," is an academic surgeon carrying out clinical surgery, research, and teaching (much as his father did) at the Brigham and Women's Hospital and Harvard Medical School, where he is an associate professor. After divorce, Chip remarried. He and Carla Dateo Moore together have six children.

There is no predicting a happy marriage. The premarital state seems to have nothing to do with it. In our day, virginity was the rule; marriage was a prerequisite to marital togetherness, to sexual union. One evening my children, in a gale of argument, asked me, "Why did you marry Mother?" I answered, "Lust." Despite their supposed sophistication and age (they already had several children) they were surprised if not shocked. Children have a hard time realizing that their parents can be passionate lovers. They do not consider that anything as dignified as their parents' marriage could be contaminated by any such earthy sensations.

What are some of the components of a happy marriage? To

Laurie and me, analyzing ours and the marriages of children and friends, it seemed clear that, after the basics, conflict resolution is one of the most important. The basics certainly include the continued expression of mutual physical and intellectual attraction, congeniality of interests, and fidelity.

Many young couples break up over their first serious argument. We were married for 53 years. Five children. Is there any way of calculating how many serious arguments we had? It was clear to us, among other things, that a double bed is a good means of conflict resolution. You can't go to bed together if you're still mad.

BOOK ❦ THREE

First Years in Clinical Surgery

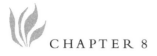

CHAPTER 8

Surgical Residency at the Massachusetts General Hospital

(1939-1943)

At some point in the spring of 1940, fully scrubbed and suitably attired, I stood a few paces back from an operating table on which lay a naked boy of about 10, anesthetized. One of my colleagues was sponging off the patient's abdomen with little gauze sponges soaked in an iodine solution. The drapes were then firmly set in place, with a small opening over the bare skin where I planned to make the incision. I can remember thinking how remarkable it was that institutions in our society could set things up so all the pieces would fall in place and I, then less than a year out of medical school and only 26 years of age, might have the immense privilege of relieving the pain, anguish, and threat to a wonderful small boy by making an incision in the right lower quadrant of his abdomen and taking out a pus-filled appendix skillfully and safely. Only 5 years previously I had greeted that smelly collection of organs in the anatomy laboratory, and it was only 3 years since Mrs. Szintax had been warned of our arrival. Now here I was, with skilled nurses and an experienced anesthetist, shiny sterile instruments at hand, ready to operate, with all the protection given the patient by a venerable institution. I felt that this was both a miracle and a privilege. I still do.

Young Professionals

In those years we learned surgery by doing, and we also learned some of the ethical values of a professional. During my internship and residency years I did my surgical firsts—operations done by each of us for the first time from the surgeon's side of the table. These operations were performed in the care of charity patients on the public wards. The patients were charged no professional fee, and their hospital bills were minimal or forgiven. We, in turn, were paid a pittance after one year of zero-pay internship. Those patients on the charity wards held our loyalty and devotion. They were ours; we knew it and they knew it.

The essence of professionalism is that the servant, the caregiver, the professional, values the interest of his client or patient above his own. Patients can never acquire the knowledge to make basic decisions about their own care or negotiate costs intelligently. They want their doctor to do these things on their behalf. Even when physicians find themselves as patients, they experience great difficulty in joining in medical decisions outside of their own field. The compact of care is taken on faith and given in trust. Although in so doing the professional makes a living, his income includes no capital gains from his work. He derives no unearned income from his work. He cannot sell at a profit. Personal inconvenience is assumed in professional care: midnight calls, long operations.

During our residency years we learned these values, almost unconsciously it seems now, without preaching or sermons, just by the behavior of our peers and the example of our teachers. We cared for the charity-ward patients in a clearly professional setting. Senior surgeons saw patients with us, advised us, and scrubbed in to assist us on difficult operations. The challenge in surgical residency training is for the young learner to gain skill by taking responsibility without jeopardizing the safety of the patient. To attain this ideal requires a special organization and a strong tradition of interpersonal trust. The Massachusetts General (MGH) has been a leader in achieving this ideal now for the better part of two centuries.

Medical students and young physicians are native idealists. They are also bright. At one time almost a third of entering Harvard freshmen listed medicine as their future career. People often ask, "Why do so many young people want to enter medicine?" My reply: "Offer the most fascinating and rapidly advancing field of science (biology) and join it with the most gratifying of human instincts (giving care to the suffering) and you are bound to get a lot of takers."

Filled with idealism, students nowadays are plunged into a gaudy and greedy commercial world of corporate profit and personal wealth. They see the huge earnings of insurance companies, hospitals (even the "nonprofits"), administrators, and doctors. They are not blind to the million-dollar incomes of many physicians and surgeons today, shocking though they may be to us old-timers. Everyone wants to make a buck out of the medical monster. That is why it costs so much to keep it alive.

What is needed is a return to the charitable purpose of all of medicine, to the church ancestry of all the great hospitals of England and France, our progenitors. The "family values" of medicine are as real as ever, and they are still out there, epitomized by care of the sick poor. But they are also experienced when the affluent suffer and need help. The poor sick. Huge corporate profits (dividends to stockholders) and personal aggrandizement are foreign to this tradition. Commercialism and professionalism are parallel streams in our society that can coexist in peace. When they start to get mixed up with each other, beware. Teaching hospitals of the 1930s—such as the MGH—indoctrinated their interns into a down-to-earth and old-fashioned professional ambience of hard work and few or no material rewards.

The Pup Enters the Pack

At the MGH and the other Boston teaching hospitals in those days, the process of applying to the internship-residency system in the spring of our fourth medical school year was a chancy business. The Boston hospitals held off on their internship appointments until all the other hospitals in the country had made theirs. In waiting for a Boston appointment you were therefore taking a big risk. Out on a long limb. If you missed, you had nowhere to go except the "Radcliffe Infirmary," the joke for a worthless appointment. Years later when I was visiting professor at Oxford, where the principal teaching hospital is the ancient and honorable Radcliffe Infirmary, it became clear that our sarcastic joke was strictly local, not to mention displaying male chauvinistic snobbery of the least politically correct variety.

On July 1, 1939, I started surgical internship. Two of us started every 3 months, for a total of eight beginners each year. For the first 3 months of internship we were called "pups," and this first period of servitude was known as the pupship. The pup begins by analyzing effluvia. During pupship we were assigned several important tasks involving the analysis (in the early hours, 6:00 to 6:45 AM) of all the urine and stools of patients for whom such analyses were deemed necessary by the more superior interns who had been pups fully 6 months before.

Our equipment for this simple but important (albeit odoriferous and inelegant) task was primitive in the extreme and left an unmistakable mark on the decor of our tiny attic laboratory in the Bulfinch Building. Urinalysis consists in part of spinning down the urine in a centrifuge and examining the sediment under a microscope for signs of infection. This required a small centrifuge, with little pointed tubes that were apt to break at the tip if dropped too heavily into the centrifuge. If a tube filled with urine had a tiny hole in it and was twirled at a rapid speed, the walls of the room and everything at a certain height around the wall would be decorated with a narrow brown stripe, this being the even distribution of urine around the room at the precise level of the spinning centrifuge. I wore an apron.

While neither of these activities could be considered complicated, one or two unsuspected cases of bowel cancer (by stool blood test) or diabetes (by measuring urine sugar) were discovered each year thanks to the humble labors of the pup. There was the constant suspicion among the older interns that the pup might be goofing off on his marvelous job. It was therefore their practice to add a little sugar, protein, or bile to the occasional sample of urine or to put a tiny drop of blood in the occasional fecal sample. Such "plants" would keep the pup fully alert, because he would be expected to detect and report these important (if intentional) abnormalities accurately. If these spurious samples (what we might now call "stings") were not discovered, the pup was to be relegated to an even more humble role. It was difficult to conceive exactly what that penalty might be.

Having performed this vital function, the pup would wash up and make himself socially presentable, as well as surgically acceptable, to join ward rounds about 7:00 AM. As pup on rounds, I walked appropriately a few steps behind the more advanced interns and those two or three austere surgeons known as residents, one of whom (the chief resident) led the parade. The most senior residents were about 30, fully 4 years older than the pup. The pup was supposed to trail behind the residents and interns (and even the students) with his little pup list, on which he would note which patients were to have chemical tests, intravenous infusions (becoming rather frequent at that time), blood transfusion (still rather rare), or those vital 6:00 AM analyses of excreta.

The Pup Transfuses

By 1939 the method for transfusing blood had improved somewhat over the two decades since 1914, when Landsteiner described the blood groups, making blood transfusion at least a reasonably safe procedure. Transfusions had been done by the direct method—literally letting the blood flow arm to arm in a series of tubes from donor to recipient. This system involved awkward and complicated paraffin-lined tubes. I carried out only one or two of these direct transfusions in my early days. Since the equipment rarely worked, and none of us understood it very well, a good deal of very precious blood wound up on the floor. Any blood that finally reached the patient was assuredly warm and fresh.

By the time I joined the scene, the method used for blood transfusion had advanced perceptibly. Most blood transfusions were carried out by the pup, drawing blood from family donors into a bottle containing citrate solution to prevent clotting. In due course (1 to 3 hours) it was given to the patient. Fresh. The pup himself, unassisted, did the blood typing (known then as grouping) and cross-matching (under the microscope) to ensure compatibility, much as we had been taught in medical school.

Furthermore, it was our job as pups to ring up the patients' families, ask for volunteers to give blood, get them in, do the typings and cross-matchings, find those with compatible blood groups, draw the blood from the arm vein at the elbow, and supervise the infusion of the blood personally. As I look back, it is remarkable that we gave as many blood transfusions as we did during those pre-war years. That we accomplished this quite successfully with very few adverse reactions is not surprising. When one person carries out a complex procedure himself, it is done carefully because his personal reputation is on the line. Severe reactions to blood transfusions, such as mismatch or the growth of bacteria in the blood, were infrequent. While it seemed that we transfused a lot of blood in those days, it was but a drop in the bucket compared with the gallons of banked blood that would be used only a few years later in taking care of severe war wounds, extensive injuries, and radical operations.

Pups also had duties that more glamorously resembled operative surgery. After the matins in the lab and the ceremony of rounds, we would proceed to the operating rooms to assist our elders. But there would come a time, usually at night, anticipated for weeks or months, when an emergency "acute belly" would come in, and a junior intern (possibly, in rare instances, even a pup) might be permitted to remove an inflamed appendix. In a crowded surgical life, few operations would seem more important than this, as described at the start of this chapter. The older residents, despite a gruff exterior, took a sort of avuncular pride in the progress of their pups, and after such an operation (strictly routine in any larger sense) they would give a handshake and a "Good job." "Nicely done."

The Pup Anesthetizes

In certain cases the pup also administered anesthesia. This was a duty with which I was very unhappy because, without suitable training, it obviously posed a hazard to the patient. I considered it a breach of professionalism in surgical training. If a patient with a relatively simple fracture (such as a fracture of the wrist or of the bones just above the ankle) was admitted to the emergency ward at night, the broken bone was set right then and there in the emergency ward. That is, it was manipulated and drawn apart by traction so it could then assume (and ultimately set in) its normal position. This nocturnal setting of fractures was usually done by a young resident just completing his internship (after 12 to 18 months in the hospital) or possibly by one of the more senior residents 2 or 3 years out of medical school. When properly done, such immediate setting of fractures gives the ideal result for the patient. But there was a catch. The anesthetic—essential not only for the patient's comfort, but also for the relaxation of spastic muscles around the fracture—was administered by the rawest intern, the pup.

It was shocking to me, and I still look back on it as a dereliction of the high standards of our surgical education at the MGH, that I was suddenly confronted late at night with an anesthesia machine, valves, cranks, and canisters of nitrous oxide and oxygen, and was expected to proceed, untutored, to induce anesthesia and put the patient "to sleep." At night, hurried, harried, and tired, with no help. That I and my fellows got through this without causing any deaths (at least none of which I was aware) was pure luck. Indeed, it was the death of a patient in just such a circumstance as this in Harvey Cushing's hands (when he had been a Harvard medical student about 40 years previously) that led him to revolt against the lack of supervision in "simple" (but dangerous) anesthesia for minor procedures. As a result, Cushing devised the type of anesthesia chart now universally used throughout the world to monitor the patient's course under anesthesia.

My own revolt against this practice as a pup was simply to state clearly—after my first frightening experience—that I would never give another night emergency anesthetic unless I (and the other interns to come) could do it safely under experienced supervision. By the look in my eye, that hospital administrator must have realized that he was dealing with the bark of a fairly determined pup. After that we enjoyed better help and fewer brushes with disaster. The bark must have had a little bite.

I devote so much of this account to the pupship because it was our introduction to those crucial 3 to 5 years spent in finally becoming full-fledged surgeons. It was a sudden deep plunge into the world of the sick, injured, and powerless. Or, to change the metaphor, kind of a trial by fire. Almost a hazing.

The Residents Operate ... a Lot

In subsequent months and years I climbed up the ladder. In those days at the MGH, removal of the gallbladder, known as cholecystectomy, was the bellwether operation for the first couple of internship years. By the end of 24 months, I was doing much more complex procedures, including the removal of diseased intestine (usually for cancer) or the uterus (hysterectomy, usually for benign tumors), operations for injury to the tendons of hand and arm, and extensive procedures on the veins of the leg.

The following (third) year, we undertook more complicated operations, such as subtotal gastrectomy. The safe and expert performance of this operation was the criterion of operative experience in advanced residency training. Subtotal gastrectomy involves the removal of about two-thirds of the stomach either for duodenal ulcer or for cancer. Although not a completely forgotten operation now (since we still use it for patients with stomach cancer), the tens of thousands of subtotal gastrectomies previously done for duodenal ulcer each year in hospitals throughout the United States and Europe have today been reduced to only tens or hundreds with the introduction of vagotomy (in which the vagus nerves to the stomach are severed) or by the use of acid-reducing drugs or even antibiotics in the treatment of ulcer.

I carried out many subtotal gastrectomies for duodenal or gastric ulcer. Like most of my operations, they seemed to go easily and well, and like most of my fellows, I gained in self-confidence. I felt secure and knew that the weeding-out process would leave me intact. Every couple of years an intern would be found to be clearly unfit for surgery, though possibly perfectly suited to some other field of medicine. Such miscast trainees either resigned or were not promoted, often moving on to distinguished careers in other fields.

In the final years of residency, our repertoire expanded to include operations on the liver and bile ducts and the pancreas; those done for cancer of the colon, rectum, or breast; and procedures for disease of the adrenals, thyroid, and parathyroid. The MGH provided an absolutely remarkable experience.

One of the key assignments, usually coming about 2 years after medical school, was that of being in charge of the emergency ward. There were two surgical services (the East and the West) and they alternated nightly coverage of the emergency ward. When you had that duty, you were on the job all night on alternate nights for several months. The MGH always had a very busy emergency ward, caring for accidental injuries, bullet and stab wounds, burns, fractures, infections, gangrene. Only the Boston City Hospital cared for more emergency patients. On one particular night, that of November 28, 1942, several hundred casualties, many already dead, were brought into the emergency ward within an hour, and I was to witness one of the most lethal civilian disasters in our history.

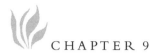

CHAPTER 9

Death After the Game: The Cocoanut Grove Fire

(1942)

Charles Burbank and I were the two surgical residents in charge of the emergency ward on the night of November 28, 1942. Charlie was a year senior to me. We worked together days and nights for many months both in the operating room and in the emergency ward. We had known each other in college and medical school, were good friends, and worked well together even in tough and demanding tasks.

It had been a quiet evening, just after Thanksgiving, the time when those final football games were settling championship titles. We were up in our rooms listening to football games on the radio. At around 10:30 PM, over the noise of the crowd on the radio, we heard the whine of an ambulance outside on the street. It did not stir us much because such whines were commonplace. But then came another and another. So we donned our white coats and ran downstairs gripping our pockets so our stethoscopes wouldn't fall out.

We got to the emergency ward pretty fast. More ambulances, trucks, and cars were moving in and out of the entry circle. By the time we arrived, dead bodies were lined up in rows in the hall. The smell of burnt clothes and hair permeated the entryway and the hall. Obviously, there had been a major fire with many deaths. Where and why we would not know for several hours.

The Cocoanut Grove was a large nightclub situated not too far from the center of downtown Boston: near the Common, just off Charles Street. Under new management, it had recently been redecorated with groves of imitation palm trees, paintings, hangings, and drapes. Designed to handle about 600 patrons, the club was overcrowded that night. Almost 1,000 people were packed in for drinks, dinner, and a show. The place was popular with the young. Officers recently inducted into the armed services were there (now one year after Pearl Harbor) looking handsome in their new uniforms and with their best girls in their finest dresses. An autumnal scene of youthful beauty and vigor having a big time after the big game.

At about 10.15 PM some of the drapes and decorations suddenly caught fire, followed by a rapid, almost explosive conflagration. According to survivors, within 5 minutes the entire nightclub was filled with flames, especially high in the drapes. Just where the fire started and how it all got going no one was quite sure at the time. Recent analysis confirms the story that it started in a basement lounge in the drapes, possibly from a match or a cigarette.

The fire department put out the flames within 30 minutes. By 10:45 PM the structure was a smelly, smoldering hulk with a pandemonium of ambulances, fire trucks, hundreds of dead, and a few severely injured in the streets, where there was a strong smell of burning clothes, hair, food, and maybe flesh, described by onlookers as sickening.

Fire Kills in Several Ways

The burning (oxidation) of the decorations and drapes had three chemical consequences. First, the oxygen inside the tightly closed restaurant was rapidly used up, so there was little left to breathe. Many died of suffocation, their skin and lips deep blue because their blood lacked oxygen. For some, death from suffocation was so sudden that they were found sitting at their tables, unburned, rigid in death, fingers clutching glasses. Others were crushed or smothered at the blocked exits.

Second, when oxygen runs out, carbon dioxide cannot be produced from the carbon in all the wood, drapes, and paint. The fire cannot breathe, either. Carbon dioxide—a carbon atom with two oxygen atoms attached—is, in itself, quite harmless. We produce and exhale a good deal of it every day. It is the fizz in fizzy water. But when there is not enough oxygen to feed a fire, many carbon atoms are incompletely oxidized; only one oxygen atom is attached to it instead of two, and it is transformed into carbon monoxide, the deadly substance abundant in automobile exhaust. In carbon monoxide poisoning, blood forms a special kind of hemoglobin that is bright cherry pink rather than deep crimson red. This abnormal hemoglobin is itself too thirsty for oxygen to relinquish its precious cargo to the tissues crying for it, causing a sort of chemical asphyxiation. The face of a person dying of carbon monoxide poisoning is often rather cherry pink. Some of the dead, and a few of those who reached the hospital alive, had that ominous and sometimes deceptively healthy-looking cherry-pink color.

Third, combustion of the paint on the walls and the dyes in the drapes produced irritant poisonous gases. Some of these were like the mustard or phosgene gases used to poison soldiers during World War I. People exposed to these gases cough up frothy, bubbly, sometimes bloody secretions. In severe cases their lungs fill up with this liquid, and they drown in their own secretions. It takes a bit of time for irritant gases to fill the lungs with froth. One naval officer actually got to the MGH and ran from room to room and down the hall of the dead, looking for his family. Then he fell, gasped, tried to cough up the secretions that were drowning him, and died.

Many people were trapped in the club because of locked exits or doors that opened only inward. Such doors still kill people every year in theater, restaurant, and factory fires. At the Cocoanut Grove there was also a large revolving door. When masses of people hit both sides of a revolving door at once, it becomes an impenetrable wall. Those who got out included some who were badly burned, others who had been severely poisoned with carbon monoxide or phosgene-like gases, and some who were unlucky enough to have both kinds of injuries. Many died within minutes of arrival at the several hospitals to which they had been taken.

When Charlie Burbank and I arrived in the emergency ward, we could see that a lot of the bodies in the hall were those of young people whose skin was either deep blue (suffocation) or cherry pink (carbon monoxide) or they had froth emerging from lips and mouth (irritant gases).

Many victims of the fire showed no burn whatsoever; skin and clothes were not burned at all. We began looking for, and soon found, patients still living but in need of our help because of lung problems, burns, or both.

Respiratory Tract Injury; Morphine and Tracheostomy

Morphine can be a problem as well as a mercy. Burned patients experience both pain and anxiety. Giving them an injection of morphine is a safe enough way to reduce pain and anxiety, so long as they are not given too much. Too large a dose of morphine interferes with breathing, which is especially dangerous when there is lung injury.

In any sort of a mass disaster and in the clearing (and sorting) of casualties, it is important to attach a label or a tag to each patient on which the doctors or nurses can record exactly what measures have been taken. Then, when the patient is moved, the new team will know what has gone before. In the first hours after the Cocoanut Grove fire, patient tags were not used. Sometimes the nurses used lipstick to mark an "M" on patients' foreheads, signaling that morphine had been administered. But this was not always clear, and sometimes a second or even a third dose of morphine was given. One or two may have died of this overdose. We never knew. But many others were deeply anesthetized by it, and for the rest of that first night, each of these patients was assigned a doctor whose job it was to keep the patient breathing until the morphine wore off and the patient woke up.

A total of 490 people died in the fire. The Boston City Hospital and the MGH received most of the casualties. It was estimated that 440 survived, making a total of 930 at risk and a mortality of about 55%. The largest number of dead and injured (about 300) were taken to Boston City Hospital. Of these, 132 were alive when they got there, 36 soon died. The MGH received 114 casualties of which 39 were still alive after the first few hours. Ten had severe burns while 29 were largely lung injuries. Two months later (late January 1943) there were still nine severely burned patients in the hospital receiving care and grafting. By April, all had been discharged. Some returned later for plastic surgery. I remember one in particular, a naval submarine officer whose hands and forearms I resurfaced when I first entered practice the next fall.

In seven of the patients suffering from inhalation of the toxic phosgene-like gases or severe respiratory tract obstruction owing to neck swelling from burn, we carried out a tracheostomy. An incision is made surgically in the neck and a tube is placed in the trachea so air and oxygen can be delivered directly to the lung, permitting the patient to breathe more easily. Many other patients were placed in oxygen tents.

Deaths from respiratory tract injury occurred within the first day or two. These patients often had telltale soot stains on the nose, lips, and mouth. Some had burns around their head and neck that within a few hours caused a grotesque swelling, making tracheostomy much more difficult. One or two died while a tracheostomy tube was being inserted. I lost one such patient, literally in my own hands, because we had waited an hour or two too long before deciding on tracheostomy.

Since the late 1960s, tracheostomy and oxygen tents have virtually disappeared from the scene, replaced by direct intubation of the trachea through the nose or mouth (less injurious to the trachea) followed by automatic machine-assisted respiration. Oxygen tents never accomplished much anyway. The oxygen concentration in the air we breathe normally is about 20%. An oxygen tent—even with all the leaks tightly closed and oxygen being delivered at full throttle—could push that up to maybe 25 or 30% at best. With the oxygen stream running directly into the tracheostomy tube (or, nowadays, an endotracheal tube), the concentration of oxygen can be much more enriched, sometimes dangerously so.

In those first agonizing hours after the fire, the scene in the emergency operating rooms and in the halls and nearby wards was wild. Many relatives were panic-stricken and screaming, desperately searching for their companions. This was during the early years of the war. I remember one handsome young naval officer in full uniform, severely burned, also lung-injured and short of breath, lying restlessly in bed and repeatedly calling out the name of his girl. Although we did not know it at the time, she had been found in the pile of dead behind the revolving door. There was one suicide, attributed to despair at losing a beloved person.

Settling Down to the Task

Within a couple of days after the fire, things began to stabilize. Several floors and operating rooms were reserved exclusively for the Cocoanut Grove patients. New supplies of blood plasma for transfusion and of dressing materials came in from all over the city. Some disaster-readiness drills had recently been conducted because American cities expected to be bombed, so the city and the hospitals were not caught unprepared. In fact, our hospital had gone through a disaster drill only a few days before. There were extra burn dressings available and a stockpile of fluids for intravenous infusion. Blood banking as we know it today had not yet been developed. But within days donors across the city had given 3,800 units of blood, largely processed into plasma by removing the red cells.

We treated the burned skin surfaces by wrapping them in a thin greasy gauze sheet covered with bulky dressings to soak up the body fluids that exude from burns. While this covering protected the burn from the outside atmosphere and made the patients more comfortable, it required a lot of dressing changes. These were so difficult and painful that in many instances we used a general anesthetic.

It was 1942, the year that penicillin was first being tried in tiny quantities as an experimental drug, soon to be supplied in larger amounts to our army and navy surgeons. At the time of the fire itself we did not have penicillin, but within a few weeks some became available and we were able to give small amounts to our patients. We did have the sulfa drugs, sulfanilamide and sulfadiazine, but not the bacteriologic methods for assessing the sensitivity of bacteria to these drugs. All these burns became infected, but the patients survived their infections. Probably the most important precautions were gentleness in handling the burned surfaces, changing the dressings often enough, and placing skin grafts at the right time. Bradford Cannon (son of Walter Cannon, our professor of physiology [Chapter 2]), a skilled plastic surgeon, was in charge of the skin coverage procedures and later plastic repair of these severe burns. He set a high standard that few of us could emulate.

Everything done in the early care of burns is designed to keep the patient as healthy as possible in spite of the severe physical insult. This involves keeping the burn wound reasonably clean and then covering the burn with new skin grafts just as soon as possible. This is a long, arduous, painful, and exhausting process. Final skin replacement with skin grafts that take (i.e., grow and cover the raw areas) is the ultimate achievement that lets the patient get up and go home. All the severely burned patients who weathered their lung injuries ultimately got well and returned home.

We lost no patients after the first week, when lung damage took its heavy toll.

For part of the year before the Cocoanut Grove fire, I had been studying burns as a junior collaborator with Oliver Cope, a senior member of the staff particularly interested in burns. He had primary responsibility for care of the Cocoanut Grove patients, and we were indebted to him for developing the type of dressing that was used (boric-petrolatum gauze) and for elucidating the nature and treatment of lung injury in fire victims.

The understanding and care of patients with severe lung injuries was revolutionized by this disaster, a direct result of the work of Oliver Cope, surgeon; Tracy Mallory, pathologist; and Richard Shatzki, radiologist. The entire team was under the direction of Edward Churchill, who was soon to leave for military service in charge of the care of the wounded in the Mediterranean theater.

Lessons

The two major lessons from the Cocoanut Grove fire pertained to safety laws and to the treatment of the lung injury in burns. The threat of death from fire in public buildings can be reduced by the installation of battery-illuminated signs and fail-safe exit doors that can be opened from the inside. This fire had been in a closed space; there was no escaping the smoke and fumes. The problem posed by fire in closed spaces is especially severe on ships and in tanks in battle, largely because of suffocation and lung injury. The care of such patients was important to both army and navy surgeons. Over the next 5 years Oliver Cope and I did research on burns for the Navy (and I later for the Army), much of it to describe the disordered physiology in burned patients and to improve treatment for burn shock and severe respiratory tract injury. In the treatment of the latter—pulmonary injury in burns—the Cocoanut Grove was a turning point thanks to Oliver Cope.

And yet the central problems of burn injury and the subsequent causes of death remain unchanged. As long as there are fires in which people are trapped and severely burned, these problems will persist. The three leading causes of death from burns have always been infection, direct lung injury, and organ failure (kidney and liver) if there has been burn shock. Use of any one of several present-day treatment procedures has made burn shock a rarity. But in the wild, away from organized hospitals, or in combat, burn shock is still a cause of early death.

Many other lessons were learned from the Grove, possibly less spectacular. One was a reemphasis on the importance of overall organization of the hospital for disaster, as well as organization of the surgical and medical staffs under the clear authority of senior members who had done research in the subject and were interested, experienced, and competent to care for such patients.

While there were few civil suits for damages, there were two public hearings. Finally, 10 men were indicted for negligence, one of them a fire inspector who had declared the decorations and drapes non-combustible because he could not light them with a match. Later it was declared that the fire inspector, without malfeasance, had merely applied the usually accepted test. It was wartime. Many more had died at Pearl Harbor a year before. At that time, exorbitant damage claims, bitter battles over insurance settlements, and incarceration for involuntary man-slaughter were rare. There were some criminal indictments. One busboy was made a scapegoat by the media when he testified that he saw the fire start but failed to put it out. He was indicted but later acquitted and released. One of the owners was judged guilty of negligence and served 3 1/2 years in jail.

The cost of caring for these patients was borne by the hospital through its endowment. To my knowledge no money from public sources ever found its way to recompense either the hospital or the surgeons for their services.

Now, more than 50 years later, I am one of only a small group of physicians, surgeons, and nurses still alive who were there, hands-on, in the emergency ward that night and on the burn floors through the weeks of travail. I never lost my interest in burns, nor my concern for the safety of public places, many of which still pose a hazard, nor my respect for how the people of the MGH rallied to deal so effectively with this sudden, unexpected, and overwhelming challenge.

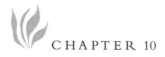

CHAPTER 10

Defeats and Triumphs: Residency Is Not All Smooth Sailing

The realities of human injury and illness, of birth and death, were commonplace in our lives as residents. Part of our education was in learning to make our peace with these realities, or at least accommodate our lives to their impact.

The first patient who died after an operation I had carried out myself was a woman of about 62, suffering from breast cancer. I had performed a radical mastectomy, the only operation used for treatment of the disease at that time, about 1940. She was doing very well when on the 10th day (note that she was still in bed in the hospital) she got up to walk to the bathroom. While on the toilet, she fell to the floor, dead. Autopsy showed a massive clot in the artery to her lung, a pulmonary embolus. A pulmonary embolus is a clot dislodged from the legs that travels to the lung and plugs a major artery there. This dangerous and sometimes lethal event is especially apt to occur after injury or surgery. In this case the clot may have been dislodged by changes in intra-abdominal pressure associated with straining on the toilet. That was not an unusual sequence of events.

When, after the war, we began to get patients up out of bed and walking sooner, such clots and the resulting emboli became less common, though they were still a threat in many situations. Had I been a little bit more sensitive to the slight rise in her temperature and pulse the day before, I might have suspected the large clot lodged deep in the vein of her leg that was the source of the fatal snakelike embolus (almost 6 inches long). Despite her husband's distress when I told him of his wife's death, he granted permission for the autopsy. He did not resent the request and appreciated my attention to his wife. He wanted to try to help others by consenting to the postmortem examination. The families of most patients are trusting and grateful. Even though this event took place before the anticlotting drug heparin was available and before the technique of deep venous interruption (in which the veins of the leg are closed off so a clot cannot migrate to the lungs) was accepted as an emergency procedure, somehow I felt her death was my fault. Maybe young surgeons always feel that way about their first deaths.

A few days later another patient of mine died after an operation performed by one of the senior surgeons. I was only the second assistant at the operation, but the patient was on my floor, so I was responsible for her daily care. I knew her well. She had undergone an exploratory operation to examine both sides of her neck in search of a tumor of the parathyroid gland. Possibly the operation was not as expertly done as it should have been. Had the chest been opened (which later became common practice), the operation would have been safer, because the anatomy of the upper chest, the great vessels, and the lungs and their coverings (the pleurae) could have been more easily and safely exposed. Often, in surgery, the bolder, seemingly more radical step is the safer one.

After the operation, the patient never looked quite right. Because this was before hospitals had recovery rooms or intensive care units, the patient was returned directly from the operating room to her regular ward bed even though she had not yet recovered from all the effects of the anesthesia. This was the usual practice. Her blood pressure, breath sounds, and heartbeat were as expected at this stage. An hour or two later, I was up on that floor seeing nearby patients when the nurse called and said this patient was breathing hard and was very blue. A moment later when I got there on the run, she was indeed dark blue and almost dead. By stethoscope I could hear the last few distant beats of a laboring heart. No breath sounds. No reflexes.

Air had accumulated under pressure in both the pleural cavities that line the lung and are normally free of air. This caused both lungs to collapse. During the operation her surgeon had inadvertently entered the chest cavities and nicked the lung on both sides without knowing it. The tiny leaks had not become evident until the trapped air built up pressure that prevented her from breathing normally. Such events were preventable and diagnosable. Although we placed drainage tubes in both sides of her chest to let some of the air rush out, it was much too late. The patient died of a bilateral pressure pneumothorax.

Sensitivity Among Surgeons

Among surgeons there is a variation in sensitivity. Every doctor is shocked by the first few deaths close to his or her daily work. For the surgeon they are especially close. Once an internist said to me, "You surgeons take death so damned seriously." What did he expect? If he was the patient, he would certainly like us to take any threat quite seriously. Somehow he seemed to be implying that we cared too much.

Because the surgeon is so close to the reality of life in the balance and of death, he needs to develop skin of exactly the right thickness. If it is too thick, he is resistant to learning, too resistant to feeling the death of a patient, a little bit slow to seek the autopsy permission, his mind closed to new ideas. Sometimes he may even tell the family some blarney to spare them the truth about why the patient died, a truth that families thirst for and deserve. But if the surgeon's skin is too thin, then he is whipped by death, he broods and worries, cannot sleep, learns little, and is not ready for the next day's operation. Like a cowboy thrown from his horse, the surgeon, although hurt, must be able to get back on his horse and ride again.

That middle ground of sensitivity is something that is either inborn or acquired from parents, probably in childhood. While it cannot be created, it can be strengthened by example. And it must be sought in the young. In later years I saw interns and residents I considered too tough and hard-boiled, big talkers, and I was not impressed. But I also remember one or two who were just the opposite: too sensitive, too worried, too introspective. I was concerned about their future in surgery. One of these later became a leader of research in heart disease at the National Institutes of Health. A better niche for him.

Sometimes the heavy blows of a surgical career do not come from the death of patients but from some other miscarriage of medical care that has resulted in complication, misunderstanding, or litigation. In my early days as intern, resident, and practitioner, malpractice suits were almost unheard of.

Senseless Things Can Happen

Severe injury, life-threatening diseases, and the very act of surgery itself come close to the essence of life. The circulatory system, the bloodstream, the heart, the brain, the kidney: all are vulnerable, exposed to the possibility of injury in many operations and affected by drugs, including those used for anesthesia. Surgeons should constantly be reminded that the state of patients under anesthesia is not sleep, it is drug-induced coma. Despite our use of the blissful word "sleep," the anesthetized state bears little resemblance to normal sleep, in which the blood is free of sedatives or hypnotic drugs, arousal is immediate, and the brain is resting, idling in a state of near-readiness. Under anesthesia, the bloodstream and the brain are affected by depressant drugs that profoundly alter sensation, tissue irritability, thought, consciousness, and arousal. These drugs of course affect other organs, particularly the liver and kidney. Research and development in anesthesia are devoted to making these drugs less harmful. In case some anesthesiologist might be offended by a surgeon writing about how dangerous is the state of anesthetized coma, he should be reassured. I am emphasizing my admiration for those colleagues who can induce, manage, and achieve arousal from this drug-induced coma as smoothly as they do.

The death of a baby boy born with a faulty stomach shows how dangerous anesthesia and even simple operations can be and how events sometimes defy us. He was a precious and appealing baby suffering from a narrowing of the stomach outlet called pyloric stenosis, usually due to overgrowth of the muscle. This overgrowth impedes emptying of the stomach and results in severe and repeated vomiting. The disorder develops rapidly in infant boys (very rarely in infant girls) and, if not treated, soon leads to dehydration and death. The diagnosis is not difficult to make if you suspect it, because the little olive-shaped enlargement impinging on the stomach outlet can be discerned by gently feeling the abdomen.

I operated on this little boy while I was a senior resident. The operation is not a difficult one, but it is potentially dangerous and is sensitive to accuracy in detail. If by accident the incision made to open up the thickened muscle bundle is a millimeter too deep, it opens the mucous membrane lining of the intestine, releasing the bowel contents and producing peritonitis. Prevention of such a catastrophe is the major precaution of this operation.

The operation had gone well and took only a few minutes. The nurse who gave the anesthesia was someone with whom I had worked a lot in the care of infants and young children. I trusted her. The baby had been deeply anesthetized with ether and nitrous oxide. The operation over, I checked a few details of the child's condition, as well as the orders to be carried out by the nurses. We agreed to meet in a few minutes back at the infants' ward, a few hallways down from the operating room, to which the infant would usually be trundled, still asleep, in a small, wheeled crib. As mentioned earlier, there were no postoperative recovery rooms or intensive care units in those days.

As I left the operating room to go the surgeons' dressing room, I noticed out of the corner of my eye that the nurse lifted up the unconscious baby as a mother might, draped his head on her shoulder, and clasped him firmly with one arm, holding the record sheets in the other hand. She set off through the swinging doors of the operating room to go down the hall and around a few corners to the infants' ward to place the child back in his crib. The nurses there would take over.

After a change of clothes, I started off for the infants' ward to talk with the parents. This would probably be one of those reassuring conversations accompanied by a hand clasp and maybe an embrace from the mother. "It all went well...he'll be fine." As I turned through the door into the infants' ward, my calm feeling, that pleasant feeling of assurance and confidence that surgeons have when operations go well, disappeared in a blinding flash of suspicion. It was replaced by a full alert.

A small group was gathered around the baby's crib. The anesthetist was there, the head nurse, a pediatric intern. The infant's mother, who was still wearing her overcoat, had come in from the waiting room a few steps away. The atmosphere of the normally quiet infants' ward with the late-morning sun streaming in the windows was somehow different, ominous.

My walk changed to a lope, and I was at the bedside in an instant. The whole scene could be taken in at a glance. The pink, lovely infant was now ashen pale, deadly white, and absolutely still.

"He's dead!" the mother shrieked and held a handkerchief to her mouth, her fists clenched and white.

The nurses, anesthetists, and pediatric intern had all been trying to revive the child. Breathing mouth-to-mouth. An intracardiac injection. A quick look under the bandage to see if there was hemorrhage, but there was none. I just watched, somehow knowing it was all futile.

In tiny children, the events of life and death progress very fast. After a moment or two the child's face and head were already cold. I took the weeping mother, who was still crying aloud and calling out, to the waiting room. I tried to find some words somewhere. There were none. There are none now. Some things in life simply do not translate into language.

If some specific memory of a life in surgery could somehow be wiped out in one stroke, it would surely be my memory of those few moments with that mother. Suddenly she had changed from a young Italian girl from the North End into a distraught, protective animal, fighting for her young.

What had happened? It is only a guess. The deep anesthesia paralyzed the infant's poorly formed blood vessel reflexes that, when we stand up, keep the venous blood flowing against gravity, up from the legs and lower part of the body to nourish the brain and the heart itself. In an infant just beginning to stand upright and walk, these reflexes are not yet strong. When the nurse anesthetist so lovingly picked up the child and held him against her shoulder, she unwittingly restrained him in the upright posture. If a person is forced for long periods of time to maintain this position, the stagnant blood pools in the legs. The brain, robbed of blood, starts to die, and with it the drive for respiration. And then the person dies. Death by crucifixion occurs because, when the body is held helplessly upright, all blood flows to the feet and legs and stays there. Fainting is soon followed by death. While the nurse anesthetist held the baby with

73

his head on her shoulder, she could not see his face. For this little boy, deeply drugged with anesthetics, lying down in his wheeled crib would have been safe.

Nothing since then has changed my interpretation of those events, now more than 50 years ago. This was not of any interest to the mother, only to those of us who went over the details again and again, hoping that it would never happen again. Whose fault was it? Mine, of course. The surgeon, like the captain of a ship or the pilot of an aircraft, is responsible for everything that happens. His word is the only one that cannot be gainsaid.

I never spoke harshly to the nurse anesthetist or blamed her. I knew how she felt. She later volunteered that she shouldn't have picked the child up. I agreed, and asked her if she had ever done that before. She did not respond. Criticism was not necessary, nor were false reassurances.

In the long pace of days and weeks and the long years of human life with remembrance of things past and apprehension of things to come, it is hard to remember that in preserving human life there are occasions when seconds count, minutes are too long. This is especially true in infants. A single minute of poor blood flow to that tender brain, a single moment of open bleeding from the heart or a major vessel, may spell the end of a life.

Surgery has plenty of hidden dangers for the unwary. I enjoy a rather mixed metaphor about surgery, the sea, and flying: Surgery, like aviation, is in itself not inherently dangerous. But to an even greater degree than the sea, it is terribly unforgiving of any carelessness, incapacity, or neglect.

Severe Infection

Sir Berkeley Moynihan, the great British surgeon who helped perfect abdominal surgery, said: "Every surgical operation is an experiment in bacteriology." The skin is our barrier against surroundings that teem with bacteria: a microbiological world unfriendly to large animals like us. Once the skin has been breached, by accident or design, infection can occur. This has been a cause of death after battle wounds since the dawn of time or after surgical operations since a sharp knife was first used to make an intentional incision.

Besides the threat of bacteria from the outside world, there are viruses, fungi, and parasites out there seeking admission. We also harbor billions of bacteria inside us, mostly in the lower intestine, the colon. These bacteria are called *Escherichia coli* in honor of Theodor Escherich, a scientist of the nineteenth century. This name is usually abbreviated *E. coli*: Theodor's germs from the colon. Our normal intestinal tract excludes these *E. coli* from the true interior of our bodies or the bloodstream. During intestinal surgery and in infections such as acute appendicitis, there is always the threat that these usually cohabiting bacteria, if given a chance, will leak into the peritoneal cavity where they wreak havoc only a half-millimeter away from where they usually reside in peace. Some of these *E. coli* secrete potent toxins that can kill if they grow in food that has spoiled. Or if they grow in the peritoneal cavity or in abscesses.

Despite antibiotics, infection remains the bane of surgery. Most surgical patients who die after severe injury or with complications after major surgery still die because of infection. Our intensive care wards save many lives, but we still lose patients to multiple infections caused by organisms that are either resistant to antibiotics or, like some of the fungus infections, enhanced or worsened by antibiotics. In such multiple infections, many of our vital organs fail in sequence: first the kidneys, then the liver and brain, and finally the heart. The term multi-system organ failure describes these troubles. Without antibiotics many of these patients would have died of their injuries 1 or 2 weeks previously. Some survive because of antibiotics and intensive care. In some cases these infections are, in a sense, the byproduct of antibiotics. Sometimes, as in acute appendicitis, the surgeon actually removes the infection along with the infected organ. And then there are other situations in which the infected tissue is surgically removed but under more perilous circumstances.

The story of a teenager dying of colitis is a case in point and emphasizes some of the challenge and human satisfaction of surgery. The patient was a young man of 16. Before his illness he had been robust, healthy, and athletic. He played tackle on the high school football team. But in the 6 or 8 months before I saw him in the hospital, he had become increasingly ill with intestinal bleeding and diarrhea due to a dangerous disease of the large intestine—ulcerative colitis. For the past 6 weeks he had been wildly, dangerously, and overwhelmingly ill with a rampant form of the disease. He was given large doses of cortisone. In ulcerative colitis the colon seems to infect and literally digest itself with its own bacteria, those same colon bacilli with which we usually live in peace. The colon becomes swollen, and bacteria spread to the lymph nodes near the bowel. Over time, the patient's immune system fails and other commonplace bacteria become involved in the infectious process. The bowel disintegrates and then perforates, producing a foul, stinking peritonitis and death. This condition is called toxic megacolon, and it was frequently associated with cortisone treatment.

In the realm of surgery, there are a number of operations wherein the procedure itself solves most of the patient's most urgent problems. Recovery starts immediately and dramatically. The surgical act can cure the awful wrongs that the body has been suffering. The recovery mechanisms of the body easily accommodate to the relatively minor stress of the operation itself. Stopping a major hemorrhage, removing a piece of food from the trachea, relieving a blocked kidney, draining an abscess, restoring blood flow to a blocked coronary artery early in a heart attack, transplanting a new kidney or liver to replace one that is failing, setting a painful and shock-producing break in the thigh bone are examples of some of the most dramatic effects of operation itself. Sometimes these rescue procedures are rapid and simple, such as removing a ruptured spleen in an athlete hurt in a football game or removing a ruptured tubal pregnancy in a young mother.

Although the removal of the infected, decaying colon in toxic megacolon is more complicated and more time-consuming than the operations mentioned above, it has the same dramatic effect on the patient. The colon must be gently dissected out, blood vessels and lymphatics ligated to avoid bacterial spill into the general circulation, and the entire length of the colon (often 3 or 4 feet) removed. No bleeding can be left behind. A new intestinal opening (an ileostomy) is made. The abdominal cavity is washed, rinsed out, and returned to its normal glistening appearance. The rectum is then removed and these two large incisions are closed.

In this teenage patient, infection and fever had made him delirious; in the last hours before operation he was hallucinating, his pulse racing. His blood pressure was edgy and falling, his kidney and liver function were deteriorating. A positive blood culture showed that *E. coli* bacteria were growing in his bloodstream.

The operation I performed, although done as an emergency, was deliberate. It took over 3 hours. Within minutes after his colon was removed, his pulse slowed down and became steadier, his blood pressure became stable and normal. Kidney and liver function soon improved. And his brain, once cleared of the anesthetic, was soon back to normal. In a short time the blood culture became sterile. The students who helped with this surgery were immensely impressed with how this long, difficult operation, requiring several blood transfusions, could produce such an immediate improvement.

When I next visited the patient, a few hours later, he was coming around from his anesthesia. One might think that just the pain of those incisions and the worry about the new intestinal opening on the abdomen would overwhelm any feelings of relief or improvement. This boy had lived for some time with raging infection and the pain of spreading peritonitis, not to mention the dread of what might come next. Relief from this suffering was evident. The clearing of his mind, reduction of the work of his heart, and the new ease of his breathing were evidence of how rapidly and completely a sturdy young person can recover from severe disease and an extensive operation when it has abated the crisis. Somehow the survival responses of the body were able to reach down into evolutionary processes, some very ancient, and summon recovery once he was relieved of the infected tissue of his colon.

The following day when I visited him on rounds, his face broadened into a smile of joy, relief, and a kind of bodily animal pleasure that is difficult to describe. The ordeal was over. He could distinguish the pain of a healing incision from the anguish of infection. He was safe and he knew it without anyone telling him.

"Hey Doc! You saved my life!" Sort of a teenage greeting-shout, one of joy. A bit corny, but from the heart. My only answer, with a squeeze of the hand, was the usual mumbling of something along the lines of, "Hell, you did most of it yourself."

How true. His body was already back at work, returning to tissue growth and synthesizing new proteins for healing. Little cells—fibroblasts that heal wounds and are the surgeon's best friends—were already moving in to restore his tissues to their normal strength.

Every student of medicine, everyone concerned with what medical treatment is about and how the body can respond, should join in the care of a patient like this every now and then. It is good for understanding what doctoring is all about. We were looking at the remarkable combination of modern surgery in a vigorous youngster and the truly marvelous primal recovery mechanisms deep within his body. We were witnesses to mental and physical processes that are inseparable.

A few days later, "Say, Doc, when can I start eating? I'm starved! They haven't given me anything to eat for weeks."

"Wait a while. Another day or two until you get settled down, and then we'll give you a turkey dinner."

Another squeeze of a newly strong young hand, no longer sweaty, but pleased and confident and grateful.

"See you tomorrow."

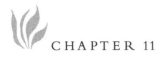

CHAPTER 11

Finishing the Wartime Residency; White Suit to Civvies

(1942-1943)

In learning the surgical care of the sick, we were most influenced by the practicing surgeons of the attending staff. Arthur W. Allen in abdominal surgery, Joseph Vincent Meigs in gynecology, and Richard Sweet in thoracic surgery were national leaders in their fields and typical of the senior surgical staff at the MGH in those days. For me, the most influential was Leland S. McKittrick. He was a middlewesterner, hailing from Wisconsin. Maybe this Illinoisian intern was drawn to him by that background. He was plainspoken and clear thinking, his eye on patient welfare and clinical teaching rather than social status, hospital hierarchy, or national medical politics. When I finished the residency, I became his private assistant for 2 years before devoting all my time to academia, to the university in research and teaching. The academic surgeons to whom I was closest were Edward Churchill and Oliver Cope.

Teachers

The MGH had a large surgical staff rich in talent of all ages. George Washington Wales Brewster was, for me, quite special as an example of the most senior group, after retirement. His son Henry had been a classmate of mine at college, and the father, a legendary old-time surgeon, took an interest in both Laurie and me. He and his wife often

79

treated us to Sunday dinner in their brownstone townhouse at 213 Beacon Street. It was typical of the Boston doctor's house of that day. His office was on the first floor. The living quarters were on the floor above. The food rose from the cellar kitchen to the upper floors on a dumbwaiter. Patients and social acquaintances came in through the same door, but the latter walked up a staircase or took the ramshackle elevator.

George W.W. Brewster was an old man by the time I knew him, an old-school cutting surgeon of the most pragmatic type, often given to pithy opinions, many unprintable. Maybe this time-honored toughness was a sort of bluff protection against newfangled surgery; the more precise, slower, meticulous operations; research; elaborate x-ray diagnosis (to him always a newfangled gadget); and academic concerns of the younger surgeons. Brewster had been active in surgery when the x-ray was invented. He did not always trust those strange pictures. Early x-rays were taken on glass plates rather than films, hence the term "plate" for an x-ray picture. The Brewster treatment of fractures consisted of making rounds, seeing an x-ray plate that did not agree with his perception, breaking it over his knee, throwing the pieces into the wastebasket, and making it clear that the patient was progressing just fine despite that damned x-ray.

One of the younger clinical surgeons who influenced us was Claude E. Welch, the Nebraskan assistant to Dr. Allen. He later became the senior clinical teacher for generations of surgeons and was the acknowledged leader of MGH surgery for years, even after his retirement. Then there were Marshall Bartlett, Horatio Rogers, Langdon Parsons, Bradford Cannon, Richard Wallace, and a whole group of clinical teachers who, with boundless energy and good humor, shepherded all of us fledgling surgeons through innumerable operations and made a profound imprint.

The youngest member of this group was Fiorindo A. Simeone. He had been my chief resident when I first started as pup and it seemed certain that he was the greatest of Italian surgeons! He looked, acted, and talked like New York's feisty mayor, Fiorello La Guardia, and came from the same part of Italy. Simi, as he was known, later became Professor of Surgery in Cleveland (at Western Reserve). Then he moved to Providence (at Brown University) where he found a large Italian clientele and continued to operate on patients and play the role of a sort of father figure in surgery until his death, when he was almost 80.

During my time at Harvard Medical School, a subtle change was taking place in the home origins of staff and faculty in surgery and indeed throughout Harvard University as a whole. While George Brewster may have epitomized the old Boston lineage, tracing his line straight back to an elder on the Mayflower, Allen (Kentucky), Welch (Nebraska), and McKittrick (Wisconsin) hailed from other parts. Churchill was from Illinois. Cope from Philadelphia. At one point six of the senior university full-time professors of surgery at the Harvard Medical School came from the middle west: Churchill, Gross, Russell, Austen, Folkman, and Moore. In fact there was an article in *The Atlantic Monthly* not long after the war about how the center of gravity of faculty leadership at Harvard was shifting westward and away from the Charles River tidewater; the blue blood was beginning to run pretty thin with the outgoing tide. To me— and I think to most of the interns and residents—this did not make any difference whatsoever. A remarkable group of men constituted Boston surgery, and many of the leaders were at Harvard, the Brigham, and the MGH.

The Lighter Side

Simeone and Welch were involved in one of our rare hospital pranks. In the surgeons' room there were a lot of stuffy old pictures of stuffy old surgeons: formal pictures of the hospital staff that went back at least to the invention of the photograph if not back to the daguerreotype, the tintype, and the discovery of ether anesthesia. Under the stimulus of Claude Welch, some of us dressed up in frock coats, glued on stage mustaches and beards, and stared seriously at the camera. We wanted to see if anyone ever really looked at all those old pictures. We hung our phony photo in the surgeons' room. It was several weeks or months before somebody gave away the secret. No one ever noticed that the picture showed a bunch of young upstarts dressed up to look like old Boston Brahmins.

Then there were the "change parties." Every 3 months the resident staff changed. That is, the various members were rotated upward to a more advanced position. Every year or so the change might involve a new man at the top in the form of the chief resident. These milestones were marked by events known as change parties, at which the off-duty staff became especially cheerful after a few drinks. A bit rowdy. It had long been noted and was a source of some humor that a surgeon should not wear a long tie that could dangle embarrassingly and dangerously down into the wound or incision while he leaned over the patient. Our white uniforms did not include ties or even shirts with collars. But the change parties were mostly for the off-duty residents who attended in their rarely used civvies (i.e., charcoal grey suits with neckties). So it became a custom during change parties that a few of the white-suited on-duty troops (cold sober) would invade the party for a few minutes, bandage scissors in hand. Now bandage scissors can cut through almost anything, including plaster. So cutting off the necktie just below the knot, thus in effect defrocking the rowdy civilian-clad celebrants, became a customary activity at change parties. If you wore a tie at all, it had better be a bow tie or a very old one.

In spite of all our work and many duties, there was also time to do some writing and begin some clinical research. As mentioned earlier, I had, while still a medical student, done research on a placental hormone. In 1941, 2 years after medical school and during my junior residency, I applied for a fellowship from the National Research Council to learn how to use the then-new radioactive isotopes in research. To my surprise and delight, the fellowship was granted for a year starting in July 1941. During that time I carried out research using radioactive isotopes under Joseph Aub and Waldo Cohn and began the study of the chemical anatomy of the body, otherwise known as body composition (described in Chapter 14). A year later, in July 1942, my research fellowship being over, I returned to the residency, operating on many patients, serving in the emergency ward, applying dressings, setting fractures, making rounds, and teaching students.

Pearl Harbor: "Your Job is Right Here"

The war in Europe had begun on September 1, 1939, with the German invasion of Poland. This was the start of our third month of internship. It was clear that a terrible event, long anticipated, had now

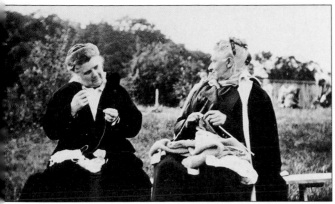

Harriet Seymour Daniels (*left*) and Sarah Tompson Moore (*right*) — two grand-mothers (in their 60s), knitting in the sun, Grafton, Vermont, about 1915.

A young family strikes a Victorian pose in Evanston, Illinois, about 1916: Philip W. and Caroline D. Moore with their children (*from left to right*), Philip Wyatt Jr. (age 6), Harriet Lucy (age 4), and Francis Daniels (age 3).

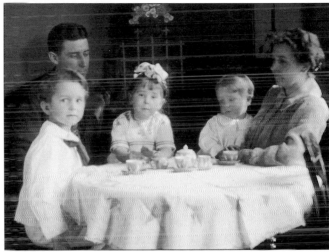

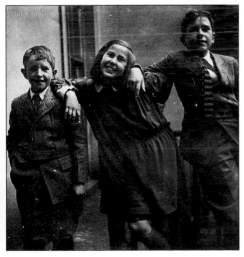

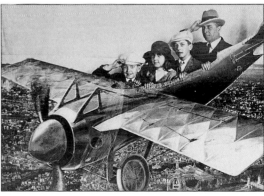

Flying over the Eiffel Tower in a photographer's pasteboard airplane in Paris are Francis in front, with sister, brother, and father behind, about 1923.

Three supportive siblings: FDM (age 10) holding up his sister (age 11) and brother (age 13), about 1923.

Plate 1

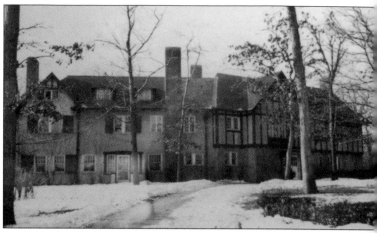

Family home in Hubbard Woods, Illinois, where FDM lived from 1918 (age 5) until departure for college at age 18.

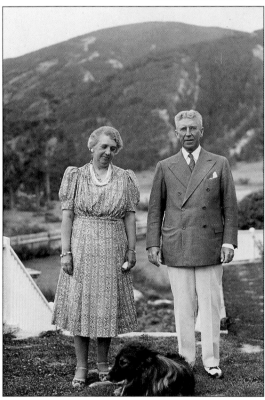

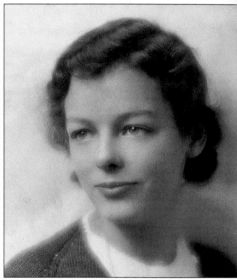

Laura Benton Bartlett as a high school girl, age 17 in 1932.

Philip and Caroline Moore (at 55) on the terrace at Horseshoe Ranche in Wyoming, about 1934.

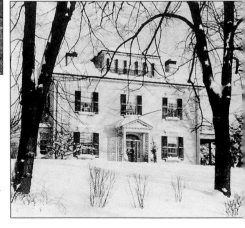

Home of FDM and family from 1944 to 1974; 371 Walnut Street in Brookline, Massachusetts, wintertime, 1950.

Plate 2

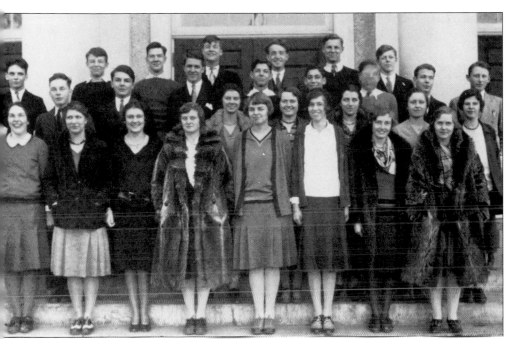

Class of 1931, North Shore Country Day School. There are 15 boys and 13 girls. (FDM is in the back row, fourth from left.)

THE

HASTY PUDDING CLUB
of HARVARD University

PRESENTS AS ITS

Eighty-Eighth ANNUAL SPRING PRODUCTION

The Extravaganza

"HADES!
The LADIES!"

in TWO ACTS *and* SEVEN SCENES

1795   1934

at the *Club House* in the city of
CAMBRIDGE

March 28th and 29th, 1934

The PLAY

The LANGUAGE is the collaboration of J. PARTON '34, L. P. HOWARD '35, C. F. HAAS '35, and F. D. MOORE '35. ~ The MUSIC is by E. E. STOWELL '34, F. D. MOORE '35, and G. SHAW '34. ~ The LYRICS are by E. E. STOWELL '34, F. D. MOORE '35, J. PARTON '34, L. P. HOWARD '35, C. F. HAAS '35, and A. M. JONES '35.

THE PRODUCTION was staged under the direction of Alistair Cooke. The dances were arranged by William Holbrooke.

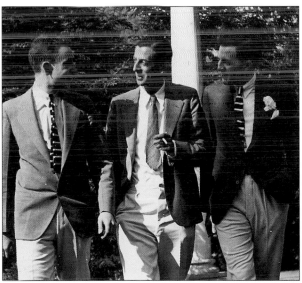

Alistair Cooke, Director of the 1934 Hasty Pudding Show "Hades! The Ladies!," is flanked by FDM (*left*) and Matson Holbrook (*right*) between rehearsals at Pinehurst, North Carolina, April, 1934.

Playbill for the 1934 Hasty Pudding Show at Harvard College, listing the authors, composers, and the Director.

Plate 3

The Great Picture of Handsome Dan II, pedigreed "By Harvard, Out of Yale," licking John Harvard's boot, as it appeared on the cover of the March 1934 issue of the *Lampoon*. This picture was also printed on a deck of cards that sold widely among alumni.

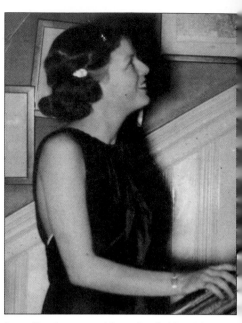

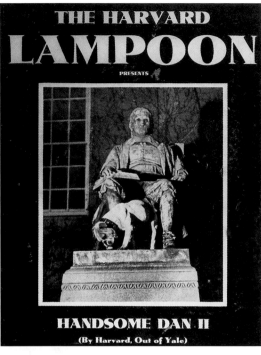

Laura Bartlett on a visit to Cambridge, 1934. She is standing on the stairs of the Hasty Pudding Club at the Annual Dance before the opening night of the show.

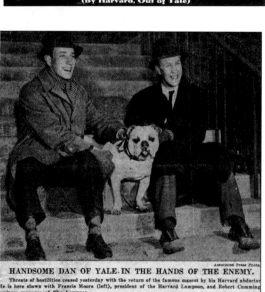

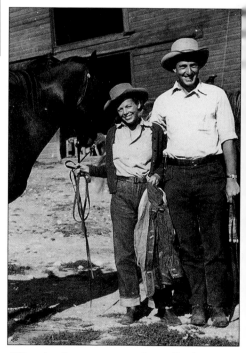

The New York Times photo of FDM (*left*) and Robert Cummings (*right*) getting ready to return Dan to his rightful owners in New Haven and only too happy to reveal The Great Secret to the press.

Wyoming honeymooners. Laura Bartlett Moore and FDM in front of the barn at Horseshoe Ranch, August 1935.

Plate 4

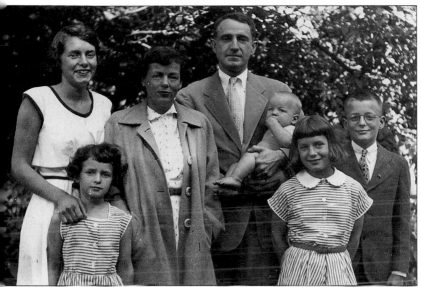

he family is complete. On the lawn of the Bartlett
ome in Winnetka, Illinois, are (*from left to right*) Nancy
ge 14), Caroline (age 6), Laura (age 35), FDM (age 37)
olding Chip in arms (FDM, Jr., age 6 months), Sally
ge 9), and Peter (age 11), in spring of 1951.

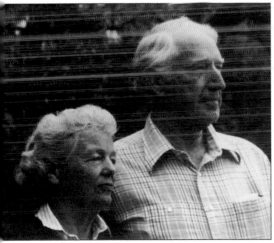

he same honeymooners nearing their 50th anniversary
hile on vacation, March 1983.

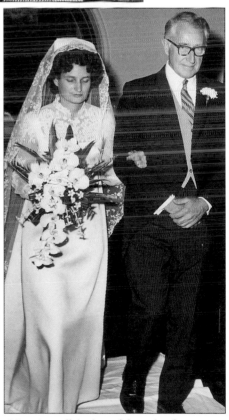

Marrying off the last of three daughters.
Caroline, on FDM's arm, starting down the
aisle for her marriage to James Tripp, First
Parish Church, Brookline, Massachusetts,
October 14, 1972.

Plate 5

Ticket admitting "Mr. Gray" to the Lectures on Anatomy presented by Professor John Warren in 1811. Note use of the term "Cambridge University," a designation for Harvard that was occasionally used in those days.

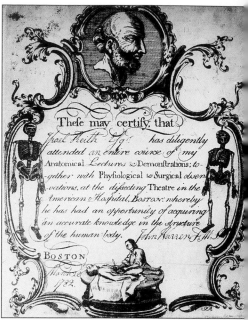

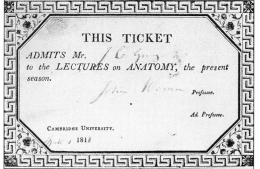

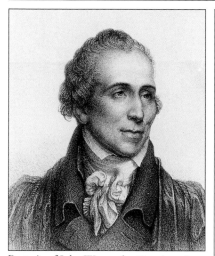

Certificate of Attendance at "an entire course of my Anatomical Lectures and Demonstrations," signed by John Warren and dated March 28, 1782.

Portrait of John Warren by Rembrandt Peale. John was the first Professor of Surgery (and Anatomy) on the medical faculty of Harvard College.

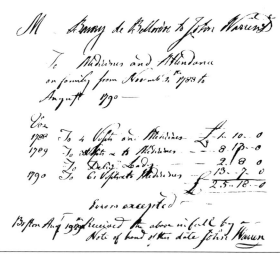

Bill for professional services rendered by John Warren to an officer of the French Navy covering the period from November 1788 to August 1790. Note obstetrical charge for "Delivery Lady." Next to his signature, Warren has certified that the bill was paid in full. Since he was a physician, not a Doctor of Medicine, there is no "M.D." after his signature.

Plate 6

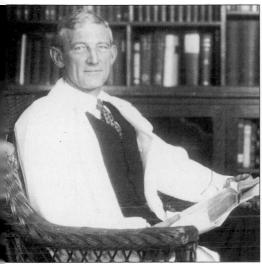

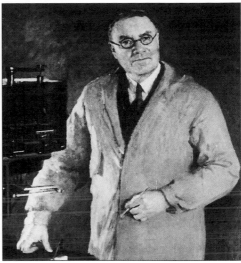

Elliott Cutler, Moseley Professor of Surgery and Head of the Department of Surgery at the Brigham during FDM's medical school years. Cutler was the fourth Moseley Professor and the seventh Professor of Surgery in the direct line from John Warren.

Walter Bradford Cannon, George Higginson Professor of Physiology during FDM's years at medical school. Cannon's studies of the function of the adrenal glands demonstrated an integrated and highly evolved response to injury.

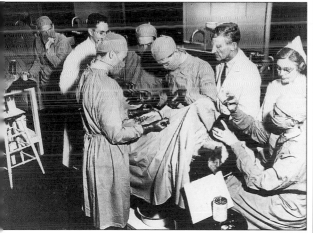

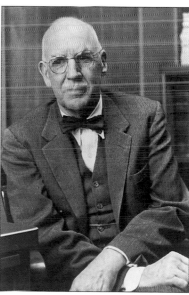

Student surgery course, 1938. At right is Miss Gertrude Gerrard instructing the student anesthetist Branch Craige; to their right is Elliott Cutler, making suggestions to the student surgeon Eben Alexander and his assistant John Brabson during an operation on a dog. The second assistant is Charles Jennings. In white surgical garb, standing at the end of the table to the left, is Carl Walter, instructor. Behind him, chin in hand, is FDM about to anesthetize another animal.

C. Sidney Burwell, Dean of Harvard Medical School during FDM's student years. In 1950, Burwell was succeeded by George Packer Berry.

Plate 7

FDM as a third-year student carrying out his first research project, evidently weighing something as accurately as he can on an old-fashioned balance.

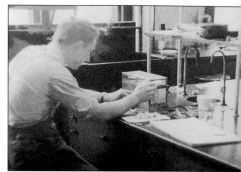

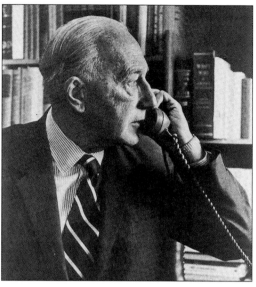

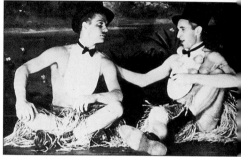

Claude E. Welch, surgical instructor during FDM's early years and later a colleague at the Massachusetts General Hospital (MGH).

Annual medical student spoof of the faculty, 1939. Set in the South Sea Isles, this scene shows two natives clad in remnants of a tuxedo over grass skirts: Donald D. Matson (*left*) is having an argument with Alexander H. Bill (*right*). Both men later became eminent surgeons.

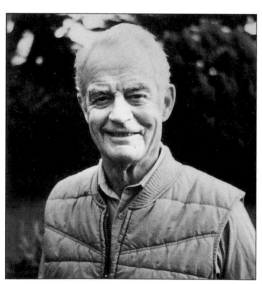

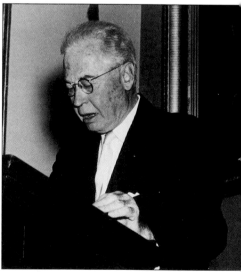

Richard Warren, surgeon of the MGH and the Brigham, descendant of the Warren surgical lineage, and close friend of FDM. His son, Richard Agassiz Warren, married Sally Moore.

A. Baird Hastings, Hamilton Kuhn Professor and Head of the Department of Biochemistry at Harvard Medical School during FDM's student years and a source of inspiration to FDM's later work.

Plate 8

arrived. Then, in December 1941, in the midst of that research year, came the attack on Pearl Harbor. Now we, too, were at war.

By spring 1942, every aspect of the hospital and our surgical work, as well as research and teaching, had become part of the war effort. Because of bronchial asthma I was classified 4F in the doctor draft and declared essential to the home front. I was told by Dr. Nathaniel Faxon, the hospital director, "Your job is right here." I finished up my junior residency, became senior resident and then chief resident, and finished the whole span of residency in November 1943, 4 $1/2$ years after graduating from medical school and starting internship. Actually, this amounted to only 3 $1/2$ clinical years because of the year taken off for research. During this time I gained expertise and a fair load of confidence. But 42 months was quite a speed-up over the 50 or 60 months many of my predecessors had been able to spend covering the same ground. While I might have enjoyed a longer residency and felt more confident, I was glad to get out of a white suit and join the MGH attending staff in surgery as its most junior member, on November 1, 1943.

Almost immediately after the attack on Pearl Harbor, the surgical residency plan at the MGH was changed around to adapt it to wartime, shortening surgical training from the former 5 or 6 years to a basic 9-9-9, or 27 months. This involved giving very young physicians lots of surgical responsibility, which meant they would require lots of supervision. It soon became my job to help make this supervision effective. This is when I came to feel most keenly the obligation to emphasize professional conduct, ethics, and honesty—as well as surgical skill—in the residency years. For those young wartime surgeons required to finish their residency in only 27 months after medical school, it was a severe challenge. The appetite of the army and navy for surgeons seemed insatiable. The teaching hospitals of the United States turned them out by the thousands.

Job Offers

In November 1943, Oliver Cope called me to his office. Edward Churchill, then head of the West Surgical Service at the MGH, was away at war. In his absence it fell to Oliver Cope to discuss career plans with the residents. Because he had been party to my classification by the hospital as essential to the home front and was aware of my asthmatic status and 4F classification in the draft, he knew he could count on my availability. He offered me an academic job at the most humble Harvard faculty level, as instructor in surgery, and a staff appointment at the MGH. Most important, he generously offered me a laboratory—at first, to share his own laboratory quarters—and money to buy biophysical apparatus not then available at the MGH, such as those used in radioactivity measurements (Geiger counters, electrometers), special handling equipment, and storage facilities for radioactive isotopes. I accepted his offer of an academic position but asked if I might also help one of the senior surgeons in practice. It was evident that my own ambivalence remained, that I was part surgical practitioner, part surgical scientist. I always remained so, never wishing to abandon completely the joy of surgery despite the pull of the research laboratory.

Cope assented to this plan, muttering that there wouldn't be much time for both academic work and practice. At the same time, as the end of my residency approached, Arthur Allen also considered me for a position. He was one of the most active of the senior surgeons at the MGH and headed up the East Surgical Service. His assistants, among them Claude Welch, were away at war. Dr. Allen asked Laurie and me to dinner one evening at his home. The next day at his office he discussed his practice arrangements with me. After our talk he said, "Franny, you are an academic, a professor, at heart." Yet he offered me the possibility of working with him for a year or two to help out while others were away. Although I was grateful for and flattered by Dr. Allen's offer, I turned it down. I felt that he should look further, that my commitment to research would interfere too much with my work as his assistant.

Within a few days Leland McKittrick, in a sense Allen's rival in Beacon Street practice, called me to his office and asked me if I would assist him in his practice. His most recent assistant had been Richard Warren, who was away at the war with the Harvard unit in Ireland and southern England, soon to go to the Continent after Omaha Beach. Warren and I were close friends and had done some work together. Dr. McKittrick's practice was situated at the MGH as well as at the New England Deaconess Hospital and its older branch, the Palmer Memorial Hospital. Leland McKittrick was understanding of my irregular hours in the lab, away from the office, so I chose to work as his assistant. Thus, for about 2 years I led a whirlwind existence including both research and practice, tolerable only to one of irrational ambition, unforgivable ego, and insufferable determination—possible only for one with a supportive wife who possessed an inexhaustible reservoir of forgiveness.

White Suit to Civvies

Thus, I became Leland McKittrick's assistant in November 1943. I had enjoyed my progress through the residency and the contacts with colleagues and senior surgeons of the staff, many of whom became close friends. I especially appreciated the chance to take a year off for research (Chapter 13) and even to do some clinical studies. But most of all I enjoyed my patients, many of whom followed me—or rather I followed them—over the years. They and their families were my contact with the continuing warmth and shared trust of surgical care.

Laurie and our family surely suffered a good bit with my constant absence during those residency years, though they never complained. Usually I was off to the hospital between 5:30 and 6:00 in the morning and didn't get home until quite late. The residents remained on duty in the hospital alternate nights. We also worked on Saturdays, Sundays, and holidays every second week.

A few days after entering practice in November 1943 and becoming a staff member at the MGH, my first private patient was referred to me, a woman with a small thyroid tumor. All surgeons remember that moment, a sort of debut after white-suited years in training. From that time forward my practice thrived, waxing and waning with the press of other responsibilities in teaching, in running a department, and in research. I always enjoyed the personal practice of surgery and that very special relationship with my own patients.

During those years as a beginning instructor and then as assistant professor at Harvard and as Leland McKittrick's private assistant, I did quite a lot of surgery. I enjoyed the art of surgery and my practice grew as McKittrick referred many patients to me. McKittrick himself practiced general surgery, that is, operations involving the abdominal cavity, the gastrointestinal tract, liver, and pancreas. He also did thyroid and breast surgery, as I did. I operated on the parathyroids and adrenals and the autonomic nerves, but he did not. We both were interested in ulcerative colitis and cared for many patients with that disorder. I became surgical director of the ulcerative colitis clinic at the MGH.

McKittrick was especially concerned with vascular surgery because he was the surgical consultant to the Joslin Diabetic Clinic. Diabetic patients are prone to severe obstructive disease of the arteries of their legs, which eventually leads to insufficient flow of blood (ischemia) and often to amputation. While I was with McKittrick, we took care of many diabetics. Unfortunately, without the benefit of present-day x-ray techniques for visualizing the arterial blood flow and with no means of restoring blood flow to previously closed arteries, we had to perform hundreds of amputations. McKittrick used to say that if he were shopping in Brookline and saw somebody coming toward him on crutches, he was pretty sure he was going to greet a patient. While this is not a happy situation for any surgeon, we were doing what was needed to save lives. That old-fashioned, long, sharp, amputation knife and the bone saw, depicted in cartoons of "Old Sawbones" since the days of Napoleon, saw lots of use in our hands in those hectic days during and right after the war. Today, with arterial reconstruction and better management of diabetes, such amputations are much less frequent.

My own health was at its worst with asthma and pulmonary infections in the 1940s and 1950s. After age 40, and thanks to good care, this drain on my time and energy gradually decreased. If age helps asthmatics, Mother Nature has smiled on many of those who began young. I seemed to have been an example.

I am grateful to those physicians who kept me going through the most severe years of asthma. Both at that time and up to the present, they have carried me through my many medical crises: Francis Rackemann, long-time MGH physician, and now Albert L. Sheffer, head of the allergy and asthma unit at the Brigham. Dr. Sheffer is an authority on asthma, which has become an increasingly prevalent problem in our society. He sets an example as one who provides personal attention, a caring about detail. This was not lost on his surgical patient.

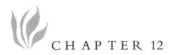

CHAPTER 12

Patient Outcomes, Ernest Codman, and Clinical Research

There are three ways by which one person, the physician, can help another person in distress: words, drugs, and hands.

"Words," although the easiest to administer and seemingly the least expensive, are of immense importance. While psychiatrists use words as their main weapon against disease, some of the worst mistakes made by surgeons, internists, and pediatricians arise from the misuse of words, and some of their clearest triumphs in human relations come from saying it right. The role of the mind in healing seems to be rediscovered by every generation. Words are the pathway to the mind.

"Drugs" encompass the whole range of chemical compounds used to treat human illness. While all physicians use drugs to some extent (even psychiatrists and radiologists), the use of chemical medicines is most clearly the province—indeed the main weapon—of those in internal medicine and pediatrics. Today surgeons and psychiatrists use drugs more than ever before. In their overuse and misuse lie many of the misfires of all medical care.

"Doing with the hands" is latinized as "manipulation" and enshrined in the Greek root of the word surgery, *chir-urgie*. But the laying on of hands is not solely the domain of surgery. Every doctor should use his friendly touch. Any physician worth his salt carries out a physical examination that goes beyond shining a light and asking the patient to say

"Ahhh." A common criticism of internists is their failure to examine the breasts of their female patients or to perform pelvic and rectal examinations. The gentleness with which any physician carries out those examinations (doing with the hands) is an important aspect of his empathy with the patient.

For the surgeon, this laying on of skilled hands is sometimes accomplished without any sharp instruments, as when he sets a simple fracture, or it may involve extensive sharp dissection under anesthesia in the familiar setting of the operating room. And then there are those severe injuries, such as burns, and diseases such as acute pancreatitis or advanced peritonitis, in which the responsibility of the surgeon extends over many weeks or months without any operation at all or with the selection of the right moment for operation as the key surgical decision.

If medicine is applied human biology, then surgery is its engineering arm. Surgery is based on the same corpus of human knowledge as the rest of medicine, but to this is added a craft, a skill with the hands. Surgery has no independent existence. It has no value *sui generis*, no existential component, no intrinsic message for the beholder. Surgery exists solely for the care of the sick and by that alone shall it be judged.

Forgive, But Do Not Forget

In internal medicine, pediatrics, and psychiatry, it is often the doctor's job to enroll the patient for continuing care. It is the surgeon's job to release the patient from care by definitive treatment and then return him to normal life. Sometimes—increasingly often—we succeed. Our failures have many causes, some of them preventable. Some of the deaths that occur on a general surgical service (including thoracic and vascular/ cardiac operations) are potentially preventable because they result from errors in diagnosis, judgment, or technique.

The other deaths are due to the progress of disease, advanced cancer, old age, hopelessly severe injury, or a combination of factors that defeat the surgeon's best efforts. In some cases a skill factor might have been sharper. Matters of skill are never quite so clear. Only to the experienced realist is it evident that when an elderly woman with gallbladder infection dies after operation, it might have been wiser to wait another few days before the operation, letting her stabilize after a simple drainage procedure. Then she might have made it through removal of the gallbladder or that procedure might even have been avoided. Sometimes a surgical error is very clear-cut. In cardiac surgery, for example, a single suture placed in error can be fatal. After any operation, failure to reoperate promptly for delayed hemorrhage can be disastrous. Recognition of error, of mishap, fostering rigorous honesty in the face of adversity, is essential to good surgery.

The assumption of risk is intrinsic to surgery. When you are experiencing the crushing chest pain of a severe heart attack, you want a surgeon willing to take risks, who might be willing to put his reputation on the line with an emergency bypass operation. You don't want a surgeon too proud to lose, too timid to accept a postoperative death. But you certainly want a surgeon, a department, a hospital that has done everything possible to reduce those risks. You want a surgical team that faces each error, each mishap, straight up, names it, and takes steps to prevent its recurrence. While this is the essence of a teaching hospital, any hospital can maintain this standard if it so chooses.

Judith Swazey and Renée Fox, who have written on the ethical aspects of surgical teaching and clinical research, inspire the phrase "Forgive, but do not forget" to describe the attitude shown by conscientious teachers of surgery. This attitude was evident in the weekly review of deaths and errors conducted by our chief, Dr. Churchill, using a system developed 25 years before by a surgeon named Ernest Amory Codman.

Codman's Classification

Ernest Amory Codman was born in 1869 and graduated from Harvard College in 1891 and Harvard Medical School in 1895. He was, rather characteristically, both a Bostonian and an iconoclast. He felt that hospitals were not sufficiently concerned about the quality of the outcomes they produced and that, like a factory, a hospital should evaluate its product critically—its product being the welfare of its patients. Since he believed this evaluation was not properly done at the MGH, he started his own hospital in protest. When he found that it too was flawed, he closed it down.

Codman introduced a system for classifying imperfect outcomes, complications, and deaths. His missionary purpose was to ferret out human error and distinguish it from the inevitable downswing caused by disease itself. Complications, deaths, or other faulty outcomes were rigorously classified as being due to errors in diagnosis, technique, or judgment. These were differentiated sharply from a group identified as patient's disease. Examples of the latter would include the continued growth of late cancer, unchecked by whatever treatment was carried out (or intentionally withheld); deaths from severe injuries; or massive burns in which the surgeon would be powerless. Such a system of classification is a good discipline for anyone in any field of medicine, especially when it is supplemented by a frank and full discussion of all the details by those most intimately involved in a patient's care.

In considering errors in diagnosis, technique, or judgment, it is important for the individual surgeon to stand up and be counted. At our weekly service meetings we were asked to give our own account of events—often a frank statement of error—before a group of our peers and teachers. Such meetings are often called morbidity and mortality conferences, or M&M.

As playwrights look back on the ones that "bombed in New Haven," so also a surgeon maintains a mental catalogue of the things he did wrong at various times in his career and tries never to repeat them. And if he is also a teacher, it is his job to tell his students about them. The memories always remain; some are pretty painful and are rarely brought up after that first meeting. On one occasion I left a strip of gauze in an obese woman who had undergone a mastectomy. A few days after she had returned home, it poked its tip out through the incision. I removed it under local anesthesia. I made no excuses to her husband. The hospital paid the bill. He said, "Thanks, now she's better." And she lived for at least two decades, a cure by most criteria.

On another occasion, I failed to drain a colostomy correctly. A severe infection followed and the patient died. Had I handled this correctly she probably would have lived. Despite my efforts to explain my own misjudgment in this complex bit of surgical technology, the family never really understood its import. I appreciated their continued expressions of gratitude for the care I had given and my concern over their tragedy.

M&M meetings might seem impossible and inadvisable in today's era of malpractice litigation, but they are conducted in most hospitals. The recognition of error and its open discussion by the surgeon are intrinsic to honesty in surgery. A young surgeon's life should not be ruined when he discusses an error he has made, for everyone else to hear and hence to learn. "Forgive, but do not forget." What better way of stating the philosophy of honest surgery?

The thrust of a conference on morbidity and mortality—identifying errors and the ways to avoid them—should permeate any surgical service, as it should permeate hospital departments of medicine, radiology, pediatrics, or any others that deal with the sick. Without this point of view, this self-searching honesty, medicine is somehow fraudulent, just as caring for pain and illness without a firm basis in the medical sciences is quackery.

Outcomes; Clinical Research

Early in my medical school years I was impressed by the forthright habit of surgeons in analyzing and publishing their results. These clinical papers often report on a series of patients (sometimes only one patient) and describe what was learned. They constitute clinical research. Many deal with outcomes. In my experience, good clinical research is as difficult to do as good laboratory science, although the latter may require more specialized education and skill. In both, the challenge is to meet a high standard of honesty and excellence. Research of both kinds can be sloppy, dishonest, self-serving, or fraudulent. Clinical research can be marred by biased statistics or by gathering cases by computer and giving them to someone unfamiliar with and inexperienced in the field to be written up for publication. Advertising on glossy paper.

My first clinical paper, on the study of a single patient, appeared in *The New England Journal of Medicine* in 1943. The patient was a gardener who had an open sore on his chest and developed high fever, pneumonia, and a destructive local infection that looked for a time as if it might spread and kill him. We considered several bizarre diagnoses: anthrax, tuberculosis, actinomycosis, black widow spider bite. Nothing showed up on cultures of the ulcer. Just on a hunch, I requested a blood test for tularemia. It was positive. Tularemia (a disease primarily of rabbits) was first described in Tulare County, California. This was one of the first proven cases of tularemia in New England. There was no antibiotic for this disease. After a long illness, the patient recovered completely. I was pleased at having made this diagnosis, piecing it together, and describing its significance in public health and epidemiology. When the galley proofs came back from the journal, I enjoyed the smell of printer's ink. That first article, "Tularemia in New England," is still quoted in reviews of that disease. It gave me pure joy and provided a special kind of excitement. As to writing, I was hooked.

In my early staff years at the MGH, I carried out several other clinical research projects in the fields of thyroid disease, duodenal ulcer, and ulcerative colitis, interests I had developed during residency.

The Thyroid and Antithyroid Drugs

Another of my early papers (1946) was on the treatment of thyrotoxicosis. The term "thyrotoxicosis" refers to overactivity of the thyroid gland, also known as hyperthyroidism. The former term accentuates the toxic nature of overproduction of thyroid hormone. When I was a young surgeon, we treated almost all such patients by removing most of the thyroid gland, an operation known as subtotal thyroidectomy. In the patient with severe thyrotoxicosis, this could be a hazardous procedure. Oliver Cope guided us in carrying out this operation safely. During my residency a new drug for thyroid disease, thiouracil, was introduced. This was the first of the antithyroid drugs. At first, such drugs were used primarily to make surgery safer by temporarily reducing thyroid overactivity.

As a junior member of the staff, I worked in the thyroid clinic under the leadership of Howard Means. We used thiouracil to reduce the hazards of operation. Because I felt that what we were learning could be of value to others, I corresponded with other surgeons in hospitals throughout the country and published a summary of this wide experience (theirs and ours) in using thiouracil for the preparation of patients for surgery. The paper was accepted by the *Journal of the American Medical Association* and was also published in 1946.

While my paper on tularemia was of interest to me and maybe a dozen people who were concerned with such epidemiology (and hopefully to a few more who were seeing such cases), the thyroid paper attracted wide attention. Lots of patients had thyrotoxicosis. Safe surgery was hard to come by. With the tularemia article I had smelled printer's ink, but with the thyroid article I experienced for the first time a widespread response: the medical public in this country and throughout the world was interested in an article on an important new topic. Any young person (I was about 32 at the time) would get some sort of a bang out of receiving a lot of correspondence and invitations to speak at medical meetings. I was no exception.

Duodenal Ulcer and Vagotomy

Duodenal ulcer is a painful disorder of the duodenum, the intestine just beyond the stomach. It is due in part to acid. The underlying cause is unknown. Two of our senior staff, Arthur Allen and Leland McKittrick, were very active in treating this prevalent disease. In the 1930s, hundreds of patients were treated surgically for duodenal ulcer every year at the MGH. When other treatments failed, the usual operation for duodenal ulcer was the subtotal gastrectomy. In this operation about two-thirds of an essentially normal stomach is removed to treat the disease next door in the duodenum. It was like taking out the engine to decrease noise in the gear box.

In the spring of 1943 it occurred to me that dividing the vagus nerves (vagotomy) might decrease the secretion of gastric acid and help the patient. The vagus nerves run from brain to stomach and activate gastric secretions. They were later dubbed the "worry nerves," because emotional stress sometimes made ulcer symptoms worse. I read up on the matter and discussed it with several physiologists and neurologists. There was a small literature on the effect of vagotomy in experimental animals. Although this procedure had been carried out in a few patients in Italy, it had been done for other diseases. From what little was known, vagotomy markedly reduced the acidity of the stomach without too many side effects.

It was February 1944. I had a patient with duodenal ulcer all lined up for vagotomy. His name was Barstow. He had been treated by internists with powders and pills for many years and had consulted several psychiatrists—all with little effect. His main problem was pain in the upper abdomen after meals, made better for a little while with alkali pills but always coming back. X-rays repeatedly displayed an unhealed ulcer and much scarring.

With the blessing of Chester Jones, who at that time was in charge of medical gastroenterology at the MGH, we had scheduled Mr. Barstow for the operation later that spring of 1944. One day in April or May, Chester Jones called me up and said, "Franny, Lester Dragstedt has just reported several vagotomies for ulcer." Dragstedt had been working at the Billings Hospital (at the University of Chicago) where I had taken my third-year medicine course 6 years earlier. I had met him but did not know him well. After discovering our common interest in vagotomy, we became fast friends.

The fact that he had already done the operation did not make a great deal of difference to our plans, except to remove from me the onus of doing the first one. It never occurred to me that this news meant that I could no longer claim priority for this new operation. In fact, I didn't consider that at all, because I had long since concluded that, in scientific work, true priority does not go to the person who does it first, but to the person who understands it and exploits it most effectively. What better example than the discovery of ether anesthesia? Crawford Long used it first, but Morton, at the MGH, and his surgical colleague Warren more clearly understood its meaning and awoke the world to its use.

I operated on Mr. Barstow on August 1, 1944. The patient got along very well. His pain disappeared completely while his stomach remained in place and intact. He continued as a grateful patient and friend of mine, and I followed his medical progress for years. He was a brilliant result from this operation, the first such performed outside the Billings Hospital.

For quite a few years many patients with duodenal ulcer were referred to me. When I published my first paper on vagotomy in *The New*

England Journal of Medicine with Chester Jones as coauthor, Arthur Allen quipped, "Franny, I saw your local advertising." We laughed about it. Both he and Leland McKittrick sent me several patients for vagotomy. I was delighted and flattered to have my own senior teachers as patrons of my new art, not to mention the many patients thankful for being spared a gastrectomy.

For about 25 years (from around 1950 to 1975) vagotomy became the standard fixture, virtually replacing gastrectomy. But now the disease itself (duodenal ulcer) has almost disappeared from the scene, the surgeon has disappeared from the setting, and a bacterium (of all things!) may be part of its cause. Other methods of treatment, especially drugs that diminish gastric acidity and now antibiotics, are less dangerous and sometimes equally effective. And as for the use of words in the treatment of duodenal ulcer, psychiatrists attest to the fact that they do not accomplish much

While I enjoyed this foray into the upper gastrointestinal tract, it never became a part of my research life. I was never a serious research scholar of duodenal ulcer (as Lester Dragstedt was) nor of diseases of the gastrointestinal tract in general, particularly the hormones that affect those diseases, subjects in which many of my colleagues soon became expert.

BOOK 🔥 FOUR

Basic Research and Academic Life

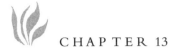

CHAPTER 13

The National Research Council and Isotope Research

(1941-1942)

S tarting back in high school, I had been interested in science and research. Several of us dreamed up an elective course on psychology that we asked one of our senior tutors, Mr. Jones, to teach. We were curious about how scientists designed experiments to study psychological reactions, whether they be of mice in a maze, pigeons in a box, or people in trouble. When someone did something stupid, kids used to say, "A crayfish learns in three lessons." This individual must be dumber than a crayfish, an allusion to those experiments teaching crayfish how to negotiate a maze.

Then, in college, I did absolutely no research other than figuring out how to get to New York as inexpensively as possible to see Laura. Now in medical school, happily married to Laura, I could broaden my research horizons. As a student I had investigated the decline in placental gonadotropic hormones immediately after delivery, as recounted in Chapter 2. More important than that, I was fascinated to learn at first hand the researches of people like Walter Cannon and A. Baird Hastings. Most of all I admired Fuller Albright. He presided over Ward 4 at the MGH, an area in the Bulfinch Building where there were four or five research beds.

The nurses on Ward 4 were especially trained to measure carefully everything their patients took in and to collect everything they put out. This was necessary so that metabolic changes could be measured accurately. Ward 4 was one of the first metabolic wards in the country. It was later endowed by the Mallinckrodt Company and was called Mallinckrodt Ward 4. Some years later—and now I am skipping ahead—the National Institutes of Health, inspired by such research units, granted funds to support clinical centers in many teaching hospitals. These were greatly expanded versions of the original Ward 4 at the MGH.

A Choice, and the Two Paths

While working at the MGH and attending Fuller Albright's research seminars, I developed a desire to learn more about metabolic research. In the winter of 1940-1941, 2 years out of medical school, I decided to spend a year in research. My life as a university surgeon, using quantitative biology to study surgical illness, began at that moment.

In many ways my decision to acquire some basic research skills was more crucial in changing my life than was the decision to go into surgery. Coming from a nonmedical, nonacademic background, I did not recognize this choice for what it really was: a branch in the roadway for a young doctor. At the time I did not even realize I was making a big decision. I just wanted to get involved with science.

I set out on this branch in the road when in January 1941, as a junior surgical resident at the MGH, I applied for a fellowship of the National Research Council. Dr. Frederick C. Irving wrote the necessary sponsoring letter. He was the obstetrician who had delivered Nancy and Peter and was soon to deliver Sally, and I felt closer to him than to any other member of the Harvard Medical School faculty. Some time in April, I learned to my delight that I had been awarded this fellowship. I was going to be paid $1,800 for that year—more than I had ever earned before.

When I embarked on that fellowship year in the laboratory, and later spoke of my research, senior members of the faculty began to think of me as a research academic, a potential university surgeon. By contrast, my own plans were to go into clinical practice in Chicago after completing my residency. Dr. Vernon David, a prominent surgeon at the Presbyterian Hospital in Chicago, was a close friend of my father. I had been a patient of his only a few years previously. Before I completed my residency, Dr. David had offered me a job with him in Chicago. The offer included a small corner of his office in the Loop. As a matter of some note, many of the doctors' offices in Chicago were situated in the People's Gas Building. It would have been in this appropriately designated sky-scraper that I would have settled.

After I published some research papers, the few members of the surgical community who knew of me at all certainly thought of me as an academic. Ironically, only a few years after Vernon David first talked with me about a job, and after I had published a few papers and made some presentations at national meetings, I was offered a position as the new academic professor of surgery at Presbyterian Hospital. Whether I knew it or not, I was heading on a route toward academia, with signposts clearly visible.

The two paths—clinical practice and academic work—do not have many crossovers. By the time a young surgeon is 3 years out of his residency in private practice (meaning that he is somewhere around 32 to 35 years old), it is almost impossible for him to make the change to academia. He will not be offered an appointment. Such young clinicians, no matter how brilliant or able, will not have the list of publications in basic science journals, the beginning of a reputation in research, the knowl-edge and know-how, and the concepts and methods of quantitative biol-ogy related to their clinical field. They will not have had the experience in laboratory design, administration, and finance required to make the change. They will have gained no funds to support whatever research they might plan. To enter the academic world of American biomedical research, you must start young, by studying and learning the methods of science in a laboratory.

Once in academia, if the call of research fades and young doctors fail to have new ideas, yet wish to continue clinical care of the sick full time, they can always change back to a life in practice. Whatever the connection between these two career pathways, it is a one-way street.

A Year at the Huntington

For my fellowship year in biophysics, I joined the research group at the Huntington Memorial Hospital under Joseph Aub. This small hospital was on Huntington Avenue, not too far from Brigham Circle, the Peter Bent Brigham Hospital, and the Harvard Medical School. The Huntington, the only hospital Harvard University ever owned, was devoted entirely to the study and care of cancer. Joseph Aub, as Physician-in-Chief, was working on the definition of abnormal growth. He was also interested in metabolic disease and was a pioneer in the application of isotopes to research, the newest and most rapidly growing hybrid of biology and physics, only then becoming known as "biophysics."

Bringing that National Research Council fellowship stipend with me meant that Aub would not have to pay me even though he paid for my equipment. Waldo Cohn and Austin Brues were the two scientists who introduced me to isotope research. I was assigned a Geiger counter and the job of calibrating it each morning. For a whole year I saw no patients and did not scrub on any operations. I took a course in nuclear physics. I learned by direct observation that the amount of a radioactive substance present is proportional to the number of nuclear disintegrations per second, some of which made a click on the Geiger counter. A curie of any radioactive substance yields radiation at the rate of 3.7×10^{10} nuclear disintegrations per second. I had entered the world of applied physics and isotope research.

Isotopes and Biophysics; A Radioactive Dye

We had learned in medical school that certain dyes concentrate in abscesses. It was my plan to make one of these dyes radioactive so that when it was injected it would collect near the abscess, and its location could be detected from outside the body with a Geiger counter. Much as I would like to claim originality for this concept, the idea came from Valy Menkin, one of our teachers in pathology. In his writings Menkin stated that if this dye could somehow be made detectable, it might be useful as a way to diagnose and localize abscesses. That was 8 or 10 years before radioactive isotopes became available.

An isotope of an element is its twin sister, having identical chemical properties but a different atomic weight. The number after the name of the element indicates its weight relative to hydrogen. Some isotopes are radioactive, some not; most are natural, some manmade. The nonradioactive isotopes of some common elements (deuterium for hydrogen, heavy nitrogen) differ by weight only. They can be measured by mass spectrometry.

Tracers are spies, informers. If radioactive, they announce by their radiation where they are and therefore where their compatriots are, like a bellwether that tells where the flock is. Radioactive isotopes have the additional feature that they can be detected from a distance by their radiation, such as from outside the body with a Geiger counter, or with a gamma camera, which takes a picture showing the "hot spots." Radioactive isotopes make ideal tracers. I was to learn how to make use of this wonderful new scientific method, first used only a few years earlier, after Lawrence of Berkeley, California, invented the atom smasher (as the newspapers called it), or cyclotron.

To accomplish our mission of finding abscesses by means of radioactivity, we needed to make a radioactive dye. For this synthetic challenge I was fortunate in enlisting the aid of a young organic chemist, Lester Tobin. He had been studying under Louis Fieser, our teacher of organic chemistry, an expert in organic synthesis (making new compounds such as drugs). Tobin synthesized the radioactive derivative of a dye called trypan blue by linking two radioactive bromine atoms to its phenyl groups. We obtained the radioactive bromine by bombardment at the cyclotron either at Harvard or at MIT. In his book *Why Smash Atoms?*, Arthur Solomon explained how cyclotrons worked and how this all came about and thus helped our generation grasp the physics involved.

To make bromine radioactive, we placed an organic fluid, bromoform (the bromine analogue of chloroform), in glass bottles for neutron bombardment. Two physicists, Leo Szilard and T.A. Chalmers, had described this nuclear reaction. When a bromine atom in this fluid was hit by a neutron, it would be knocked off the bond attaching it to the bromoform molecule and be rendered radioactive. These radioactive bromine atoms would then become soluble in water. The radioactive bromine could therefore be separated from the bromoform by using an ordinary separatory funnel (high-school chemistry). This yielded highly active radiobromine. Szilard later became famous as a pioneer in the development of the atomic bomb.

As junior-grade researchers working closely with the group at

MIT under Professor Robley D. Evans (Chairman of the Department of Nuclear Physics), we occasionally attended biophysics seminars. I had taken some physics courses. One toe was immersed in nuclear physics. Later that year, MIT held a meeting on practical applications of nuclear physics. To my delight, I was invited.

The last speaker was a man I had never heard of before. His name was Enrico Fermi and the title of his talk was "Uranium Fission." He made it clear that the atoms of certain heavy elements (that were unstable and spontaneously radioactive) would be split apart when hit by neutrons, causing them to release an immense burst of energy. Uranium was one such element. I listened with some interest because I had been using a uranium salt (uranyl zinc acetate) in my job with the Geiger counter. In his lecture Fermi was describing the basic nuclear reaction of the first atomic bomb. The term "uranium fission" was not mentioned again in public nor published in any form until after the war. About 2 years earlier, in 1939, Albert Einstein, in collaboration with Szilard, had written his famous letter to President Roosevelt about the military potential of Fermi's discovery of uranium fission. Get enough of the right isotope of uranium in one clump—a critical mass—and it would touch itself off with its own neutrons, causing one hell of an explosion. At that time no one knew of the letter; few even in that audience grasped the implications of Fermi's talk. Certainly not I. But after that moment the whole concept became highly classified, and those of us who worked with radioactive isotopes and nuclear physics were required to have security clearance, even including this young surgeon who was learning biophysical techniques to locate abscesses.

Lester Tobin and I went ahead with our work, but we were very careless with the everyday hazards of handling radioactive materials. We did not even wear exposure badges when working around the cyclotron. The only precaution we took was to remove our wristwatches, since the extremely powerful magnets of a cyclotron would ruin a watch forever. We even carried those big bottles of radioactive bromine under our arms and out to the car! Fortunately, neither of us has (as yet) suffered any consequences. And I fathered three more children. Maybe we were lucky as well as careless.

Once we had figured out how to produce sterile abscesses in the bellies of anesthetized rabbits, Lester and I injected some of the radioactive dye and mounted a Geiger counter over the animal. To our delight (but surely no surprise) we could tell where the abscess was by the counts per minute. It took us about 7 months of hectic work to arrive at this point.

Later that spring (at the urging of Dr. Aub) we submitted an abstract of our work to the Society for Clinical Investigation. This was the leading organization of young medical scientists (known as the Young Turks) who were turning over new ground. We were thrilled to be given a place on the program of the society's meeting at Atlantic City in April 1942. I was given 12 minutes to describe our research and demonstrate the localization of abscesses with a Geiger counter. In addition we showed that this dye tended to concentrate in tumors and theorized that a technique like this might be used to diagnose abscesses and treat tumors. We submitted three articles (on the radioactive dye synthesis, the abscess work, and tumor localization) to the *Journal of Clinical Investigation* and were pleased (and this time we *were* surprised) when our manuscripts were accepted and then published.

What we were doing, without having a word for it, was to stir around at its very beginnings in the field later called "nuclear medicine." Nowadays, radiologists use radioactive isotopes for diagnosis and treatment daily in all major hospitals. I am proud of these early ideas, of Tobin's organic synthesis, and of our early successful application of nuclear physics in the laboratory.

Our radioactive dye had other applications as well. In his lab at the MGH, Oliver Cope was examining changes in the permeability of capillaries in burned animals. By injecting the radioactive dye into these experimental animals, we could discern minute changes in permeability produced by even a tiny burn because we could detect a few molecules of the dye leaking out of the bloodstream into the lymph. This led to a better understanding of the fluid leak in burn injury, which requires plasma and fluid replacement. By then (1942) we were working under the wartime Office of Scientific Research and Development.

About that time I conceived the principle of diluting isotopes in the body to measure the body's chemical components. By injecting minuscule amounts of isotopes into the body and measuring the extent of their dilution, we could determine how much there was of the substance in which they were diluted. We first applied this principle to burns, and it became the basis of our treatment of burn injury, providing a way of measuring the fluid requirement of burned patients and representing the beginning of a study known as "Body Composition," a term we later used to describe this rapidly growing area of knowledge.

Academia Beckons

Upon finishing the residency in November 1943, I could return to serious research along with the clinical tasks of assisting Leland McKittrick. I was very busy, but it was wartime and so was everyone else: some at home, others abroad fighting the war.

After a couple of years of riding the two horses of clinical practice and academic work, it became obvious that my heart was in academia and, as Oliver Cope had warned, there was not time for both. By now my career ambivalence was vanishing. After the war, and with the return of many staff colleagues, I concentrated entirely on my academic and surgical work at the MGH. A couple of years later, the Barnes Hospital and Washington University in St. Louis offered me a professorship. They had read my papers and knew of the direction my work was taking. Surely this was yet another clear sign that the surgical establishment had made a choice of which way I would go. I thanked Bob Moore, the Dean at Washington University, who had come to visit and tried to recruit me, but told him I wanted to stay in Boston.

Those wonderful years at the MGH following my residency, from 1943 to 1948, were vital not only to my clinical development but also to my long-range plans in biological science and surgery. I am grateful to Edward Churchill and Oliver Cope for giving me so much help in those crucial years—crucial for all young doctors starting out either in practice or in academia—and to Leland McKittrick for giving me such a joyous introduction to the private practice of surgery. My debt to the MGH is boundless.

In 1947 I sent a review article to *Surgery, Gynecology & Obstetrics*, a major surgical journal with an international circulation. Entitled "The Use of Isotopes in Surgical Research," it was given the leadoff position in the

January 1948 issue. To me it was old stuff going back 8 years. But for many of the surgical readers, it contained new ideas and attracted a lot of attention. In it I described in understandable terms, without physics or formulas, the principle of isotope dilution, the meaning of body composition, and their potential for improving surgical care.

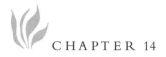

CHAPTER 14

Body Composition and the Stuff of Which We Are Made; The Body Cell Mass

Some of the most pressing problems of surgery in the 1930s and 1940s were the dangerous inaccuracy, inadequacy, and often disastrous ineffectiveness of supportive care for patients who had sustained severe injuries, burns, or major operations. These problems of midcentury surgery came into focus as anesthesia, asepsis, the increased range of surgery, and two world wars had brought surgery to greater prominence in the treatment of a remarkable range of illnesses. This change in the scope of surgery was to be expected in historical terms about the time our generation entered the field. We did not invent it. Maybe our generation was acutely aware of the need for greater accuracy and depth of knowledge as we saw the methods of surgery spread to patients in every specialty of medicine.

Supportive care might include intravenous infusions of water, salt, or sugar; transfusions of blood and plasma to replace lost fluids or blood; and nutritional (dietary) support by mouth or vein. The amount of fluid given often missed the mark by a wide margin. While flying blind can be a problem in internal medicine, it is in surgery that such inadequacies are especially dangerous. This is because of the responsibility of surgeons for the care of massive injuries, wounds, burns, and major operations, all of which produce abrupt and potentially lethal changes in the bodily economy.

I saw many burned patients go into shock or die in the first 24 hours because of inadequate fluid treatment. Sometimes I was guilty of the same errors because there were no reliable guides. If the surgeon could have estimated a patient's blood volume from simple age–sex–weight tables (not available at that time) and could assess the degree of plasma loss based on the blood cell count, he could have done a more accurate job of estimating how much replacement fluid was needed. I recall a patient having an adrenal tumor removed—a dangerous operation at that time because of sodium loss from the body—who was literally drowned by saline infusions that greatly exceeded any rational need. Such deaths were often termed postoperative pneumonia because the extra fluid in the lungs was audible by stethoscope, as in pneumonia. But it was not pneumonia in any sense of that term. Nor was it infection. It was simply too much fluid. Pulmonary edema.

These treatment errors came about because no one knew how much fluid there was in the body to begin with, in its various fluid compartments, or pools. No one could appreciate the meaning of the extent of water or sodium losses without knowing the normal baseline values. Some of these losses could actually be due to relocation within the body: from the blood plasma to the lymph in burns, for example. Using isotopes, we solved the mystery of the whereabouts of the lost plasma of burns. It was in the body but in the wrong place. This loss of plasma could be lethal without a drop of plasma escaping from the body.

Until several years after World War II, even such matters as avoiding dehydration in intestinal obstruction or vomiting, or managing an imbalance of chemicals in the blood, were dangerously mishandled. Today, these are simple, even routine problems, easily corrected. Disasters could have been avoided had the surgeon known normal body composition and the meaning of fractional gains and losses of tissue and fluid. Our studies of body composition led to a definition of the biochemistry of surgical illness as well as a sounder estimate of the most urgent needs of sick or injured patients. They also led directly to research in the biology of surgical convalescence, the chemistry of getting well.

Chemical methods for measuring blood volume had already been developed and exploited by Magnus Gregerson, the physiologist at Columbia, and had been extended to other aspects of the bodily economy by

John Stewart, an MGH surgeon a few years ahead of me in the residency. My special opportunity arose from the ability—gained in that glorious year as a National Research Council fellow at the Huntington Hospital— to use isotopes (both stable and radioactive) for this work. Through isotope dilution we could get a better handle on body composition, on the needs of sick surgical patients, and how to treat them more accurately.

We measured total body water, extracellular water, blood volume, the total mass or weight of body cells, total sodium, and total potassium. From these we could accurately estimate total body nitrogen and hydrogen, body fat, and the weight of the skeleton. The stuff of which the body is composed could be measured accurately and without pain or inconvenience in the living by using new biophysical tools: isotope tracers. In this work we were lucky in being able to do the whole job with tiny doses of radioactivity.

The principle of isotope dilution is disarmingly simple. To measure an unknown volume of water, put a known bit of salt in it and find out how much it is diluted. This is a familiar chemical principle. If you have a bucket of fresh water and you don't know how much is in it, put in a gram (1.0 gram) of salt. Stir the salt around and let it equilibrate, that is, come to rest fully diluted and distributed. Then take a small sample. If there is 0.001 gram of salt (1/1,000th of a gram, or 1 milligram) in each milliliter of the water, then the salt must have been diluted in 1,000 milliliters (i.e., 1 liter) of solution. You have measured the unknown volume of water in the bucket by adding a known amount of tracer to it and measuring the extent of the tracer's dilution.

We adapted this principle, using radioactive isotopes, to measure several key elements of which the body is composed: water (using heavy hydrogen, or deuterium, and later hydrogen of weight 3, or tritium), potassium (using ^{42}K), sodium (using ^{24}Na), and chloride (using radiobromide, ^{36}Br, which behaves like chloride). Later we used heavy nitrogen (^{15}N) to measure the rates of protein synthesis. We used radioactive chromium, as developed by Seymour Gray in the Department of Medicine, for measuring the red cell volume and Evans blue dye (Gregerson) for the plasma volume. A small sample of blood was all that was required to measure the extent of dilution and the total body composition.

In explaining the measurement of volume by dilution, the drink-of-whiskey model is a good one. A jigger of whiskey in a small glass of water is harsh stuff. Put it in a quart of water, well... lots weaker. The taste (i.e., concentration) of the whiskey reflects the volume of water you have added. You are measuring a volume by dilution of a tracer. By the same token, the density of dye color is inversely proportional to the volume of water added to soften the color.

We live on a planet constantly bombarded by radiation from outer space (cosmic rays and solar flare emissions). We have a naturally occurring radioactive isotope of potassium (^{40}K) in every cell of our bodies, mixed intimately with the chromosomes and genes that guide our growth and behavior. We are also hit by radiation from the Earth itself (uranium, radium) and from medical tests (x-rays, nuclear medicine). When radiation doses are increased far above this natural background level, cancer and other diseases can result. Genetic changes are sometimes produced. Therefore, in our studies of body composition we were careful to see to it that the total dose of radiation did not exceed that from a one-shot diagnostic x-ray. In pregnancy, even very small doses of radiation are dangerous to the unborn child, so we did not use radioactive isotopes in studying the body composition in pregnant women or in young children.

How Much Water Is in a Rabbit?

It is said that Archimedes first conceived of the physical principles by which some things float and others sink while he was floating in a bathtub. I can claim a certain kinship with the great floater, because it was while taking a bath that I first conceived of the idea of measuring the amount of water in the body by diluting an isotopic tracer for water. An isotope of either hydrogen or oxygen would be required to measure the total amount of water, which is a compound of these two elements (H_2O). Isotopes of each element differ in atomic weight but not in chemical properties. Hydrogen (H) has an atomic weight of 1. Deuterium (D), as one might guess from its name, is an isotope of hydrogen of weight 2. It is also called heavy hydrogen. Deuterium is not radioactive; it is a stable isotope. When combined with oxygen, deuterium makes heavy water.

Ordinary water is H_2O. Heavy water is D_2O. Tritium (the hydrogen isotope of weight 3) is radioactive.

For isotope dilution of a water tracer, heavy water certainly seemed the way to go. It can be detected because of the tiny difference in its weight or specific gravity. Needless to say, like all young scientists, I thought my idea of measuring total body water by deuterium dilution was original. I therefore wrote to Professor Harold Urey (who had discovered deuterium), told him of my idea for body water measurement, and asked if I could obtain some of this isotope. He replied helpfully, sending me a little test tube of deuterium (as heavy water) from an atomic reactor. I still treasure this gift in my personal museum.

More important, in his reply Professor Urey told me that the idea would certainly work and that a Hungarian scientist living in Sweden, Georg von Hevesy, had considered this possibility a few years before. There is nothing new under the sun. I then wrote to von Hevesy, who told me this story. While having tea in the Rutherford Physics Laboratory in Cambridge, England, in 1934, he and his partner (H.J.G. Moseley, the physicist) mused over the fact that, "If there were a little heavy water in this tea, we could measure how much water was in our own bodies." They had not done the experiment. It remained for us to accomplish this in our laboratories in the next few years and to define the normal total body water content in human beings of both sexes and all ages as a basis for studying changes in body water content in disease. Georg von Hevesy became a friend and to him we later dedicated our book on body composition (*The Body Cell Mass*).

But first we had to prove that the method really worked. Start simple. So we began by measuring the total body water of rabbits by deuterium dilution, injecting heavy water as normal saline solution. After we had finished the measurement (which required two or three blood samples over the course of an hour), we killed the rabbits by injection of an anesthetic. After weighing each carcass carefully, we took each to absolute dryness in a vacuum desiccator and weighed it again. This may sound complicated, even bulky, but it was a simple principle. Kitchen chemistry. A bit smelly. I had as assistants two young women, Margaret Ball and Caryl Magnus, who did the hard part, the analytic steps. If you weigh something while it is wet (a sponge, let us say), then take it to absolute dryness so that it won't lose any more weight with further drying, the difference between the wet weight and the dry weight will equal the weight of water that was in the sponge at the start. Same with the rabbit.

You can imagine our elation when we found that the amount of water in the rabbit's body, as measured by drying, correlated perfectly with the total body water, as measured by heavy water (deuterium) dilution in the living animal. Our new and elegant isotopic method, based on nuclear physics and chemistry, really worked.

From this beginning, we developed methods for measuring some of the other substances in the body using radiobromide for the volume of extracellular fluid, a principle based on studies done a few years before by our chemistry mentor at Harvard Medical School, A. Baird Hastings. We also measured the total weights of sodium and potassium in the body by dilution of their radioactive isotopes, an entirely original idea. And it worked, as proven again by analysis of the whole rabbit. We were on our way. The dream was to analyze the human body while the patient lay quietly in bed, reading the morning paper.

On to Our Own Species; The Body Cell Mass

Once assured that the low doses of radioactivity were safe and that the method was accurate in laboratory animals, we studied people. To begin with, we studied ourselves, our wives, and our families. In the women and children we used only nonradioactive deuterium and the blue dye, so as to avoid even tiny doses of radiation. Because we were interested in changes throughout the age groups, we measured the total body water in our children and enlisted willing patients who were compositionally normal or awaiting study or operation. With an able team and laboratory staff we could get the job done. We perfected the method to the point of a single injection of several tracers and simultaneous measurements of equilibrium concentrations, all in 2 to 3 hours: "one-shot" body composition. James D. McMurrey, later a surgeon of Houston, Texas, was a leader in the development of the multiple simultaneous compositional methods.

We had shown that all the potassium in the body exchanges with the radioactive tracer (unlike sodium, about a third of which is trapped in bone). About 98% of body potassium is within cells, at a chemically constant concentration in normal health. In disease, this concentration fluctuates with the osmotic strength of the plasma and can be estimated accurately. Thus, in measuring total body potassium we were, quite directly, measuring the total mass (weight) of all the cells of the body. The total body cell mass is the engine of the body that needs fuel and oxygen to keep going, since it does all the work of exercise, secretion, and thinking (the brain is a very active tissue metabolically). It is the central core. All else (skin, bone, tendons, fascia, cartilage, joints) is chassis and is, interestingly, sodium-rich, while the cells are potassium-rich with (normally) only tiny concentrations of sodium.

The concept of the body cell mass was a major fruit of our findings and our thinking and became the title of the book we published in 1963 describing the findings of almost 20 years of research.

From such data we could define normal values for human body composition as well as growth and aging in those terms. We found sudden changes at puberty for both sexes. When a girl reaches puberty she gains fat that helps form her breasts and the curves of her feminine figure. This is fatty or adipose tissue deposited in characteristic locations. At puberty the relative amounts of water and potassium (muscle) therefore fall. Meanwhile, her figure changes from that of a young girl to that of a mature woman. Her male counterpart at puberty does just the opposite, losing notable amounts of fat, gaining water and potassium (muscle), looking less chubby and more angular, lean, and muscular, as he matures into an adult man. The male has a larger body cell mass than the female—a larger total metabolism—but is often less resistant to hardship and starvation.

From time to time we published our findings in both the clinical and the scientific literature. This had a remarkable effect. Doctors began to think more clearly about the body composition of their patients and how it was affected by disease and treatment. Many young scientists were attracted to our laboratories from several different disciplines and from foreign countries. Within a few years similar work was undertaken in other labs, often by our pupils. The exact composition of the human body and the effects of disease on body composition are of interest and importance to cardiologists, internists, pediatricians, nutritionists, dietitians, and even veterinarians.

To finish this job, measurements in hundreds of sick patients before and after treatment now became our task—one that was to occupy our laboratory staff and successive groups of young physicians, surgeons, and scientists for many years. We started this task at the MGH but then moved to the Brigham. These results, too, were published in the scientific journals as well as in clinical papers and chapters in textbooks. This work was to lead to my recognition as a scientist not only among surgeons but also by scientists from other fields. Many other laboratories here and abroad took up the work, and it remains a lively field of study 50 years after our first start. The findings have made surgery safer and have assisted in the care of medical and pediatric patients everywhere.

Within a year or two of starting these studies of human body composition in health and disease, we broadened our focus to investigate the forces that drive convalescence (described in the next chapter). Changes in the human body after severe injury involve characteristic alterations not only in body composition, but also in metabolism and in the hormone secretions of the endocrine glands.

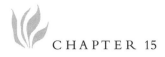

CHAPTER 15

Getting Well;
The Response to Injury and
the Nature of Survival

To discern the sequence of changes that occur within the human body after injury became our most important ongoing quest. I suppose this quest was born in reasonably full-fledged form somewhere around 1945, when we began to measure total body water with deuterium and to measure the loss of nitrogen and potassium after injury. Later, this work became dignified as a field of study known as "metabolism in convalescence," or the biology of getting well. Since nearly all of surgery involves the care of patients after injury or operation, this chemistry and physiology, the biology of convalescence, is central to the understanding and care of surgical patients.

You do not need to be a researcher, chemist, or biologist to be thrilled by the strong natural forces and inner drive that lead to recovery after severe injury. We all sense this when we witness the recovery of someone we know who has had a bad infection, a major operation, or a broken bone.

The Beauty of Convalescence; The Normal Sequence

At first the body is struck down. The patient is in pain and is listless, wants to stay in bed, and can't do much else. No appetite; weight and fat are lost rapidly. Precious water and salt are rigorously conserved.

Nitrogen (and therefore protein) is lost, muscles shrink, the patient feels weak and has no interest in much of anything.

Then comes a turning point. In ordinary major abdominal operations this usually comes at 2 or 3 days. After a severe burn it may take a week or longer; in multiple fractures, as seen in automobile accidents or war wounds, this turnabout may be postponed as much as 10 days. This spectacular turn of events, readily visible to all, is that suddenly the patient takes a much greater interest in surroundings, food, and people. There is a desire to get up, get eating, and get going. Patients ask for the newspaper or turn on the TV. They are once again interested in the world outside the hospital and eager to join it. In women, the first sign of recovery may be a bit of lipstick, the "positive lipstick sign." Visitors are welcomed. But the patient is still quickly exhausted because the muscles are just not there to match ambition; they take longer to rebuild. Weight loss seems to increase sharply for a day or two. If you examine this seeming enigma, you find that it is because the patient is now making more urine. A diuresis. The swelling around the burn or fracture (as an example) goes away. During this time the area of the injury itself becomes not only less swollen but also much less painful and tender. Toward the end of this phase, the stitches are removed (or reabsorbed) because the skin has gained enough tensile strength to hold itself together without the help of stitches.

Then the patient moves into the third phase of convalescence. The recovering economy of the body starts to rebuild muscles. The rehabilitation phase. The teenage football player with the broken leg doesn't need to be told what is going on. He begins to feel stronger. The body cell mass, the muscles, and strength increase with eating and intake of protein. Bones heal much more slowly than skin, and fractured bones cannot take the full load of body weight for several more weeks. Muscles rebuild at an intermediate rate. In burns, the skin covering is also slow to heal, sometimes taking weeks or months. Rehabilitation exercises and physiotherapy as well as an appetizing protein diet help muscle regrowth. Libido returns. Women usually have no monthly periods after severe injury, but a few months later the menses return. The patient who felt ready to leave the hospital some time after the turning-point phase now may feel strong enough to consider a return to work. Nowadays, doctors often permit patients to return to work too soon (at least in my opinion).

Metabolic studies show that for several weeks muscle protein is still being resynthesized. The doctor should be saying, "Don't go back to work until you feel strong enough."

Finally, starting about 5 or 6 weeks after major surgery or injury (several months after a severe burn), muscle mass has returned to near normal but body fat is yet to be regained. In the fourth phase this fat is restored, and the patient finally gets back up to normal weight. It requires calories to rebuild protein in muscle; when the muscle is rebuilt to the size needed for daily demands, those calories (now extra calories) are stored as fat.

This normal sequence of convalescence has deep roots in evolution. It is driven in part by hormones and is reflected by changes in body composition (some of them hormone-induced) and by the net balance of important nutrients such as nitrogen, salts, vitamins, and total calories.

Cannon and Cuthbertson

When we first became interested in pulling this fascinating picture together and doing the research to understand it better, it was only 8 years after I had been a pupil in the physiology classes of Walter B. Cannon, who contributed the first hormonal (endocrine) data to this field. He was the first pioneer in studying bodily changes after injury. David Cuthbertson was the first to show the protein loss after injury. I was fortunate to have known both men, one as my professor of physiology, the other as a friend whom I had met in Scotland when I was visiting professor in Edinburgh with Sir James Learmonth in 1952.

Walter Cannon spent most of his life studying the autonomic nervous system. In his book *Bodily Changes in Pain, Hunger, Fear and Rage; An Account of Recent Researches into the Function of Emotional Excitement*, he showed that certain types of stress or excitement elicited an outpouring of the adrenal medullary hormones epinephrine and norepinephrine, sometimes called the fight-or-flight hormones. Now we know that these hormones produce profound changes in the metabolism of sugar and fat, with changes in heart rate and other adaptations to a reduced circulating volume of blood. In many cases of stress or injury—and most certainly in big operations, severe accidents, or burns—this line of defense is the first evidence of the body's response to injury. It is not so much "fight or flight" as it is "hard times ahead." These same adrenal medullary hormones, acting via the pituitary (as shown by George Thorn), then activate increased secretion of their next-door neighbors, the adrenal cortical hormones, to engage the body as a whole not only in emergency damage control, but also in initiating the long process of getting well.

David Cuthbertson was a veterinary researcher in Scotland. In experiments on rats he showed that after fracture of the femur there was a marked outpouring of nitrogen, a proxy for body protein. All protein contains nitrogen, and most of the nitrogen of the body is in protein. If you are losing more protein than you are taking in, you are said to be in negative nitrogen balance. Protein is disappearing. Building directly on Cuthbertson's first studies in rats, we showed that the same thing is true in humans and that in certain types of very severe injury or infection the loss of body protein can be massive. During the nitrogen buildup phase it reloads again. Cuthbertson used the term "ebb" for the early nitrogen loss and "flow" for the resumption of synthesis. To this background we added data on many surgical patients, along with studies of water and salt balance, body composition, and the activity of the endocrine glands; it was clear that Cannon and Cuthbertson were the pioneers who had provided the basis for our emerging understanding of convalescence as an innate biological sequence after injury. In Darwinian terms its survival value is obvious: this is how the fittest survive after injury.

In those years (1946 to 1952) we were setting out to fill in this intricate picture of human survival. In 1952 I was invited to Edinburgh as visiting professor of surgery. Through the kindness of my host Sir James Learmonth, I had an opportunity to meet David Cuthbertson. We became friends, and 32 years later, in 1984, David (later Sir David) was present when I had the pleasure of giving the first Cuthbertson Lecture of the European Society of Nutrition, in Milan. Five years later Sir David died at the age of 88.

When I asserted that the whole of convalescent biology is an adaptation to injury that is important to survival, an innate chemical and physiologic process of the human body, people sometimes had trouble understanding what I was saying. Even if I stated that it is a survival mechanism, the product of millions of years of evolution, many still did not grasp my meaning. For the species to survive, individuals must survive the severe adversity of injury, fractures, and burns.

Three of Life's Sequences: Pregnancy, Growth, and Convalescence

To understand the body's program for convalescence it helps to recognize two other familiar processes or programs analogous to convalescence: pregnancy and growth. Like convalescence, each involves a stimulus, certain nerve mediators, hormone activation, massive changes in body composition, a target date for completion, and an event signalling that completion. Each is deeply programmed in our genetic makeup. Each of these basic bodily programs might be restated, in rather stilted terms, as a "sequence of changes in composition and chemistry with accompanying hormone stimuli, a targeted outcome, and a set length of time to get there," a biological process essential to survival of the species.

To gather data on this matter in the human being after injury, we studied a great many patients. To our patients, this research did not seem very remarkable or upsetting because their care was unchanged thereby. Mostly we measured their diet and their output, their gains and losses. In many instances we admitted them to a small metabolic ward, a sort of surgical version of Ward 4 at the MGH (Chapter 2). We had established this research unit in 1954 with an endowment in honor of Laura's father, Edmund B. Bartlett, given in his memory by Laura's mother and called the Bartlett Unit. In this metabolic unit we were able to measure everything we needed without running around all over the hospital. While this arrangement might have seemed at first glance to be inconvenient to the patients, actually it was not. Each patient was given a single room and had special nurses attending to them around the clock without having to pay extra. Most important were their overall surgical care, their urine collections, dietary analyses, and their one-shot multiple-isotope injection to determine body composition. The tracer dose of radioactivity was tiny and within the established safety guidelines.

We studied lesser kinds of surgical injury as well as severe, life-endangering trauma. Patients were selected who had all sorts of difficulties, including major operations, minor operations, and some severe injuries, compound fractures, total body crush (a term used by residents to denote severe injury from an automobile accident), and major burns. My son Peter came down with acute appendicitis at this time. With his informed consent (about which I was the butt of a certain amount of ribbing in later years), he was admitted for the study of the metabolic responses to a very simple operation: appendectomy.

Our studies showed clearly that in patients of all ages, of both sexes, and with a variety of injuries or operations, the process of injury and healing followed essentially the same sequence. In all instances there was the stimulus of injury, such as accidental trauma, elective surgery, or even an acute infection. This was accompanied by psychological and emotional changes, including fear and apprehension, as well as neurological responses, especially those of pain. Endocrine changes (alterations in the blood level of hormones) showed (just as Cannon had shown) that the adrenal medulla was one of the first glands to respond, followed by the outer layers of the adrenal (the cortex) with cortisone-like hormones. The pituitary gland is activated at the outset to stimulate these adrenal cortical changes and, in addition, to secrete antidiuretic hormone, which conserves body water. Since salt and water are retained, it is important not to give too much at this stage, especially in older people. The body shifts its energy source from burning carbohydrate (sugar) in food to oxidizing its own stored fat for calories. As one patient put it, "My operation was the world's most effective and expensive form of weight loss." Muscle protein is also hydrolyzed (chewed up) in this catabolic (destructive) process, the amino acids (building blocks) thus being made available by the metabolic mill from which new proteins can be synthesized and wounds can be healed. Then comes the long rebuilding phase, or anabolic (constructive) period of rebuilding body protein and finally body fat.

We began to publish some papers (occasionally a chapter in a book) about the metabolism of convalescence. Younger physicians, surgeons, and medical students who read about this work were evidently fascinated and wanted to know more about it. Many came to work with us. They understood the basics immediately. The analogy between convalescence and the bodily sequences of pregnancy and normal growth helped to explain convalescence to doubting practitioners.

In pregnancy the stimulus to metabolic change is the fertilization of the egg by the sperm. The bodily changes occur first in the uterus, then in the mother's metabolism of food as she passes nourishment along to the growing fetus. She gains water and salt, and her blood pressure rises. Her mammary glands enlarge and as she nears term her pelvic ligaments relax before labor begins. After the baby is born, her breasts continue to make milk proteins at a spectacular rate. When these protein factories are no longer needed because of weaning, the metabolic sequence is complete and her body returns to normal, though it will never be quite the same. Something has been accomplished by all these complex interlocking changes in hormones and body composition: the product is a well-nourished baby. The whole sequence is targeted for completion in about a year, including both pregnancy and the suckling phase.

The same sort of sequence occurs in the normal growth and later development of the child. After its birth and that intense protein synthesis in mother's milk, the baby picks up the synthesis of protein at a rapid rate as well as the multiplication of all the body cells and elongation of the skeleton. All these events proceed in a precisely programmed way. The sex hormones kick in with a boot at puberty and produce the fat deposition that we call curves in the adolescent girl as well as breast growth and readiness for pregnancy; ovulation and menstrual periods begin. The young man grows muscle and loses fat, the sex organs get larger, and he has a more urgent libido. These sequences finally peak out with the emergence of the finished product: an adult human being. The duration of this particular metabolic-endocrine sequence is about 14 to 16 years for girls and 16 to 18 for boys.

Convalescence from injury is a closely similar sequence. Now, the stimulus is injury itself, the sequence consisting initially of loss of body protein with retention of water and salt, followed by gradual healing and rebuilding, as mentioned above. The duration here seems to be determined by the severity and nature of the injury. When it is all over (maybe 2 to 4 weeks after an ordinary abdominal operation, 2 or 3 months after a compound fracture of the thigh), we have the final product: a convalescent person who is ready to return to society, work, and procreation. With a healed wound.

Obstetricians need to know the bodily changes in pregnancy to care effectively for their pregnant patients. Pediatricians need to know the normal sequence during growth to care effectively for their young patients. By the same token, surgeons need to know the normal changes in the body during convalescence to care effectively for their patients after an operation or injury.

Shock and Starvation

We think of convalescence as a normal sequence, that is, a predictable sequence in normal people. Sometimes the injury is too severe for the body to accommodate with a normal recovery. Shock and starvation are two special aspects of severe injury that interrupt the normal sequence of getting well and threaten survival.

The term "shock" refers to prolonged deficiency of blood flow usually due to loss of blood or extracellular fluid volume. With transfusion and intravenous fluids we can usually prevent or abate shock if we can get there soon enough. But in civilian accidents far from civilization and in combat settings, the flow deficiency is sometimes just too prolonged. Evolution has provided strategies for survival after expectable injuries in an animal's daily struggle for existence. If the injury is so severe that prolonged shock results, then the bodily response alone is not enough. Without the surgeon's help, death usually results.

As for starvation, a person can feed his body from within by oxidizing fat for calories and mobilizing muscle protein for its building blocks (amino acids). But only for a while. Meeting daily or even extraordinary expenses by drawing on your bank balance can go on for only so long before new funds and new metabolic riches are needed to replenish deposits. This means taking in fuel in the form of carbohydrate, fat, and protein, plus vitamins and minerals, somehow, by some route but preferably by mouth. The best route for food intake is that planned by nature: eating and chewing and swallowing. But when that fails, there are other ways.

During the war Fuller Albright had done some experiments at the MGH to develop means of providing the body's total nourishment through a needle intravenously. I picked this up from him and used it a good deal, describing this approach in my book on metabolic care in 1959. However, we did not study it adequately, nor did we spread the word successfully. The credit for priority in all of science should go to those who are the first not only to perceive a discovery but also to make public the message. In this case it was the group under Jonathan Rhoads, Douglas Wilmore, Henry Vars, and Stanley Dudrick in Philadelphia who did experiments of this type in dogs. They showed that giving the entire (total) nourishment intravenously could support normal growth and the ability of the bitch to whelp and nurse puppies. Since the mid 1960s the giving of total nourishment by this method has been accepted throughout the world. This is vitally important in taking care not only of certain types of surgical patients, but also of many babies born with an inability to eat as well as older patients who are wasted or starving with disorders that preclude normal food intake. This sort of feeding is called total parenteral nutrition (usually abbreviated as TPN).

From this picture of convalescence came a better understanding of a matter of major importance in surgery: the chemistry of confidence. Fear and apprehension add to the intensity of the injury. One of the jobs of the surgeon is not only to repair the injury but also to "hang in there" with the patient; explain what is going on; offer solid reassurance; do the little things that help with pain, such as morphine or special positioning and splinting; and bear with the questions of the family, as companion and mentor. When the patient enjoys the surgeon's visits, seeks his touch and his care, and rests secure in trust, a sort of stress-free basal state is established. This is why a capable and understanding surgeon (as well as nurses and hospital helpers) contributes so much to recovery. Mental stability and emotional calm are engines of recovery, just as the stressed and shocked mind is an injury in itself and continued anxiety an impediment to recovery. "Doctor" means "teacher." Part of the doctor's job is to teach patients about their troubles, what is needed, what will happen, how the future looks, and what to expect.

Support and Colleagues

During those years our research was very expensive. The institutions in which we were working—the Harvard Medical School, the MGH, and the Peter Bent Brigham Hospital—gave us the facilities, the opportunities, and the moral support. We were fortunate in obtaining generous grants from the National Institutes of Health, the Navy, the

Commonwealth Fund, the Hartford Foundation, and the Atomic Energy Commission. It was under contract with the Army that many of these studies were done and my teaching in this field extended to the army courses at Walter Reed Hospital. I became consultant to the Surgeon General of the Army. We did our best to bring the message from our whole laboratory group directly back to the cause for which it was supported: the care of the wounded. Our most intensive research covered the period of World War II and Korea, with later application in Vietnam.

Friends in other institutions worked in this field of study with us. Sometimes they learned from our example, especially with regard to isotopic methods. In other cases we learned from them. These colleagues included Henry T. Randall of New York, William Abbott and William Holden of Cleveland, George Clowes of Boston City Hospital and Brown University, David Hume of our department and later Virginia Commonwealth University in Richmond, Everett Evans at Richmond, and the brilliant group of officers at the Surgical Research Unit at Brooke Army Hospital in San Antonio, Texas. John Kinney, originally a member of our unit and later on the faculty at Columbia, was particularly interested in the energy sources and overall energetics of trauma metabolism. Because of the particularly congenial nature of this group, we formed the Surgical Biology Club in 1954 to get together and talk about these problems. This club soon expanded to include many other features of surgical biology, especially cardiac surgery and transplantation. And before long, similar discussion clubs were formed by our younger colleagues in surgical research.

Books and Honorary Lectureships

In 1947 I asked my chief laboratory technician, Margaret Ball, Radcliffe graduate and chemist, to join me as coauthor of a monograph that described the results of our early studies of water and salt changes, nitrogen metabolism, and energy exchange in surgical patients. It was called *The Metabolic Response to Surgery* and it was intended to present the plain facts about metabolic change in surgery. No pretentious conclusions.

Several years later, in 1959, the W.B. Saunders Company published *Metabolic Care of the Surgical Patient*. This also was a monograph—a clinical as and research monograph—based on our work, including chemistry and endocrinology, body composition, and certain important surgical operative steps. This became my most widely read book, translated into Spanish, Polish, and Japanese. There was said to be a Russian translation, but since the Soviets did not follow our copyright laws, we knew little about it. For a while it was one of the more quoted books in the surgical literature. We were all pleased by the interest shown in this book by the surgical public both here and abroad. I never wrote a second edition, but other authors, including particularly Douglas Wilmore (who took over my laboratory upon my retirement), published several books on these topics in collaboration with one of our graduates, Murray Brennan (now of Cornell University and the Memorial Sloan-Kettering Cancer Center).

During the war Edward Churchill, my boss during my internship, was surgical commander in the Mediterranean theater. The Excelsior Surgical Society formed by his colleagues in the war established the Churchill Lectureship. In 1952 I was asked to give the first Churchill Lecture, where for the first time I discussed publicly my theory of the four phases of convalescence and of surgical convalescence as an integrated natural process similar to pregnancy and normal growth.

Then, in 1956, I was invited by the Harvey Society to give one of their lectures. As a surgeon I was flattered by this invitation because these lectures are usually given by scientists in the basic fields such as chemistry, physiology, biochemistry, or endocrinology. It was on this occasion that I first discussed our growing knowledge of the endocrine changes after surgical operations and postulated the existence of a "wound hormone." By that I meant a circulating substance from the wound itself that could stimulate the endocrine glands directly. Many years later George Clowes showed that a newly discovered lymph-cell stimulator called interleukin-1 (IL-1) could act in exactly that way. Much remains to be learned about this wound stimulus to bodily change.

The awards, distinctions, and honorary degrees that came my way over the years were recognition of the work of our laboratory group in surgical metabolism and the biology of convalescence. As I made clear on so many occasions, this was not a solo effort. My many colleagues in the lab, as well as some of these honors and appropriate bibliographic references, are set forth in the Notes and References section later in the book.

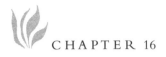

CHAPTER 16

Two Harvard Hospitals: The Brigham and the General; A Candidate for Promotion

(1947-1948)

D uring medical school Laurie and I had moved from the walk-up on Longwood Avenue to a house up on Corey Hill over-looking Boston Harbor (in the far distance). A few years later we moved down the hill to a place near Brookline Village called Griggs Road. This was a circle of small row houses, facing a central playground. In these houses dwelt several friends of ours, doctors and medical students, including, particularly, Reed and Faith Harwood, John and Sally Adams, and the older man I would come to admire so much, virologist John Enders, and his wife. All our children played together out in the middle of the playing field. I was supposed to mow the lawn in front of my house but became too engrossed with other activities to do it as dutifully as I should have. Once the grass grew so long that Henry Swan, another friend who lived nearby, came with his mower and mowed "MOORE" in the long grass as a gentle reminder that I was the owner and (delin-quent) mower of that particular bit of greenery.

By 1944, entering practice and feeling a little more affluent, and because we had three children and were about to have a fourth (Caroline), we needed a bigger house. As always, Laurie was the person who found our new house. I was too busy working at the hospital. She found a marvelous big old New England house up on the Walnut Street hill in Brookline, across from the First Unitarian Church.

In 1947 we purchased a few acres on Marion Harbor about 60 miles south of Boston, where the wind blew hard and the sailing was wonderful. The children's summers were spent in Marion learning to sail. We built a small house there to which we added another bubble every now and then. I took a couple of weeks off each summer, but Laurie and the kids lived down there all summer.

By the middle and late 1940s our work in surgery seemed to be going well, and people in other centers were interested in it. I had been elected to some surgical societies and national organizations. I was pushing along with our projects and did not worry too much about exactly where it would all lead. My practice was growing and I enjoyed the whole bit immensely: Laurie, the family, research, practice, teaching at the hospital and the medical school.

Elliott Cutler's Death and the Search

In the summer of 1947, before we built our house in Marion, we rented a small cottage in Sippewisset, across Buzzards Bay, north of a small summer colony called Quisset. One August day (the 16th to be exact), we turned on the radio for the news, as we did every morning. To our surprise, we learned that Elliott Cutler had died.

Cutler, as I have said, had been one of the most important teachers of our class at medical school. Because my internship was at the MGH, I saw him but rarely after the war, since he presided over surgery at the Brigham. I admired Cutler and the surgical tradition at the Brigham and visited that hospital occasionally, even though not many residents at the time did this sort of visiting to learn what was going on at nearby hospitals. Many friends of mine were in residency training there. When we heard of Cutler's death, Laurie and I had no idea at all that I might be asked to become his successor. Somehow the myth has been started that I was pointing for this job ever since childhood. Nothing could be further from the truth. Originally, I had planned to return to practice in Chicago. Now I was perfectly satisfied with the wonderful opportunities given me at Harvard and the MGH.

Fred Ross, our friend and classmate, was Cutler's chief resident at that time and helped care for him through his final illness. Cutler was a young man, still under 60, when he died of metastatic cancer of the prostate.

We heard little of search committees or other rumors until 7 months later, when, in March 1948, Dr. Churchill called me into his office at the MGH to tell me that I was on the list of candidates for appointment as the Moseley Professor and Elliott Cutler's successor as Chief of Surgery at the Brigham. He asked me what I would think about such a thing. I told him I hadn't thought much about it at all, and that I was very happy where I was, working in his department.

Churchill then asked me if I would like to stay on at the MGH and take charge of all the surgical research there, a sort of administrative promotion. That he should bring up such a counteroffer should have given me a hint that matters had already progressed pretty far. I told him that I appreciated this handsome and generous offer. Fortunately, I was tactful enough not to mention that I couldn't think of anything worse, since I had trouble enough managing my own research, getting the money for it, and keeping all those granting agencies happy. I had no desire to start worrying about a lot of other people's research, controversy over research space, and raising even more money.

By 1948 our four children were all in Park School, next door to our home. Our friends included doctors at all the Harvard hospitals, about our age, also with children, many of them living nearby in Brookline. From college and other associations we enjoyed friends who were in business or the other professions, especially law and teaching.

I was not anxious to change jobs, and we certainly did not want to move. I began to weigh the alternatives. If something came up that led me to be appointed to the Peter Bent Brigham Hospital, we certainly were well situated. The Brigham was only 2 miles from our house. By this time my lab at the MGH was well financed and several research grants had come through, so I no longer had to rely solely on the generosity of Oliver Cope and Edward Churchill. My private practice was coming along pretty well, aided a good deal by my interests in duodenal ulcer and burns.

MGH and PBBH

The MGH was large and strong at that time, while the Brigham was small and much weakened by the war and an aging senior staff. It had only 250 beds, compared with the 850 beds at the MGH. And the surgical department was taking some hard hits. Not only had Elliott Cutler died, but other prominent surgeons there, notably David Cheever and John Homans, were close to or at retirement age. Nobody was doing cardiac or thoracic surgery, and there was no one in charge of several of the other surgical specialties (gynecology, ophthalmology) at the Brigham. Some specialties (neurosurgery, orthopedics) were shared with nearby hospitals. Bob Zollinger had left to take over the service at Ohio State.

On the other hand, the Brigham could hold its head up pretty well. While much smaller than the MGH, it had been responsible for many advances, ranging from the introduction (under Harvey Cushing) of an entirely new field, neurological surgery, to the publication of a new, richly illustrated how-to book, the *Atlas of General Surgical Operations* by Cutler and Zollinger. This bestseller was used extensively (surreptitiously even by the residents at the MGH) and avidly read by other surgical residents throughout the world. The Brigham was a haven of learning for students and residents. And in 1948 it had a young, brilliant, newly appointed chief of the Department of Medicine, George W. Thorn. The possibility of working as Thorn's opposite number was very attractive.

Despite some reservations, I was impressed by the opportunities the position offered and was flattered to be—as Dr. Churchill told me—on the short list. I realized that now I really had to get off my chair and start thinking about this proposition more seriously. I went for a visit to the Brigham, taken there by William Quinby, the head urologist, whose assistant, Hartwell Harrison, was a longtime friend. Quinby had been acting chief of surgery since Cutler's death. We made rounds and saw the laboratories. The remarkable gap between those who did and did not go to the war was pointed up by the fact that Fred Ross, my classmate who had been away in the army for 5 years, was still the chief resident in surgery while I was being offered the professorship. He took this with good grace. I knew there were plenty of people at the Brigham who were candidates for the job. They also greeted me warmly. I told Dr. Churchill I would accept the job if it were offered.

An Offer and Its Response

In May I was told that I had been selected for nomination as Moseley Professor at Harvard and Surgeon-in-Chief at the Brigham. Dean Burwell took me to visit the President of Harvard University, James Bryant Conant. He had been our university president during my last 2 years at college and was a member of the same undergraduate club, so I knew him slightly. He asked if I would accept the offer and take on the job, offering me a ridiculously low salary. After a little bit of negotiation, I accepted the post.

The hospital board needed to approve this new joint appointment of university and hospital. I met with the Board of Trustees of the Brigham Hospital, the most vocal member of which was Robert Cutler, the younger brother of Elliott Cutler. Bobby Cutler was to become the President of the Board, later Chairman of the Board, and finally Honorary Chairman. He and I became well acquainted. I operated on him and took care of him when he was sick. A close friend of President Dwight Eisenhower, he migrated to Washington a few years later where he served in the Eisenhower White House as the first director of the National Security Council. He was also an author, a humorist, a blythe spirit, and by far the best raconteur of off-color stories that I have ever heard. The women of the ladies' board blushed and were suitably shocked but tried their best to remember the stories. The Board seemed enthusiastic about my decision to accept the job.

In June, Laurie and I went to Marion to take a vacation before the new job began. For the first time we moved into the small portable house that we had bought, to which we had added a living room and a dormitory for children. On July 1 I would take on new responsibilities. My 35th birthday was still a couple of months away.

BOOK ❦ FIVE

Professor of Surgery

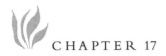

CHAPTER 17

Surgical Professors, Ancient and Modern

Professors appointed to the endowed chairs at the Harvard Medical School in the clinical fields (medicine, surgery, pediatrics, radiology, anesthesiology, and psychiatry) perform their work at one of the several Harvard teaching hospitals. Once there, they become overseers of clinical care at that hospital. Endowed university full-time professorships are critical to the advancement of academic programs, teaching, learning, and—especially in surgery—new ways of caring for the sick. Only on rare occasions in Harvard's history have such endowed chairs been transferred from one hospital to another. At whichever hospital surgical professors are situated, one of them by historic precedent becomes the chief surgeon at that hospital, as well as head of that Department of Surgery at the university.

Warrens and More Warrens; Hersey and Moseley

Harvard's first professor of surgery, John Warren, was the younger brother of another surgeon of colonial Boston, Joseph Warren. Both these eighteenth-century Warrens were at once surgeons and patriots. Joseph was a prime mover in the activist patriotic movement that led to the American Revolution. He dumped tea into Boston Harbor and wrote some of the Suffolk Resolves, a series of anti-Crown inflammatory tracts.

Joseph Warren must have been near the top of the British list of most wanted rebels. He was killed on June 17, 1775, in the fighting north of the harbor on Breed's Hill in the encounter known as the Battle of Bunker Hill. His body, buried in a shallow grave, was later found by his younger brother John and Edward A. Holyoke, a patriarch of Massachusetts colonial medicine and a Salem physician, of whom Joseph Warren had been a disciple. It is said that the decaying remains were identified by Paul Revere, who had made Joseph's denture.

John Warren was appointed Professor of Anatomy and Surgery at Harvard College in 1782. Neither Joseph nor John Warren was designated as "Doctor" because they were not doctors. Like the majority of the physicians in the Colonies at that time, they had neither attended a medical school nor received a doctorate. They never signed their names with "Dr." or "M.D." appended. Their education was by apprenticeship.

In 1770 Ezekiel Hersey, a physician of Hingham and a graduate of Harvard College (1728), bequeathed an endowment of £1,000 to Harvard College for a professorship of anatomy. This endowment finally reached £3,400, an amount equivalent to the $1.5 to 2 million required to endow a Harvard professorship today. This very generous endowment made it possible to start up a medical faculty at Harvard College, and on John Warren was conferred the title Hersey Professor of Anatomy and Surgery.

Warren took a rather radical step for Bostonians of that era when he married Abigail Collins. Not only did she come from the South (Rhode Island), but she was of a different Protestant persuasion. Their son, John Collins Warren, became the second Hersey Professor. He was the operating surgeon in the first public demonstration of the use of ether for surgical anesthesia in October 1846. This operation was conducted at the Massachusetts General Hospital only 30 years after the hospital opened and was the basis of its worldwide reputation. In addition to performing this famous operation, John Collins Warren had helped found the MGH (1811), a medical journal (the predecessor of *The New England Journal of Medicine*) (1812), and the American Medical Association (1847). The Hersey endowment helped make all this possible, and the remarkable energy of these first two Warren surgical professors made it all happen.

Upon the death of John Collins Warren in 1856, the professorship of surgery fell to his son Jonathan Mason Warren, and then in turn to his grandson J. Collins Warren, who thus became the fourth Warren surgeon to be made a professor at Harvard. By then, the Department of Surgery had generously given over the Hersey title and income to strengthen the newly separated Department of Anatomy. The Hersey endowment was later given to the Department of Medicine (Physic). So for about 70 years, three generations of Harvard professors of surgery, all of them carrying the name Warren, lacked a named chair and a suitable endowment, though they might not have put it quite that way.

In those days professors at Harvard Medical School earned part of their income by selling tickets to their lectures, which were open to the paying public. To us, this seems rather old-fashioned, even arcane. When there was no endowment, this practice helped support the senior faculty. (Those old lecture tickets are now collectors' items at antique stores.) Whatever its shortcomings, this system of payment must have provided a strong incentive to the professors. They had better be good teachers and give smashing lectures if they wished to survive.

Finally, in 1897 the long-awaited endowment for a chair in surgery was given to the university. It came as the result of a family tragedy, when, on August 14, 1879, a recent graduate of the Harvard Medical School Class of 1878 was killed in Switzerland while climbing the Matterhorn. William Moseley was 30 years old when he died. In his memory, his parents, Mr. and Mrs. William Oxnard Moseley, gave several gifts to the medical school and to the MGH. The largest gift, made in 1897, endowed the Harvard Medical School professorship that bears his name.

A few months after the Moseley endowment was accepted by the President and Fellows (the Harvard Corporation), J. Collins Warren was appointed to that chair and became the first Moseley Professor of Surgery. He held the professorship for 9 years, until his retirement in 1907. As the first Moseley Professor at Harvard, he enjoyed a notable career. He was the prime mover in establishing the new medical school buildings on Longwood Avenue in 1906. Construction had begun about 1895. A century later the medical school remains right there, where Warren and his colleagues put it, still a source of heated argument: wouldn't it be better off in Cambridge, near the college and the other graduate schools?

In addition to his local leadership in Boston/Harvard circles, J. Collins Warren was a strong advocate of Joseph Lister's system of surgical cleanliness, which was introduced to American surgery in the years between 1867 (when Lister published his first paper) and 1888 (when the practices of antisepsis and asepsis were finally adopted throughout the United States). As a young man, Warren had visited Lister in Scotland. He could clearly see the importance of Lister's new methods. For example, it enabled patients with compound fractures (previously fatal) to recover. Most important, it led to the modern methods of asepsis that enable surgical operations to be carried out without inevitably introducing infection. Old-time surgeons had borne dried blood and pus on their garments and carried more sources of infection than they realized on their hands. "Listerism" was a move from primordial filth to systematic cleanliness, and the United States trailed years behind Europe in adopting this practice. A conservative faction that now, in retrospect, seems obviously to have been shortsighted and self-serving opposed the introduction of Lister's methods. Warren led the charge for its acceptance.

The name Warren continues to be an important name in Boston surgery and medicine. The son of J. Collins Warren, John Warren, an anatomist, wrote the text we used in our anatomy course in 1935. Richard Warren, grandson of J. Collins Warren, is our contemporary. He is Professor of Surgery, Emeritus, at Harvard Medical School, a close friend, a staff colleague, and an expert vascular surgeon. Richard Warren edited a widely used textbook of surgery and was for many years Chief of Surgery at the West Roxbury Veterans Administration Hospital in Boston. An outstanding teacher and clinical surgeon who was particularly interested in surgery of the blood vessels, Richard Warren added luster to the Warren name. Some of Richard Warren's grandchildren have a double legacy of surgery: his oldest son, Richard, married our second oldest daughter, Sally. Richard and I have three Warren grandchildren: Peter, Rebecca, and Samuel. Richard Warren's nephew, Howland Shaw Warren, now carries on the Warren medical tradition in the younger generation as a microbiologist. Any more Warren surgeons? Not yet.

Cushing and Cutler

The second Moseley Professor of Surgery, succeeding J. Collins Warren, was Maurice Howe Richardson, who was later made Chief of Surgery at the MGH (the first and, as it turned out, the last to hold such a title). He was succeeded by Harvey Cushing, who held the Moseley Chair from 1912 until his retirement in 1932.

Cushing developed the field of neurosurgery and was one of its most expert exponents. He was an endocrinologist during the formative years of that field, describing the activity of the ductless glands. This work arose from his knowledge of the pituitary gland, which in turn resulted from his treatment of the many patients with pituitary tumors who sought his assistance. In 1912 the President and Fellows of Harvard College and the newly created Board of Trustees of the Peter Bent Brigham Hospital offered Cushing a joint appointment as Moseley Professor at Harvard and the first Surgeon-in-Chief at the Brigham hospital. He was on the scene when the Brigham opened its doors in 1913 and conducted the affairs of the surgical department for 20 years.

Elliott Cutler succeeded Cushing as Moseley Professor and Surgeon-in-Chief at the Peter Bent Brigham Hospital in 1932. He was a New Englander who sought to refine and standardize the teaching and performance of surgical operations. Early in his career Cutler had been interested in the surgical treatment of heart disease. In 1924 he carried out several operations to open the narrowed (stenotic) mitral valve. Only one of these first efforts to repair chronic valvular heart disease was in any sense successful. The patient lived several months, much improved. But important lessons were learned that helped Dwight Harken when he resumed this quest at the Brigham 24 years later in 1948. It was to be 30 years after Cutler before these operations became safe and widely performed. Cutler's career as the fourth Moseley Professor was cut short in 1940 by World War II. He left his professorial duties after only 8 years to help organize a base hospital, later being given theater responsibilities for the care of the wounded in Europe. He was promoted to the rank of brigadier general, one of the few medical men of the civilian establishment to reach this rank in World War II. While on active duty in the European theater, he developed some pain in his back. X-rays showed deposits of the fatal tumor that had metastasized from his prostate to his bones and led to his death on August 16, 1947.

A New Arrival in the Old Lineage

On the morning of July 1, 1948, I arrived as the fifth Moseley Professor at Harvard, the eighth surgical professor in this line stretching back to the Revolution, and the third Surgeon-in-Chief at the Peter Bent Brigham Hospital. I pulled into the allotted parking space and went into my office (Cushing's old digs) to start work.

Little of the history I have just recounted was known to me that first morning. I was not interested in history. I was mainly concerned with picking up the reins of this fine department, which included so many distinguished surgeons. It was getting started that counted.

The welfare of patients in the 140 surgical beds of the Brigham was our first responsibility. It was from their care that we were to learn so much. And it was to them that we owed our loyalty and later our gratitude. I performed my first surgical operation at the Brigham 2 weeks after I arrived. The patient was a young man suffering from severe ulcerative colitis. I carried out a total colectomy (removal of the colon) and made a new opening on his abdomen, an ileostomy, similar to the procedure described in Chapter 10.

I had already met with the Trustees of the Brigham to point out that, in addition to our long-established laboratory at the Medical School, we needed a laboratory to study patients at first hand. I was concerned about the processes of illness and of getting well and therefore requested a clinical research laboratory right there in the hospital. My work, already begun at the MGH on body composition and the biology of convalescence, needed the facilities to proceed at full speed.

The industrious and talented young Radcliffe graduate whom I have already mentioned, Margaret Ball, became my head technician and director of our laboratory staff and analytic work. I had brought her with me to the Brigham from Oliver Cope's laboratory at the MGH. She remained in this important role for 27 years. The Trustees had given me the rooms of the old blood bank for our laboratory. They were right next to my office, conveniently situated between the two surgical wards and just below the operating room. Miss Ball and I went to an abandoned fish processing plant and found some soapstone benches and sinks. We moved them to the Brigham, and the first Surgical Research Laboratory in the history of the hospital (smelling a little fishy) was ready to go.

I did not bring a large clinical staff with me to my new job. I was too young for that. But I did bring one surgeon who turned out to be tremendously important throughout the decades to come. This was John Robinson Brooks, who had attended Harvard College and Medical School ('43), served in the armed forces during the war, and took his residency at the Roosevelt Hospital in New York. Following those clinical years, he joined me at the MGH, assisting in our study of duodenal ulcer and vagotomy. He would soon become the Chief Resident Surgeon at the Brigham, later a member of the attending staff with increasing responsibility, and finally the right-hand man of the entire department.

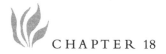

CHAPTER 18

Young Man at a Young Hospital

(1948)

My new hospital, the Peter Bent Brigham (the Brigham for short) was 35 years old when, on July 1, 1948, its new Surgeon-in-Chief arrived for work. I would be 35 the next month. The hospital and I were both opened in 1913. It was only 3 years after the war, and the surgical department was suffering from two disasters in addition to the residual effects of wartime absences. These two adversities were the aging of the senior staff and recent domination by a surgeon who was sure he could do anything and everything and therefore let the specialties wilt on the vine. In the unedited opinion of others, there was a third disaster: a callow youth taking over the department.

Our aging staff included two famous surgeons, David Cheever and John Homans, both of whom had been my teachers and one of whom (Cheever) had operated upon my wife. Another, Robert Zollinger, one of our most valued teachers, was not so very old at this time but had departed to take over the Department of Surgery at Ohio State University. Still, there was plenty of talent and young blood in general surgery, as will become evident.

As for Elliott Cutler, although an inspiring teacher who was much enjoyed by our class, he was one of the last of those who might truly be called a general surgeon. One morning (just before the war) I recall visiting the Brigham where I witnessed Cutler perform (in a single day) an operation for a brain tumor, a hysterectomy, and a colon resection for cancer. While one operative virtuoso might of course encompass these three distinctly different kinds of operative surgery, no one person could possibly keep up with the literature; master new trends; attend the specialty meetings in neurosurgery, gynecology, and surgical oncology simultaneously; or provide leadership for residency training in all three fields.

Generalists and Specialists

Everybody is against specialization except the patient. The patient always seeks the most expert care. By 1948 the surgical specialties were well developed. The events of the war had accelerated this trend because of urgent demands for expert surgical treatment of wounds involving all the organs and systems of the body.

Teaching hospitals provide the perspectives and opportunities that arise when young people work with senior specialists. This is how students get an idea of the many careers that make up the practice of medicine and surgery. Teaching hospitals should also instill, by example, the concept that you can be a specialist but still have a humanistic view toward the patient and the family, their social and emotional needs. The primary care physician or the family doctor must surely possess these empathetic traits, but he has no monopoly on them. Those specialists who are sought after by patients and other doctors exhibit these same traits.

With regard to leadership in the surgical specialties, the Brigham of 1948 was almost dead in the water. Our surgical service, which had been the birthplace of neurosurgery, the most highly specialized field of all, did not have a neurosurgeon on the staff who was entirely responsible for adult patients. But its most glaring deficiency was that no surgeon on the Brigham staff was performing adult thoracic and cardiac surgery, two fields that had rapidly expanded in scope and importance during the war. As my first major outside appointment I therefore asked Dwight Harken, then working at the Boston City Hospital, to join our service. This was November 1948. The story of his remarkable work and the beginnings of surgery within the heart is told in Chapter 23.

We had no one concentrating in gynecology, even though a half dozen of the general surgeons (including me) performed gynecological operations. None of us was concerned with the rapidly opening fields of gynecological endocrinology, fertility and sterility, and the special problems of malignancy of the ovaries and uterus. I asked Somers Sturgis, then at the MGH and one of my teachers, to come and join our service. He had a long and brilliant career as a leader in gynecology at the Brigham, which included the first attempt to transplant human ovaries and the creation of the first full-time psychiatric unit in a surgical department in the United States to examine the emotional impact on women of removal of the ovaries and uterus or of the breast.

I asked Donald Matson—another classmate—to take over neurosurgery in the adult, working closely with his professor, Dr. Franc Ingraham, at the Children's Hospital. Within a few years I asked Joseph Murray to take over in plastic surgery, Andrew Jessiman in oncology, Henry Banks in orthopedics, and Leo Chylack in ophthalmology. All turned out to be very strong appointments that led to strong divisions of surgery in those fields.

For a young man to take over leadership of a surgical department so lacking in full-time staff specialists for its 250 beds might have seemed a bad deal. But in retrospect it was a marvelous opportunity to appoint brilliant young people (only two of whom were my age or younger) to these important positions. I was repeatedly warned not to appoint anyone older (than I was); everyone thought that would turn out to be bad news. But since I was only 35 or so at the time, I didn't have much choice.

As for anesthesia, it was still a division of the Department of Surgery. In the early 1930s nurse-conducted anesthesia in this country had just begun to yield to physician-led departments. The latter were the rule in all the teaching hospitals and universities of Great Britain and for the most part on the Continent. The United States was still reluctant to make this change, despite the fact that in 1914 Harvey Cushing had appointed a physician-scientist, Walter Boothby, to lead Brigham anesthesia. Boothby was a respiratory physiologist who was also expert in anesthesia. With the appointment of Boothby, Cushing was one of the first in the United States to enhance his surgical department with an expert physician-scientist as anesthetist. After a few years, Boothby left the Brigham to head up research at an institute in the southwest. Nurse anesthetists had staffed the Brigham department for almost 30 years under the leadership of Miss

Gertrude Gerrard, who was not only a fine anesthetist but an engaging person well known to all of us as medical students.

As fine as a nurse anesthetist might be, it was impossible for a person lacking a full medical education to absorb the increasingly complicated studies of pharmacology, physiology, biochemistry, and neurology on which the practice and teaching of anesthesia were based. A full curriculum in biomedical science was required for their understanding and incorporation into anesthesia practice. After the war a flood of bright young physicians began entering the field of anesthesia. Within a few years, physician-led departments began to dominate anesthesia in this country as they had in Great Britain for almost 75 years.

Upon Cutler's death, William Quinby (the senior urologist of the hospital) had been asked by the Dean and the Trustees to take over the surgical department as acting head. It is to his credit that the Brigham moved into physician anesthesia during that difficult interim period by appointing William S. Derrick Chief of the Anesthesia Division of the Department of Surgery in 1947. And it was a credit to Bill Derrick that he accepted the job despite uncertainty as to who might become his boss as professor of surgery only a few months later.

About 5 years later, Derrick was offered a position as director of anesthesia in Houston, Texas. He accepted the offer but gave me only 3 weeks notice. I had to drop everything and undertake a search for a new anesthetist. If ever I was destined to develop a stress ulcer or high blood pressure, this would have been the moment. The search took me a lot longer than 3 weeks. For several months we had a very rough time conducting operations, because Derrick took the nurse anesthetists and most of the support staff with him to Houston. We began to use a great deal of local and spinal anesthesia (at that time administered by the surgeon himself).

I traveled far and wide, from San Francisco to New York and back again, in my search. In due course I discovered Leroy D. Vandam in the Department of Anesthesia under Robert Dripps at the University of Pennsylvania. With great good luck I convinced him and his wife Regina to join us in Boston. Within a few years he had built one of the finest teaching departments of anesthesia to be found anywhere. He later declared independence and formed a separate department of anesthesia. He remains a near neighbor and close friend.

In general surgery we were fortunate in having on the staff J. Englebert Dunphy, who had been near the top of the list of the local candidates for the job as professor and head of surgery to which I was later appointed. Dunphy and I had known each other for many years, were good friends, and got along well even in times of stress and crisis. It was a sure thing that we would be unable to hang onto him for very long. Within a few years he was appointed head of the Harvard Surgical Service at the Boston City Hospital, later becoming Professor and Head of the Department at the University of Oregon in Portland. Finally, he culminated his career by serving for 25 years as Professor and Head of the Department of Surgery at the University of California at San Francisco. He was a joyous person, filled with good humor and known the world over for his leadership in surgery.

In urology, I was also blessed in having J. Hartwell Harrison in charge, likewise an old friend and a much beloved expert surgeon. That was one area of surgery I never had to worry about. As a loyal Virginian and graduate of Thomas Jefferson's university, Hartwell's principal interest outside of Harvard was clearly at Charlottesville, where he served for many years as member of the Board.

Adding new people to the staff would have been the height of folly unless we could open more beds for their patients and broaden our internship and residency training program beyond the confines of our own small hospital. In those hectic years just after World War II, many other teaching surgical departments were learning the hard way that breadth of competence requires width of bed capacity. A few were learning that their home-grown gospel was not the only source of truth.

Farming Out a Few Residents

The concept that surgical residents might do well to expand their vision beyond one hospital was introduced soon after the war. One of the jobs Churchill had given to me at the MGH was to be in charge of the resident staff assignments. We established an affiliation with the Salem Hospital (in Salem, Massachusetts) to give our residents a chance to experience the surgical life and times of a community hospital and contrast them with those of a university teaching hospital. Churchill had a wartime friend who was in charge of the surgical department in Winfield, Kansas, so we sent some residents way out there. Our men enjoyed both these assignments very much.

Inspired by these outreach adventures with Dr. Churchill, I began several experiments at the Brigham. We sent a resident to New York to Memorial Hospital, then under the surgical leadership of Alexander Brunschwig. The object was to give our residents the opportunity to work for a while with someone who was extending the scope of cancer surgery. This did not work out very well because the residents were unimpressed with the results. Before long I came to appreciate their view. Meanwhile, the New York affiliation had given one or two people a remarkable experience. One such was Joseph Murray, who had the opportunity to see the joining of plastic surgery with cancer surgery at its inception. He brought that message back to us and made it an important part of his career.

We also initiated an affiliation with the Beverly Hospital (in Beverly, Massachusetts), again to give our men a chance to see small-town hospital life, and likewise with the Burbank Hospital in Fitchburg, Massachusetts, then under the direction of one of my classmates, Fred Ross. The latter affiliation was the most successful, lasting for about 30 years. Many of the Brigham residents looked back on the months they spent in Fitchburg as among the most rewarding of their 5 years in training. There was a substantial volume of surgery, and they were able to carry out many operations themselves. There was less of the bustle and pressure of academia. They got a taste for surgery in a smaller community, and many of those who did not feel the pull toward academia entered practice in smaller communities, in part because of their experience with Dr. Ross.

Our most remunerative training arrangement for the residents was one made with the Sun Valley Hospital in Ketchum, Idaho. This came about because John Moritz, the brother of our pathologist Alan Moritz, was in charge of surgery there. This hospital took care of all the skiing casualties from Sun Valley and was owned by the Union Pacific Railroad. They needed extra hands during the height of the skiing season and were willing to pay handsomely for them. We grabbed this opportunity. While our men were out there, they treated lots of fractures in addition to being treated to some good skiing. They were paid a rather generous salary by the Union Pacific. Several of our residents saw as many as 250 fractures during their 3-month stay. I often thought it would make a great advertisement for a skiing resort if we emphasized the tremendous experience to be gained in fixing up broken bones. One of the annual hospital spoofs of that time included the song, "O Franny! Please send me to Sun Valley!"

Through an unexpected happy circumstance we established an exchange arrangement with St. Mary's Hospital, a teaching unit of the University of London. This came about because the guiding spirit of St. Mary's at that time was Sir Arthur Porritt (later Lord Porritt), who had been a track star in the Olympics some years before and a visiting professor at the Brigham a year or two previously. A Boston financier and benefactor of many causes, Mr. J. Murray Forbes had also been an Olympic runner and had met Porritt at that time. Forbes was in charge of the George Gorham Peters Fund. With his help and this fund, we were able to bring an English surgeon to Boston and pay him with dollars while he was here, and in exchange send an American surgeon to London where he was paid in pounds by the National Health Service.

This was a pretty slick arrangement, and for many years we had a marvelous annual trans-Atlantic exchange of residents. The Bostonians enjoyed the variegated clinical work and the generality of surgery in London. As for our London visitors, young surgeons in Britain did not have an opportunity to do research, certainly not that involving large animals, which was proscribed by the antivivisection laws of the British Commonwealth. Therefore, many of those who came to our hospital worked at least for a while in our laboratories as well as on the resident service. The men who graduated from these jobs later occupied many leading positions in both Great Britain and the United States. Many years later, when I was made an Honorary Fellow of the Royal College of Surgeons of England, it was an unexpected pleasure for me to witness the formal procession being led by several surgeons—then of senior age—who had spent part of their training at the Brigham. Old friends.

Pay and Beds

Early in this period (1948-1955) our residents were paid almost nothing, enjoying the same hair shirt that had been our lot before the war. This changed rapidly after an intern strike or "heal-in" at the Boston City Hospital. By the mid 1950s most interns and residents were beginning to get a wage that, while it would not provide a living in itself, at least made it possible for their wives to take an occasional vacation! In those days, up until about 1965, countless young American residents in medicine and surgery got through their training because of the industry and earning power of their wives.

The surgical service needed more beds. Thanks to George Thorn's personal acquaintance with the Coolidge family, we were able to build a whole new wing of the hospital named in honor of Thomas Jefferson Coolidge, formerly president of the United Fruit Company. After I took care of the King of Arabia (Chapter 26), the Saudi Royal Family gave us a generous gift for some more beds. Before long we were up to about 300 beds and a higher rate of surgical operative experience for staff and residents. While this was a big improvement, it was still perfectly obvious that we needed a new hospital to break out of the confines and physical constraints of the old Brigham. That finally came, but it took many years and is another story (Chapter 30).

So, as we filled the need for more people to represent the various specialties of surgery, the hospital grew apace. With hospitals, beware of mere growth! Specialization sometimes takes hold of a hospital and the hospital cannot stop it, like an eagle flying with too big a fish in its talons. Can't let go. Domination by one specialty is not healthy for either public service or the balance of teaching. Domination becomes damnation.

That almost happened to us. Within a few years we became a center for kidney disease, transplant surgery, the care of burns, and cardiac surgery. While this was a result of the work of our own staff, specialization threatened to take over to a greater extent than we had wished. Nothing like the hardship of being too much in demand. But with lots of cooperation from the Board of Trustees, we weathered that threat and kept the balance needed for teaching.

Right from the start I took on a big load of teaching, having opportunities to teach in all 4 years of the 4-year medical curriculum. This helped interest the students in entering surgery, witnessing some of its fascinations both inside and outside of the operating room.

Back to Anatomy: A Case of Gallstone Colic

Early on, as Moseley Professor, I was asked to take over the first-year anatomy clinics. These teaching sessions took place on Saturday mornings, addressing the entire first-year class during their first 3 months of medical school. The name of the game was to present a real patient (or two) in person, discuss the patient's problem, and then (after the patient left the auditorium) describe the exact anatomical arrangements or misarrangements involved with the disease in question. And, in some cases, the students could observe the ensuing operation from the old Brigham operating amphitheater that was built for Harvey Cushing and could accommodate a whole class (at that time about 120 students).

I took over those anatomy clinics, trying to follow in the wonderful tradition of David Cheever, who had provided this combination of science and humanism for our class 15 years before. I enjoyed giving these clinics and always spent a lot of time preparing for them. The patients were carefully picked as being those who might enjoy describing their symptoms or telling (sometimes critically) about their care.

One Friday evening in the fall of 1949, while I was preparing for a clinic on the gallbladder, Laurie was seized with a severe pain in the right upper part of her abdomen. Her pain crescendoed to a high pitch and then backed off. It did not take much skill on the part of her husband to make a diagnosis of gallstone colic.

We called our family physician who gave her a suitable shot, and she had a reasonably comfortable night. The next morning was Saturday, the day of the clinic. I asked her if she would mind describing exactly what it felt like to have the pain of gallstone colic, the stone trying to get out, as it were, down the narrow ducts. This would be an experience that the medical students would remember for a long time.

So, the pain having subsided and she more beautiful than ever, Laurie was wheeled into the main amphitheater in a wheelchair with a snappy looking nurse in a crackling starched uniform at her side. I asked a few questions. The students could then ask her all the questions they wanted and ask what gallstone colic really felt like. The clinic went along swimmingly, and I do not think anyone suspected a rather special relationship between the patient and the surgeon giving the clinic, until, at the very end, one of the students asked, "Didn't you have any medicine around the house for this sort of thing?"

Laurie replied, "Well, my husband..." (and at this point she inadvertently glanced over at me) "looked in all the medicine cabinets and couldn't find anything of any use." For some reason this was both a big laugh and a giveaway. The students, realizing in a flash that the patient was my wife, howled with glee, Laurie smiled happily, and it all ended as the nurse turned and, in a very businesslike way, wheeled her out and back to her bed on the floor. A short while later she was operated upon by Dr. Dunphy, who removed a gallbladder full of stones.

The students never forgot this particular clinic. Many years later, walking down the streets of San Francisco or Chicago or Atlantic City, where there might be a meeting of the American College of Surgeons, we were sure to meet one or two surgeons who had been students at that clinic. When they saw Laurie, they would say to her, "Well, Mrs. Moore, I hope you are feeling better now." And there would be a happy laugh of recognition and reminiscence. The rumor was that at least for that period in the Harvard Medical School, this was the most famous anatomy clinic. To cap the climax of that particular Saturday morning, one of the students present at that clinic was John Mannick, who later succeeded me as Moseley Professor.

Visiting Professors and Friends From Abroad

We also kept up the Brigham tradition of visiting professor pro tempore. We arranged for a series of surgeons to come to the Brigham in that capacity. These "Pro Tems," as they were called, were selected because of their ability to teach, the fields in which they were interested, and the breadth of view they would bring to our residents and students. It was rumored that the Pro Tem tradition had been commenced by Harvey Cushing. We had many visitors who were the leaders of surgery in various cities in this country and abroad. One of the more remarkable was Sir

James Paterson Ross, head of the surgical department at St. Bartholomew's Hospital in London. He made ward rounds with the students, as did all such visiting Pro Tems. Any English surgeon who had "Sir" in front of his name always made a big hit with our patients. We later found that to many Americans the "Sir" suggests some kind of connection with the British royal family. In any event, when Sir James made his rounds, he encountered a certain talkative and friendly Irish patient who was charmed by him and talked with him at length. He examined her and then scrubbed in on her operation the next day. We later discovered that over the course of many years she exchanged Christmas cards with Sir James and Lady Ross.

During those early years we were successful in drawing a sizable number of applicants for our internship. Many young men (and a small number of women) also came to learn by working in our laboratories.

We were studying three topics that attracted people to our department. First, we were using tiny tracer doses of both radioactive and stable isotopes to discover some of the eternal verities of physiology and biochemistry. Second, we were looking at disorders of body composition, not only in surgical patients, but also in heart failure, starvation, infection, shock, and seriously overweight patients. And third, we were trying to improve physiological care in surgery, which came to be known as metabolic care, particularly after the publication of *The Metabolic Response to Surgery*. Many people from this country and abroad applied for research jobs, fellowships, and openings on the team. In all, over the course of the next 30 years, over 300 young surgeons, physicians, and scientists came to work in our laboratories. Some of those from other countries and other disciplines who came to work with us are mentioned below.

First was André Monsaingeon, who came to join our lab from Paris while I was at the MGH working on metabolic problems as well as ulcerative colitis and burns. These were problems he had confronted in Paris. Shortly after the war several large foundations made funds available for young French doctors who had been isolated (if not captured) during the war to come to this country to study. This was true of André, whose family had been involved in the French Resistance. He himself had narrowly escaped being shot by the Nazis. He came and worked with me as a Rockefeller Fellow early on. Soon Laurie and I visited him and his charming wife Geneviève in Paris. He became Head of Surgery at l'Hôpital Paul Brousse, in Paris, and Professor (later Dean) at the University of Paris. Subsequently he returned as visiting professor pro tem, and over the years we visited back and forth across the Atlantic to form one of those lasting family friendships that stem from scientific work, from academia. If I had been practicing surgery in Boston and doing nothing else, he never would have come and stayed a year. He came to study and to join in my research. An important reward of the academic life.

Next was a young pediatrician from Copenhagen, Bent Friis-Hansen. Like so many Scandinavians, he did not say a great deal but thought a lot. He made no pretense but understood everything. He worked with me in the early days of the total body water method and later became the world's expert on body composition in the newborn. One day I asked him if he would like to play some tennis. I had never been very good at the game but enjoyed trying. When we went to pick him up at his apartment to take him to The Country Club, he appeared in one of those spotless European-style tennis outfits such as you might see at a tennis club on Long Island. A white sweater with a blue V down the front. He was carrying three tennis rackets. Beware. It was evident after a short time on the court that I was no match for him and was unable to provide him with enough of a challenge even to give him exercise. When Laurie came back to pick us up, he politely told Laurie that he would like to run home in order to get some exercise. So much for my tennis. Laurie told the story to our kids and knowing my tennis they howled with glee. Despite this, he became a close friend. He and his wife Bente visited us many times since, as we have visited in Copenhagen, where he became Professor of Pediatrics.

Also among my early afficionados in research was a brilliant young biochemist, Isidore Edelman. He was sent to me by the Atomic Energy Commission, who wished him to obtain some grounding in isotope research. He stayed with me for a couple of years and helped in some of our early basic work on deuterium disappearance curves in humans, demonstrating the half-life of the water molecule in the body. He then worked with Arthur Solomon, Professor of Biochemistry, on developing the mass spectrometer for deuterium measurement. In 1950 he joined me in writing a review of the status of body composition and soon became the expert in internal medicine and biochemistry in this field. After leaving us he went to the University of California and was a key figure at the Cardiovascular Research Institute before being made Professor and Head of the Department of Biochemistry at Columbia University.

Paul Schloerb of Kansas and Rochester, New York, was a native son, a surgeon, and also an important early collaborator in isotope dilution studies. Recently he has improved on our ancient methods using modern biophysical methods. Graham Wilson of London was one of several men in internal medicine and cardiology who came to work with me because of the importance of body composition in heart disease. He later became Regius Professor of Medicine at Oxford.

Martin Moore-Ede, who was interested in the daily flux of body potassium, came to us from his studies in England. He later became an expert in biorhythm physiology and the need to plan the work of human beings according to their circadian (daily) rhythms. He was founding president of the Institute for Circadian Physiology in Boston.

Hugh Dudley, a surgeon of Aberdeen and of Edinburgh, came to our laboratories for 2 years and was one of the prime exponents of metabolism and metabolic care in surgery, in both Australasia and the British Isles. He became Professor of Surgery in Melbourne, Australia, and then moved to London as Professor and Head of the department at St. Mary's.

It would have been impossible to attract people with such a range of interests had it not been for the breadth of these studies and financial support from many sources. Some brought fellowships with them from abroad; others I was able to finance with my own research grants. The special fellowship programs of the National Institutes of Health and the American Cancer Society supported our people right from the start.

Because of our work on shock and burns, the Army was among our strongest backers. The Atomic Energy Commission took over funding of our isotope program from the Navy (which had picked it up right after the war). The Commonwealth Fund supported David Hume's work on the pituitary gland. The Harvard Medical School and the Brigham continued to be mainstays of our support by providing space and administrative backing as well as a hard-money budget. Within a few years a similar network of support would develop for organ transplantation and the several other fields of study being pursued in our department.

But first, how did we get started on the study of organ transplantation? This was to become the most extensive area of clinical research in our department and the largest entirely new field of medicine and surgery in this century.

BOOK SIX

Transplantation

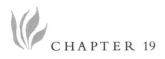

CHAPTER 19

Rejection, the Twins, and Radiation

(1950-1961)

rgan transplantation came to our department—or rather, patients in our department came to transplantation—on March 31, 1951. On that day David Hume transplanted a perfectly healthy normal kidney (which had to be removed from its host because of nearby cancer) into a 37-year-old man suffering from chronic kidney infection with severe high blood pressure and advanced renal failure. His demise was imminent. The donor kidney was sutured into place in the left renal fossa (the normal position of a left kidney). Its blood vessels were joined directly to the blood vessels of one of the patient's nonfunctioning kidneys, both of which were removed. After the transplant he was treated with adrenocorticotropic hormone (ACTH) to stimulate his adrenal glands and with heparin to prevent clotting, as well as the male hormone testosterone and antibiotics. Even so, the operative incision became infected. The kidney never functioned satisfactorily, and the patient died of renal failure on the 37th postoperative day. In present-day parlance, this would be referred to as a "random, unmatched, living-donor kidney, in the orthotopic position without immunosuppression, rejected." Immunosuppressive drugs to prevent rejection were still unheard of (but in fact were only 8 years away). None was used here.

The David Hume Series

The significance of this operation lay in the fact that it was the first ever to be performed for kidney transplantation according to a carefully planned research design, in which a surgical department committed to this study was joined to a medical department that included some of the world's experts in kidney disease and, again for the first time, with the availability of an artificial kidney. All this in a university teaching hospital equipped with top-flight consultants and a superb pathology department under Gustave J. Dammin, who was destined to become the world leader in the pathology and microscopic appearances of organ transplantation.

This particular operation had another unique feature. It was one of the few kidney transplants in which the organ was placed in the normal position of the kidney, alongside the aorta and the vena cava. Such a position for a transplanted kidney is anatomically difficult and surgically almost inaccessible. Only someone with the determination of David Hume could and—encouraged by me as his chief—would undertake such a procedure. The lesson was learned. No more kidneys were put there, even though that was where they ordinarily lived and seemed to belong.

Only 23 days later the second patient of this group was operated upon. Again, the patient had no significant kidney function. The donor, however, had suffered from high blood pressure. This time the new kidney was placed on the patient's right thigh, its artery joined to a branch of femoral artery (the main artery to the leg) and its vein joined to a vein of the leg. The ureter (draining conduit for the urine) was brought out through the skin. This same technique, developed by Dr. Hume, was used in the remaining patients of this series.

The third patient was a woman of 43, operated upon on April 24, 1951. The donor had died during operation for advanced heart failure due to mitral stenosis (a narrowing of the mitral valve of the heart). Although the donor's kidney function was subnormal because of her heart failure, her kidneys were judged to be in reasonably good shape. The kidney was placed in the thigh. ACTH was given in abundant doses as well as heparin to prevent clots, and, again, testosterone, with penicillin as a shield against infection. For the first time, the transplanted kidney functioned well. It continued to put out urine for 53 days. Even as late as the 70th day, with some real but diminishing urine output, the kidney looked almost normal on biopsy. The patient was dialyzed three times on the artificial kidney and lived until the 99th day, not bad for those primitive times and a harbinger of better times ahead. She was up and about, doing well, for that blessed but short time. In retrospect, and based on a guess that could not be corroborated in those early days, this was a happenstance close match.

George Thorn and I had planned this series of procedures (dialysis and transplants) together and had asked David Hume to carry out the operations because of his experience with experimental kidney transplantation in the dog and his enthusiasm, surgical ability, and remarkable determination. The ethical basis for such a human experiment lay in only two components: first, the patients selected were going to die shortly unless they could get a new kidney, and second, this experiment was being undertaken under the most ideal and favorable circumstances, with conscientious recording of every detail and the availability of the artificial kidney as standby.

Whatever the merit of this series of patients might be, whatever criticism we have endured regarding the ethics of these early efforts as viewed in terms of present-day mores 40 years later, whatever the troubles, difficulties, and expense we encountered, the fact is that if nothing is ventured, nothing is won. As it turned out, lots was ventured, and, finally, something remarkable was won. Late in this series of operations occurred an event the effects of which are still to be seen in every country where organ transplantation is being carried out.

A South American Doctor

The big break came in the case of a 26-year-old South American doctor who was dying of chronic glomerulonephritis (generally known as Bright's disease) and its lethal complication: extremely high blood pressure (210/120). The donor kidney came from a woman who had died on the operating table during surgery for a narrowed aortic valve. Her kidney function was quite good despite late-stage congestive heart failure. Dwight Harken, the operating heart surgeon, asked the family to donate the patient's kidney. The transplant operation was done on February 11,

1953. As in the previous case, the kidney was placed in the thigh. No ACTH, cortisone, or heparin was administered, but some testosterone and antibiotics were given. David Hume had suggested that the kidney might be enclosed in a small plastic envelope to keep the patient's white blood cells away from the outer part of the kidney. It seemed to me this was a good idea, though none of us knew enough about it to make a sage judgment. So we watched and waited. Somehow we were filled with optimism about this patient.

On the 19th day (March 2, 1953), nature smiled on kidney transplantation—and, as it turned out, on all organ transplantation—when the patient began to have a massive output of urine, a diuresis that persisted for almost 20 days. He required large amounts of intravenous fluids to compensate for the unregulated loss of fluid through the recovering transplanted kidney. After that outpouring of urine, the kidney resumed normal function that persisted almost 6 months, and he recovered from uremia (the bloodstream disorder seen in kidney failure). His blood pressure remained elevated; his own kidneys had not been removed. The patient returned home to South America. Five months later he returned, his kidney now failing. He knew that he was going to die, but like so many patients who have had some but not complete success with surgery at the frontier of knowledge, he was grateful for the 6 months of life he had been given. The magnificent human spirit of such patients cannot fail to impress everybody who sees them. He had a sort of calm assurance that the experience in his case would help others. Little did he (or we) know how right he was and how soon his prediction would be borne out.

He died on the 175th postoperative day, 5 months and 25 days after his operation. He had received a random, unmatched, fresh cadaver kidney. Under the microscope there was little evidence of rejection—another happenstance close match.

Our experience with this patient as much as any other single factor led to the successful initiation of kidney transplantation a little more than a year after his death, when Joseph Murray (David Hume's successor in the lab) transplanted a kidney from one identical twin into his brother. Clinical transplantation was born. Because of Hume's work, Joe Murray, George Thorn, Gus Dammin, John Merrill, and I felt assured that the identical twin experiment would be successful and should be undertaken.

In addition, we suspected—as Thorn had so often emphasized—that to control blood pressure, both diseased kidneys should be removed. In retrospect, it is possible that our failure to follow this course was responsible for the ultimate loss of this patient.

George Thorn, the Artificial Kidney, and the "Arm Kidney"

While kidney transplantation had a beginning at the Brigham and the Harvard Medical School, it soon spread widely and eventually led to the transplantation of other organs and tissues. This came to pass because of the work of many people, but especially because of the interest of George Widmer Thorn in kidney disease as well as his remarkable ability to foster innovation. George Thorn was born in 1905 and was appointed Hersey Professor of the Theory and Practice of Physic at Harvard on July 1, 1942, taking over the medical department of the Brigham Hospital following the death of Soma Weiss, the Hungarian physician who had been so inspiring to our class. George Thorn had a remarkable career, fostering new knowledge about the use of adrenal hormones, new approaches to high blood pressure, and perfection of the artificial kidney— a necessary prelude to kidney transplantation.

When the Dutch physician Willem Kolff visited the Brigham in 1947, he brought with him the design for his invention, the artificial kidney. He thought that of all American physicians, George Thorn might be the one best able to make good use of his new device. In that thought Kolff had one of the great insights of his brilliant career.

Not only was Thorn a physician steeped in knowledge about kidney disease and about the kidney's next-door neighbors, the adrenal glands, he was also a surgically minded physician. It has been my good fortune to work with several other surgically minded physicians, notably James Howard Means and Fuller Albright at the Massachusetts General and later John Merrill at the Brigham. Though an internist, Thorn was always thinking of things in surgical terms, that is, how can it be done, what will be its effect, and when can we get started? Some years earlier he had demonstrated this approach in his development of the treatment of adrenal failure by surgical implantation of adrenal hormone pellets. Later, it was evident in his surgical approach to the adrenal glands themselves in certain cases of high blood pressure. But in kidney transplantation, his idea was clear-cut. He wished to remove both kidneys in some instances of hypertension in which his studies showed that kidney disease was the cause. Clearly you could not remove the kidneys without putting a new one back in. The artificial kidney made it possible to think along these lines and, indeed, to temporize in acute kidney failure, sometimes long enough for the kidney to heal itself.

George Thorn and John Merrill, a young man appointed by Thorn to help in this project, supervised the use of the artificial kidney for dialysis (washing harmful waste products out of the blood) in patients with acute, reversible kidney failure, thus keeping them alive long enough for their own recovery processes to heal the kidneys. Back in 1948, the patients who recovered completely after dialysis (in the treatment of renal shutdown) were truly medical miracles and proof of the effectiveness of modern biological science.

Based on the ability of the kidneys to heal in 14 to 16 days in certain types of acute renal failure, a remarkable operation had taken place a year or two before. The artificial kidney was not yet available, and this operation was an attempt to keep a patient going those few extra days so her kidneys could heal and open up. It was a temporary transplant, the case of the "arm kidney."

To place the arm kidney episode in its historical context, it was possible because of a British physician-scientist named Bywaters, who had clearly described the temporary nature of acute renal failure in casualties of the bombing of London in World War II. Patients crushed under collapsed buildings often developed shock and renal failure (the crush syndrome). Bywaters had shown that if, by miraculous good luck, they lived 14 to 20 days, their kidneys would open up and they could survive. The arm kidney was also in a sense the parent of the Hume series and all that followed. I like to tell the story because it demonstrates George Thorn's unique innovative gift and his surgical imagination.

The patient who received the arm kidney was a 29-year-old housewife who was admitted to the hospital in 1946 with acute renal failure. About a week before, in her fourth or fifth month of pregnancy, she had undergone an illegal abortion without sterile precautions (as usual). Sometimes these procedures included the administration of large amounts of quinine or the instillation of tap water into the female reproductive tract, with leakage into the circulation. Either or both of these events will result in massive destruction of red blood cells (known as hemolysis) followed by renal failure. This was the case here. Hemolyzed blood is toxic to the kidney, and her kidneys promptly shut down.

Two or 3 days after admission, with conservative treatment, she began to look a bit better but was still not making any urine and had a dangerously high level of free hemoglobin in her blood. The artificial kidney, although on the drawing boards, had not yet become available. All the doctors who saw this patient knew that if they could keep her alive a few more days she might make it. Why not use a real kidney instead of an artificial one?

Encouraged by George Thorn, a young surgeon named Charles Hufnagel (then a surgical assistant resident) and David Hume, with the help of the urologic resident Ernest Landsteiner, offered to obtain a fresh kidney from a recently deceased accident victim and attach it to the arm vessels of this patient. Hufnagel had been a research fellow in vascular surgery and was expert in blood-vessel surgery. Both Hufnagel and Hume had already demonstrated their skill in research. They were able to suture the blood vessels successfully, giving the kidney its blood supply from the major vessel of the arm without endangering the hand.

The new kidney thus received its blood supply from the artery in the arm and drained its venous blood into the corresponding vein. The kidney was kept outside the body, lying on the arm, covered with moist gauze and secured to the arm with tape. The ureter—the duct that carries the urine to the bladder—was allowed to drain freely into a laboratory flask while the kidney was kept warm by the heat from a gooseneck lamp. The whole procedure was done on the ward under local anesthesia and did not involve taking the patient to the operating room. As I later found out, somewhat to my chagrin, this fact was not even mentioned in the subsequent abstract of the case; possibly a few conservative senior surgeons were opposed to such a bold and unprecedented step.

Subsequent events led to a happy outcome. The kidney certainly put out some yellow liquid, shown on analysis to be reasonably good urine. Maybe it did not make a great deal of urine. Maybe the urine was not very concentrated. Those figures are lost in history. But a few days later the patient's own kidneys began to open up, of that we are certain. She recovered completely. Here, a real kidney was being used to do the job later done by the artificial kidney. After about 48 hours the arm kidney was removed, as had been the plan in the first place. The patient recovered and went home. This was a temporary transplant to tide her over. A "bridge transplant," as it would now be called. Was it responsible for her recovery? Well, it was done and she recovered. Can we always identify cause and effect?

This patient was fated to receive two terrible strokes of fortune. First from an illegal abortionist (which led to her kidney failure) and then from the primitive knowledge of blood banking and plasma pool transfusion in 1946. During her acute illness she had been given plasma from a plasma pool that was later shown to carry the hepatitis virus. She developed a severe case of hepatitis and died about 3 months after the arm kidney episode. At autopsy examination both her kidneys were almost normal. The patient's case was reported in the literature as an example of the potential for complete healing of the kidney after total renal failure.

Surgery has been defined as "organized optimism" and research as "organized play for grownups." For those many members of our medical and surgical departments who knew about this patient, this procedure and its interpretation had certainly been optimistic: the arm kidney appeared to help her recover. It was one of those background events that strengthened our resolve 5 years later when George Thorn and I planned to treat a few cases of kidney failure by implantation of a new kidney, the operation carried out by David Hume. And as for organized play... well, yes, I accept that definition of research. Games include skill, attention to detail, enjoying the struggle, getting the right team, planning to win, and exhaustive exertion in a single-minded purpose. What better?

Ancient Dreams and Alexis Carrel

The idea of transferring a tissue from one place to another in the same human body was first realized with the grafting of skin in the hospitals of Paris early in the nineteenth century. By grafting skin it was occasionally possible, successfully, to cover over the defect produced by a wound or burn. Heroic methods were described 200 years ago for trying to make a new nose or a new thumb this way, by moving skin around. I am not sure any of these operations were ever accomplished. They made interesting pictures in history books. In all cases the skin was to be taken from the same patient, not another donor.

Before an organ could be taken from one person and put into the body of another person, obstacles in two critical areas had to be overcome: suturing (stitching) of blood vessels together and the problem of individual uniqueness. It was one man, Alexis Carrel, around the turn of the century, who surmounted the first obstacle. Although he witnessed rejection (the second obstacle), he did not recognize it for what it was, and he never tried to overcome it.

Carrel came to the United States from the University of Lyons in France in 1905 at the age of 32. After working briefly in Chicago, he joined the staff at the Rockefeller Institute in New York, where he was active in surgical research from 1912 to 1939. Carrel perfected the method of suturing blood vessels end to end. Like so many things in science, it was extremely simple: he used fine needles and very fine suture material to join the ends together, turning them outward a little as he did so.

Carrel's experiments in transplanting kidneys were carried out in cats. After removing both kidneys from one cat along with the large blood vessels (aorta and vena cava) above and below the kidneys, he placed them in another cat from which both kidneys had been removed. The vessels were sutured by his new method, and the ureters were sutured into the bladder.

These operations were considered technically successful. This expression is ominous, sure to be followed by "... but the patient died." And so it was here. At that time, transplantation alone was a triumph if the kidneys worked at all. The cats lived through the procedures, got along well, and made normal urine for a while. But within a few days they died. The kidneys had failed but did not seem to be infected, and blood flow had not ceased. Carrel was witnessing the process we now call rejection, but he had no word for it nor even a concept to dignify and identify it. He said it was neither infection nor infarction (loss of blood flow). It was something else that caused failure.

For his research on blood-vessel suture and transplantation, Carrel was awarded the Nobel Prize in 1912. He is usually referred to as the first

American to win the Nobel Prize. In fact, he was a French surgeon working in the United States, so perhaps it would be better to say that he was the first surgeon working in America to win the Nobel Prize.

Wartime Science: Kolff...

During World War II transplantation science made two great leaps forward: the artificial kidney (Kolff) and immunogenetics (Medawar). These leaps were scarcely evident at the time—just little jumps—because at first they did not appear applicable to organ transplantation.

In the Netherlands during the war and under the eyes of the Nazis, Willem Kolff had the idea of treating patients who were dying of kidney failure by a new method: passing their blood across membranes that were permeable to small molecules. His first membrane was made of sausage casing (wound around tomato cans). This was immersed in a sterile salt-water bath so the poisonous substances of kidney failure (chiefly urea, potassium, and certain other waste products) could pass from the patient's blood out through the tubing into the bath. The chemical name for this is dialysis; the popular name was blood cleansing or blood washing. A more sophisticated engineering version of Kolff's original device was the artificial kidney.

Many years later Kolff wrote to me describing how he had worked on this project while his professor was away. It was he who mentioned the tomato cans. According to Kolff, the professor would have told him to cease and desist because all his patients died after treatment. So it was a good thing the professor was away.

Kolff's patients were already fated to die because they suffered renal failure. Treated by dialysis, they got better, but for various reasons it did not work out as well as Kolff had hoped. He could see clearly from blood-chemical changes that the process of dialysis was doing its chemical job and that under ideal circumstances it would save lives. Kolff was convinced that the artificial kidney machine could temporarily take the place of a kidney and keep patients with acute renal failure (such as those with the crush syndrome) alive long enough for the injured kidneys to heal and come to the rescue.

... and Peter Medawar; The Birth of Transplant Immunology (1944-1954)

The other wartime advance, seemingly far removed from organ transplantation, was the development in England of a new field of science: immunogenetics. During the Battle of Britain many aviators were severely burned around the face when they bailed out of burning Spitfires. A zoologist named Peter Medawar was assigned by the Medical Research Council of Great Britain to improve the grafting of skin for these burned aviators. He chose Thomas Gibson of Glasgow, a plastic surgeon, as his collaborator. Over the course of a few years Medawar made two brilliant discoveries for which he later received the Nobel Prize.

Using skin from one animal grafted onto another, Medawar established that the first set of skin grafts was rejected in 7 to 10 days, that is, the skin became discolored, began to degenerate, and was shed from the recipient animal's body surface, leaving an open wound. Then, if a second set of skin grafts was put on, it was rejected much sooner than the first. This more rapid rejection suggested that an immunological response was involved, that the immune system was throwing off the skin as it might have thrown off an invading bacterium or parasite to which it had become partially sensitized by previous exposure. Medawar's "second set" response, as it came to be known, provided an entering wedge to the understanding of tissue rejection after transplantation. The interaction of an individual's inherited protein structure (genetics) and the rejecting foreign protein of the host (immunology) became known as immunogenetics. This is the science underlying tissue and organ transplantation. It is uniquely Medawar's field, defined by him but now pursued by thousands of scientists all over the world and defining a whole new realm of discoveries in genetics and immunology. Whole departments and textbooks are now devoted to this field of study, so new in 1945.

Medawar's second triumph was the demonstration of a "privileged time" for transplantation. It had been known for several years that there might be certain places within the body (such as the anterior chamber of the eye) where the immune process could not get at a transplant. Could not reach it. These were "privileged sites." In 1953, Medawar, working with Rupert Billingham and Leslie Brent, described a privileged time for transplantation in mice.

This privileged (safe) period for exchange of tissue occurs just before or around the time of birth. Medawar found that just before or at birth, skin from an unrelated donor could be placed on the newborn fetus without rejection. But then something unexpected was discovered. It is one of the earmarks of the beauty and wonder of science that, when carefully done, it can reveal important truths that were not anticipated at all. Now it was discovered that an animal grafted near birth could, throughout the rest of its life, take additional grafts again from that same donor animal. It became tolerant of that other animal's proteins and tissues, apparently mistaking them for "self." They termed this phenomenon *actively acquired immune tolerance.*

Medawar was a tall, handsome man, part Lebanese, with a commanding presence. He was a fine scientist, charismatic, friendly, and an inspiring lecturer. Later knighted for his work, he became known throughout the world of transplantation as Sir Peter. He died in 1987, the doyen of transplantation science throughout the world. Although he was neither a surgeon nor a clinician, his warm enthusiasm and the authoritative nature of his elegant scientific experiments influenced the whole field as nothing before or since. Rather than holding himself above clinical scientists and surgeons, he came to our meetings and knew the whole surgical community of transplantation. As a scientist he worked *with* his clinical colleagues, not apart from them.

Twinning and Genetic Identity

The matter of identical twins is worth a bit of reflection. In the western European races, twinning occurs about once in 85 to 90 births. Most of these twins are fraternal, that is, two eggs are fertilized simultaneously by two sperm and are implanted at two different sites in the lining of the uterus, forming two separate embryos with two distinct placentas that grow close together, as siblings. Hence the term fraternal twin. They don't look too much alike, are immunologically distinct individuals, and can be of opposite sexes.

Identical twinning is an entirely different process. Here, one egg is fertilized by one sperm and then splits into two embryos that are supported by a single placenta. Just why this occurs is anybody's guess. Possibly pure chance. It occurs at the same frequency in all races and ethnic groups but at differing frequencies in different animals. In human beings identical twinning occurs about once in every 250 to 270 births. That is, about one-third of all human twins are identical twins.

While fraternal twinning is an inherited trait, identical twinning does not seem to partake of any genetic or familial tendency. If you have had some twins in your ancestry or in the ancestry of your spouse, your children are more likely to be twins, most likely fraternal twins. The likelihood of identical twinning is independent of ancestry.

Many years ago it was suspected that because identical twins were so much alike and behaved so similarly, often having the same diseases at the same time, they might have similar body chemistry and, when it later became understood, immunologic identity as well. Barrett Brown, a plastic surgeon in St. Louis, had shown that this was indeed the case. By cross-grafting the skin of identical twins, he showed that skin could be traded back and forth between them with perfect success. No rejection. Between no other pairs of human siblings, parent or child, fraternal twins, or unrelated individuals is such tissue transfer possible. Crossed skin-grafting has become the acid test of identity.

A Twin Dying of Renal Failure

On October 15, 1954, Daniel Miller, a physician at the United States Public Health Hospital in Brighton, Massachusetts, called John Merrill at the Brigham to tell him that he had a 22-year-old patient (R.H.) who might need dialysis on the artificial kidney. Miller was an extraordinarily perceptive physician. He knew that the patient had an identical twin brother. He understood the significance of this fact, noting in the patient's record that the possibility of transplantation should be entertained.

At first, John Merrill (physician in charge of the artificial kidney) was a little hesitant to take on a patient for dialysis who had Bright's disease and for whom dialysis would merely prolong the agonies of death. But when Miller told Merrill of the identical twin brother and the implied possibility of transplantation, Merrill assented. The ambulance carried the patient from nearby Brighton to Brigham Circle on Huntington Avenue.

When the patient was first admitted he was very sick. Because he suffered from chronic Bright's disease, he had severe hypertension, a common cause of death in such patients. He was incoherent, thrashing about and having frequent convulsions. The first thing the physicians did was to stop his drugs. Half the medication he was taking was discontinued. Soon, he got much better. It was then possible to test him and his brother to see whether or not they were truly identical twins. Such matching could be done in a variety of ways, including configuration of the external ear, fingerprints, thumbprints, toeprints, and several other tests to detect close physical similarity. Crossed skin-grafting was carried out by Joseph Murray, who at that time was concentrating on plastic and reconstructive surgery. Joe had recently completed his surgical residency and had a strong interest in research and a commitment to the study of kidney transplantation in the laboratory. The skin graft showed that the twin brothers could accept each other's skin with ease and with no signs of rejection. They were truly identical. The push to transplant gained momentum.

Joseph Murray and the First Successful Transplant (December 1954)

After patient R.H. improved a bit on simple management, he was sent home for a while. When he failed to improve any further, he was readmitted and dialyzed on the artificial kidney. On December 23, 1954, the head surgeon of our urology division, J. Hartwell Harrison, removed one kidney from the donor twin, and Joe Murray transplanted it into the patient. The only role I assigned to myself was to carry this sacred kidney from one operating room to another, from Harrison to Murray, so it could be placed in its new host. Leroy Vandam, whom I had appointed Head of our Department of Anaesthesia only a few months before, administered the anesthesia—a touchy, difficult, and critical part of the operation, especially in such a sick patient.

The operation went well. The kidney was placed in the lower abdomen, with the ureter running directly into the bladder, according to the procedure Murray had perfected by experiments on dogs. The blood-vessel suturing was done much as Carrel had taught 50 years before. The simplest of procedures was used for the recipient patient, since we were trying to avoid complicated or careless experimentation with dangerous drugs or medicines.

When both patients were taken from their respective operating tables, they were doing quite well. The transplanted kidney was making nice, clean, clear, yellow urine. Although you may never have developed any affection for urine, if you or your patients are unable to make any, you come to appreciate it.

A couple of days later the patient appeared to take a sudden turn for the worse, a bit of a nosedive. It proved to be only a temporary setback. His kidney picked up again, and about a month later he was discharged from the hospital, his twin brother pushing him along in a wheelchair toward the ambulance to take him home. This was only 18 months after the remarkably encouraging experience of David Hume with that South American doctor who hoped his treatment might help others even though, in the end, it failed him.

In this age of communication it does not take long for such discoveries to get around. Word of the discovery of ether 108 years earlier spread around the world in a few months. News of this first successful transplant took only a few days to be known wherever people were studying renal failure. Joseph Murray was soon recognized, along with his predecessor and collaborator David Hume, as a leading pioneer in surgical transplantation.

This first successful kidney transplant of 1954, although in the freak circumstance of identical twinning, demonstrated two basic truths: first, it showed that if transplantation of a kidney could be successful over time, the kidney would continue to work well, the elevated blood pressure would return to normal (usually requiring removal of the old, diseased kidneys), and the chemical imbalance would be corrected. The kidney could reside comfortably in the abdomen in that odd spot down in the pelvis, not too far from the usual site of the appendix. Second, and possibly more important, it showed that if the immune barrier could be overcome (as it was here by a fluke of nature), tissue transplantation would be here to stay.

We feared that the identical twin's kidney, put in the sick patient's body, would acquire the same disease that the patient formerly had: Bright's disease. After all, identical twins have the same sort of susceptibility to just about everything. That is exactly what did occur, and it was the ultimate cause of failure and death in that first identical twin transplant. Eight years later, in 1962, the patient, made well by the transplant from his twin brother, developed the same kidney disease in the transplanted kidney that he had suffered in his own kidney. The donor twin, fortunately, remained well and unaffected.

Even those 8 short years of life given to this young man had tremendous meaning for him. He had fallen in love with one of his nurses at the hospital. They were married and had a family. Like the South American doctor, neither of the brothers expressed anything but gratitude for the care, caring, and help they had received, even when it became clear that the outcome was headed for tragedy in the end.

If transplantation was to help the thousands of patients dying of kidney failure every year, it was necessary to move beyond the identical twin setting. This was a hard time, with black years of failure ahead.

The Seven Black Years (1954 –1961)

Tom Starzl, the great transplanter of Denver and Pittsburgh (of whom more later), feels that I should not call these "black years," even if they were plagued with difficulty. Better to call them years of hope. I will go along with that terminology, especially since Starzl was just then beginning his own transplant study, which would combine with Murray's work in bringing hope to so many more patients over the coming decades. But for us at that time, when we saw so many dying patients for whom there was little hope, "black" would do.

No matter what we call this period, it lasted 7 years and 2 months. At the end of that time, we performed our first successful immunosuppressed kidney transplant between two totally unrelated people, using drug treatment to suppress the recipient's natural immunity. Murray was again the operating surgeon with the collaboration of Thorn, Dammin, Merrill, and the whole team in the departments of both medicine and surgery. But before this could come about, we went through what was (for me at least) a period of storm and trial.

174

During these 7 years patients from all over the world were referred to our department for kidney transplantation. Most we declined. A few were identical twins, and we could go ahead. Sometimes we permitted other patients to come, thinking there might be a close enough relative in the family so we could make the transplanted kidney function. Methods for precise tissue typing had not yet been discovered, but closeness of blood relation seemed to be an obvious source of help. Usually we tried to discourage these referrals because we had so little to offer.

With the collaboration of James Dealy, who was in charge of the radiology department, we treated most of these patients with whole-body x-ray irradiation. It had been known for years that whole-body irradiation knocks down the immune system. Transplant teams in Paris were using it to inhibit rejection of the kidney grafts, hoping that patients so treated might accept the donor kidney. Despite many difficulties, they had a few successes.

On one occasion, in April 1958, a young woman was sent to us with no kidneys at all. This terrible fix was not an infrequent source of calls to us. In her case it resulted from the surgical removal, after accidental injury, of her injured kidney. The surgeon had not realized (because he did not take the proper precautions) that she was born with only one kidney. But in this case, even if the surgeon had known this key fact, he would still have been faced with a difficult decision because her solo kidney was so badly damaged that it could not function no matter what. We tried to prepare her body to accept a new kidney by giving her a heavy dose of whole-body radiation.

Because she was heavily irradiated, it was necessary to keep her in a sterile environment. In those days we did not have sterile isolation rooms or critical care units, so we just kept her in the operating room for 28 days. Alfred Morgan, one of our interns (later a surgeon in Washington, D.C.), assigned himself to her constant care. This was inconvenient—to say the least—for him and everybody else, including the nursing and surgical staffs. But in the spirit of our hospital in general and of the surgical and operating room staffs in particular, she remained in this protected environment and avoided the infection that so often followed whole-body irradiation. She died of bleeding because the coagulating power of her blood was lost—an ironic complication of the radiation administered in a vain effort to save her life. Her kidney was still working without rejection, and at autopsy the transplanted kidney appeared virtually normal under the microscope. The balance of survival was a hard one to strike using radiation. We needed to find a better way of beating rejection.

There was one very bright spot in those black years. In 1959, for the first time, a pair of fraternal twins had successfully completed the same hazardous voyage. This successful transplant was accomplished using a smaller, survivable dose of whole-body radiation to suppress immunity. Murray was again the surgeon and James Dealy administered the radiotherapy. The patient was a 23-year-old man. Because the donor was his fraternal twin brother, the smaller x-ray dose provided sufficient immunosuppression to cover this less challenging genetic difference.

J. Hartwell Harrison, who had carried out the donor operations in all our living donors, was forced to remove the patient's own now infected kidneys (leaving the transplant in, of course) as a midnight emergency soon after transplantation. Once again, as in all these early cases, Leroy Vandam administered the anesthesia for this critically ill young man. This rather complicated course of events resulted in prolonged survival for both these fraternal twins. This was really the first successful transplant in humans in which artificial means (here, irradiation) were used to reduce or suppress the recipient's immune response.

Before this black period finally came to an end in April 1962, several more identical twins received new kidneys from their twin donors in transplants done by Murray. By 1966, a total of 23 twins had received kidneys from identical twin donors. Several of the married women in that group later became pregnant and have raised families.

Earlier, in 1960, Peter Medawar had been asked to give the Dunham Lectures at Harvard. In these lectures he opened new vistas of understanding and hopefulness in transplantation. Every medical school has one series of lectures considered to be of great importance. At Harvard it is the Dunham Lectures. We had four large amphitheaters at that time, but Medawar could speak in only one. Since this would clearly be an exciting talk at an exciting time, the amphitheater where he spoke was jam full. The other amphitheaters were wired for sound (this was before theater television) and were also crowded. The scientific community knew something important was about to happen and that Medawar's work was opening up a new field. By making use of the second set response and the privileged time, one could manipulate, change, examine, dissect, and ultimately come to grips with the newly recognized immunological phenomena of graft rejection and transplant immunology.

In time, the advent of drug immunosuppression would resolve the problem of rejection. While some work had been done prior to 1960 using chemicals to inhibit the activity of the immune system, these drugs had not appeared very promising. The drug most often used was nitrogen mustard, a close relative of the mustard gas used in World War I. Other substances were known to affect the immune system adversely, but most of them were highly toxic, similar to those used to slow the growth of malignant cells. Few of these drugs seemed to be satisfactory for transplantation. When used in experimental animals, they caused severe illness. We did not use them in patients.

Emergence from these black years is worth a chapter in itself.

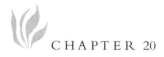

CHAPTER 20

The Advent of Drug
Immunosuppression

(1958-1962)

J ust at the height of our struggles with whole-body irradiation and its seemingly hopeless outlook, there appeared a flickering candle visible on what seemed to be the most distant scientific horizon. It is a matter of some nostalgia to all of us who saw this candle that even though it flickered faintly, we realized it could be the light at the end of our particular tunnel. It might indicate a way to suppress immunity without the uncontrollable hazards of total-body x-irradiation. Maybe the black years would give way to something brighter.

That flicker came from a point very close to us in Boston: Tufts Medical School. It took the form of an article about a new anticancer drug developed by the Burroughs Wellcome Company. The laboratories of this British-American company had a brilliant young chemist in their midst, George Hitchings. He and his assistant, Gertrude Elion, had synthesized a new drug originally intended for anticancer chemotherapy called 6-mercaptopurine (6-mp). For the synthesis of this and other key drugs based on the body's own chemistry, these two scientists were awarded the Nobel Prize in 1988.

Obtaining this new drug from Hitchings, two hematologists at Tufts Medical School, Robert Schwartz and William Dameshek, had observed its effect on the immune system of experimental animals. They had injected human serum albumin into laboratory rodents. Today we would call this a xenograft model, in which protein is traded between two different species. The animals usually rejected this very strange material rapidly and removed it from their blood. Because the protein was tagged with a radioactive tracer, the rate of removal could be measured. The tag and the foreign protein rapidly disappeared from the bloodstream of the untreated animal. Schwartz and Dameshek then gave the animals 6-mp to observe its effect on the rejection of this foreign (human) protein. The drug completely inhibited rejection, and the foreign protein persisted in the bloodstream. In 1958, these two clinical scientists published an article describing the immune suppressive potency of 6-mp. To all of us in the transplant field, this result was both important and exciting. Researchers are daydreamers at heart. It was not too difficult to imagine that this or some similar drug might be used to prevent the rejection of grafted kidneys.

Roy Calne and Drug Immunosuppression (1959-1961)

Before we could pursue this important new concept very far in the Brigham/Harvard laboratories, Roy Calne, a young surgeon in London who had also seen this report, promptly went to an animal research laboratory where he could study this matter in dogs—not too easy in Great Britain because of their strict antivivisection policies. One such lab was the Buckston Browne Research Farm of the Royal College of Surgeons in London. He performed kidney grafting from one dog to another, giving the recipient 6-mp to determine whether this drug would abate rejection. How much of importance in science is accomplished with great simplicity!

Within months Calne was able to report that dogs given kidney grafts and placed on 6-mp held those grafts very well for as long as 6 weeks (about six times longer than usual). Examination of the kidneys under the microscope showed that the usual disastrous destruction wrought by rejection was largely absent. Calne told Sir Peter Medawar about his discovery. Sir Peter suggested that he come to our department at Harvard to work on this problem. Calne wrote me about it immediately, and I encouraged him to come over as soon as possible.

So the young English surgeon took the boat to America. On the way to Boston he stopped at the Burroughs Wellcome Laboratories at

Tuckahoe, New York, to spend a day with George Hitchings and Gertrude Elion; they gave him some more 6-mp and a number of other new compounds, including 57–BW–322 (described below). At this same time, Charles Zukoski of Richmond, Virginia, who was working with David Hume, confirmed that the Schwartz and Dameshek findings using 6-mp (that is, the abatement of rejection) could be reproduced in canine kidney transplants. Things were warming up fast.

In late June of 1960, Calne walked into my office at the Brigham with his manuscript describing the latest 6-mp work he had done in transplants in dogs. He and I went over to our surgical laboratories at the Harvard Medical School, where we talked with Joe Murray. This was to be an auspicious collaboration for the future of this new field.

Within a few months Calne explored several drugs in many more animals. One of them (mentioned above) was called 57–BW–322 (i.e., drug number 322 for 1957 from the Burroughs Wellcome Laboratory). He found it to be the most effective. This drug later traveled under the chemical (generic) name of azathioprine and the trade name of Imuran.

Moving rapidly, Murray and Calne perfected kidney transplantation in dogs in our laboratories, using azathioprine to suppress the immune system. To their delight, it did not do too much other damage. We introduced the term "immunosuppression" for this action of the drug and the term "immunosuppressive chemotherapy" to cover its clinical use.

With this laboratory success in hand it was time to give the drug a try in a human patient dying of renal failure. The first two attempts (1961 and 1962) were not successful. One of these patients received 6-mp and then azathioprine. We still did not know the right dose for people sick with kidney failure. Then came success.

The First Successful Transplant from an Unrelated Donor (April 1962)

The patient's initials were M.D. Those initials were prophetic because he taught so many lessons to so many doctors. He was 24 years old when he was admitted to the Brigham on January 21, 1962, and referred to Dr. Merrill's kidney study and dialysis unit, because he too was suffering from chronic Bright's disease. In M.D.'s case, the disease had gradually worsened over many years. The reader will recall that several of the earlier transplant patients (in the Hume series and the twins) had suffered from this same fatal disease of young people.

After admission, M.D. was treated by peritoneal dialysis, in which a plastic button is placed in the abdominal wall so a small tube can be inserted and replaced without pain or inconvenience for "blood washing" on the surface of the abdominal membrane. The patient was admitted to the hospital six times during his first month to learn how to perform this type of dialysis himself so he could use it at home instead of coming to the hospital for sessions on the artificial kidney. Eventually, peritoneal dialysis became less and less effective. So the patient became a candidate for kidney transplantation. He had no twin, and no close relatives were available to act as donors. He began the long wait, knowing that he would be one of the first to be treated by drug immunosuppression for transplantation and that previous patients had not survived.

For a week Murray and two of his colleagues took turns sleeping in the hospital to keep a 24-hour watch in case some severely injured or very sick patient died suddenly, making a kidney available for transplant. The others on the kidney watch were Nathan Couch, who later helped us to preserve kidneys better, and Richard Wilson, who would within a few years take over from Joe Murray as head of the transplant unit.

There were three false alarms before they finally had their donor. On April 5, 1962, an operation was scheduled on a 30-year-old man for severe heart disease. For this particular operation at that time the patient's whole body was cooled. The operation was long and difficult, and when the patient was rewarmed his heart would not resume its normal beat. He died on the operating table despite a prolonged effort to restart his heart. After he died, his whole body was again cooled so that he could be put back on the pump-oxygenator (the heart-lung machine) to maintain his circulation artificially. His kidneys still functioned well; they were cool. And fresh. It took only a few minutes to complete the necessary arrangements with a helpful and understanding family. One kidney was removed only 40 minutes after the patient's death and was cooled further to 4°C. The total length of time from the death of the donor to the establishment of new, warm circulation in the kidney after transplantation was only 2 hours.

We knew from our laboratory work that all these circumstances were clearly favorable to the transplanted kidney. In fact, over the course of a few years it was widely recognized that this was the ideal way to preserve organs for transplantation. At the present time, whenever possible, even though a patient may have a died of severe head injury or a brain tumor, the ideal setting for donation is total-body cooling and artificial maintenance of the circulation using the pump-oxygenator. This was the first such donation.

The recipient, M.D., was placed on azathioprine. Although the kidney started to put out normal urine at the time of the operation, function soon ceased for a full 10 days. It was a puzzle as to whether this was temporary renal failure of the reversible type or prompt immune rejection of the new kidney despite use of the new drug intended to prevent just that.

On the 12th day, M.D. started to make urine again, and on the 18th day he made 6 quarts (about 1 1/2 gallons) in one day! This was reminiscent of some of Hume's early thigh kidney transplants. The transplanted kidney can get wildly out of control and make much too much urine for a while, requiring extensive fluid treatment to keep the patient from becoming dehydrated by his own kidney. Such a kidney will literally piddle the patient to death if you are too slow in replacing the lost fluids.

On the 39th day, despite recovery of more nearly normal function and despite the drug, M.D.'s immune system tried to reject his kidney. He had a typical immunologic rejection crisis characterized by high fever, severe illness, and decreased urine output. This was treated with actinomycin D in addition to azathioprine. Actinomycin, like 6-mp, had originally been introduced to treat cancer. It interfered with cell genetics and was strikingly immunosuppressive.

When this crisis subsided, the patient began to improve but his blood pressure was still elevated. On the 50th day and again on the 62nd postoperative day, J. Hartwell Harrison performed an operation to remove the patient's own degenerated kidneys. Although the patient was a sick man for two such big operations, they were essential to his survival. Blood pressure now returned to normal. George Thorn's original idea of removing the kidneys to treat hypertension was again corroborated by events, this time in an extraordinarily important patient: the world's first transplant recipient on drug immunosuppression.

Four months later M.D. experienced another rejection crisis, and for the first time cortisone was given to help get over this hurdle. While on cortisone, the patient developed pneumonia, always a frightening complication during immunosuppressive treatment. We knew from experiments in the laboratory that despite the presence of immunosuppressive drugs, such disorders as pneumonia can be treated by antibiotics without stopping the immunosuppression, a step that would endanger the kidney. We followed such a policy here. Finally, the patient was sent home doing very well. The waste products in his blood were still slightly elevated, but they soon returned to normal levels.

Then, 18 months after his transplant—as if to put the entire procedure to a severe test—M.D. developed acute appendicitis. The appendix, located right next to the transplanted kidney, was badly infected and perforated and had to be removed. Under the microscope the appendix showed suppression of its normal lymph tissue response to inflammation and infection, demonstrating the adverse effect of immunosuppression on a local infection, this one in the appendix. Over the next several years we saw a good many kidney transplant recipients with infections in various parts of the bowel, especially diverticulitis, made worse by immunosuppression.

M.D. got over this setback and went home as well as could be expected (maybe even better, considering all he had been through). He was still on the immunosuppressive drugs. But that was not to be the end of the story. That transplanted kidney, although the first ever to show long-term function after transplantation on drug immunosuppression, continued to show chronic rejection. So, on January 22, 1964—21 months after his first transplant—the patient received a second kidney. Here again, M.D. was prophetic because now, 30 years later, chronic rejection is a continuing and unsolved problem in kidney transplantation, a problem not shared to the same extent by transplants of liver, heart, or pancreas. This time the new kidney for M.D. was one removed by Donald Matson from a child undergoing an operation for hydrocephalus, during which a normal kidney must be sacrificed.

Don Matson, a classmate of mine and head of our neurosurgical division, had perfected this operation, which consisted of draining the overabundant cerebrospinal fluid into the child's bladder via the ureter so the fluid could be passed from the body along with urine. This operation was eventually performed widely throughout the world and required the removal of one perfectly healthy kidney, often useful to a patient awaiting transplant. M.D. was the first of many patients to receive a "Matson kidney."

M.D. had a hectic and troublesome time. Both he and his family, true to the stamp of these patients, remained grateful for the extension of his life. But it was not to last for very long, because on July 2, 1964, he died of generalized infection and severe liver damage. The latter may have been due to hepatitis virus from one or more of his transfusions. Also, azathioprine can be toxic to the liver. All three of these early transplant patients taught doctors important lessons that provided a model for the rest of the world. But only one, the fraternal twin, survived for a long time, remaining well and continuing his work for 25 years.

On the basis of our care of M.D., our experience grew rapidly. Of the first 13 patients operated on under immunosuppressive drugs at the Brigham between April 1962 and April 1963, 10 received kidneys from recently deceased persons, while three were given Matson kidneys. Matson kidneys are fresh when transplanted and require no preservation. Those three patients appeared to fare better than the others.

By 1963 kidney transplantation was spreading rapidly over the world. We were no longer unique. Most notably the technique was picked up again by David Hume, formerly of our department, who had become Professor and Head of the department at the Virginia Commonwealth University in Richmond; by Thomas Starzl in Denver, Colorado; and by René Küss and Jean Hamburger in Paris, where important work in transplantation had been going on for some years using both radiation and drug immunosuppression. Roy Calne had returned to London from our laboratory and then went to Cambridge, England, where he became Professor of Surgery and Head of the Department of Surgery. He was knighted by the Queen in 1986 for introducing transplantation to Great Britain.

Les Parisiens

Like transplantation in the United States, that of Calne in England clearly traced its origin back to the Brigham experience, at least in part.

This was not the case in Paris. There, over the course of several years, two French scientists had initiated a major effort in kidney transplantation that in many ways was parallel to ours. Because John Merrill spoke fluent French and was a particular friend of Jean Hamburger, one of these French scientists, we were kept pretty well aware of what they were doing. The French surgeon René Küss, senior surgeon at the Foch Hospital in Paris, had also been very active in this field.

On January 12, 1951, Charles Dubost and Nicholas Oeconomos transplanted the kidney of a guillotined criminal into a 44-year-old woman dying of renal failure. In 1955, the French surgeons transplanted several unmatched kidney grafts into unrelated recipients, much as we had done with the early Hume series at the Brigham. In Paris in those early years, about 25 patients were operated on, with no long-term survivors. Although on two or three occasions we had been offered organs from condemned criminals about to be executed, we came down hard against this practice as unethical in its unspoken bias toward the death penalty. That was our view, possibly too puritanical.

The French had perfected the use of the intra abdominal location for the transplant, as had Joe Murray in our laboratories. As we had troubles, the French also experienced severe difficulty in the early days. Starting with an operation carried out on January 17, 1960, Küss achieved increasing success using radiation in modest doses, sometimes adding cortisone and 6-mp. In 1962 six patients were reported from the Paris experience, largely based on radiation for immunosuppression. The one long-term survivor was a nonidentical (fraternal) twin, similar to our patient. Professor Jean Hamburger was an internist, a nephrologist, who had several surgeons working with him at the Necker Hospital. In the mid 1960s he reported 13 patients surviving more than a year (out of 16 operated upon) using azathioprine and cortisone but without radiation. After this, the French went over completely to drugs for immunosuppression and abandoned radiotherapy, a method with which they had far greater experience and success than we had ever achieved.

A New Star in Denver: Thomas Starzl

In 1962 Thomas E. Starzl moved from the laboratories of Northwestern University in Chicago to take a position under William Waddell,

Professor of Surgery at the University of Colorado in Denver. On November 24, 1962, 3 months after going to Denver and only 6 months after our operation on patient M.D., he performed his first kidney transplant under drug immunosuppression with prolonged survival. Starzl's work included experiments with several immunosuppressive drugs. He was a strong advocate of using cortisone to strengthen the immunosuppressive effect of azathioprine.

Starzl's enthusiastic and intensive work in kidney transplantation soon outstripped ours in sheer numbers. Within 3 years he could report 127 kidney transplants. In those involving living donors (usually family members), the success rate (survival longer than one year) was 80%.

Neither here nor in the following accounts of early transplantation is there space to give the credit they deserve to all the collaborators in this field in Europe, Australasia, and America. The earliest successes seem to command attention: in the case of kidney transplantation, our early work at the Brigham, particularly the pioneering work of David Hume and Joseph Murray; those early successes in Paris, Cambridge, and Edinburgh; and the beginning work of Tom Starzl. These were the key initial researches that explored and opened up a vast, previously unexplored territory of surgery and biomedical science.

Within 25 years transplantation was to mushroom into the largest entirely new field of medical care in this century. It involved medicine, surgery, pediatrics, radiology, and applied immunology and has been a tremendous stimulus to basic immunologic science, as stated so clearly by Sir Peter Medawar. The story of twentieth-century surgery has as its centerpiece the story of organ transplantation, which began precisely at midcentury. Forty years later, in 1990, Joseph Murray was awarded the Nobel Prize for his work in kidney transplantation along with E. Donnall Thomas (a resident physician at the Brigham with George Thorn in the 1950s) for his work in bone marrow transplantation. As I look back on the colorful years of my surgical career, few can compete with the decade 1954 to 1964 for sheer and continuing excitement.

By 1962 we had already started work on the next organ to enjoy such undivided attention, and in 1963 I performed our first clinical liver transplantation under drug immunosuppression.

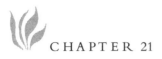

CHAPTER 21

The Liver: Transplanting the Body's Largest Organ

(1957-1965)

There were two principal reasons for us to start work on liver transplantation. First, we were interested in the immunological concept of antigen overload. An example would be an over-whelming infection in which the sheer burden of growing bacteria is more than the immune system can handle and so it retreats in disorder (as a form of immunodeficiency). The possibility of antigen overload leading to liver acceptance was part of our thinking. Transplanting the largest organ available in the body from one animal to another might somehow overcome immune rejection and enhance acceptance either of that organ or of others. The second reason was that there was an excellent team working on kidney transplantation, and it seemed important that we examine some other possibilities. For this we needed another team.

H. Brownell Wheeler was one of our residents. We had an exchange arrangement with St. Mary's Hospital in London, as described in Chapter 18. Brownie Wheeler had just returned from a year there working with Charles Rob, a leading vascular surgeon who later became Professor and Head of the department at the University of Rochester. While working with Rob, Wheeler had become expert in blood-vessel surgery. Just at this moment, sometime in the summer of 1957, he was between jobs and had a little extra time.

I asked him to come over to my office so we could discuss a new project. I told him that I was thinking of transplanting the liver in dogs. Although he was intrigued and wanted to help, he quite rightly wondered if that was going to be worthwhile. There was as yet no way to abort or abate rejection. I told him we would have a surgical problem right at the beginning, because the hepatic artery (the main artery to the liver) is complicated in the dog and does not lend itself as easily to surgical anastomosis (joining of the two severed ends) as it does in the human. So I asked him to look into this question of how we might anastomose the hepatic artery in the dog, and he promptly developed several plans.

The Laboratory Start of Liver Transplantation

A few weeks later, we carried out our first liver transplantation in the dog. These operations were long, difficult, and complicated. There was no prior experience to guide us. We had to devise new methods and new instruments. Louis L. Smith of the medical school at Loma Linda, California, was a prime assistant in this work, as was Peter Knight of Canada. Tom Burnap gave the anesthesia for these operations. We developed some special apparatus so the veins from the lower part of the animal (completely obstructed during the process of suturing in the transplant itself) could drain their blood through outside channels (shunts) back to the heart. Without this, no animal could survive the operation.

Almost immediately we witnessed some interesting things. First, the transplanted livers worked very well. We measured many enzymes and tested the liver function in these animals. The transplants did all the jobs that livers should do. Second, the operation was difficult and dangerous because of the tendency to hemorrhage with temporarily compromised liver function. Finally, the donor liver had to be handled with extreme gentleness to maintain its normal softness and circulation of arterial blood. The canine liver is much more sensitive to manipulation than is the human liver.

At that time (1958) we had no inkling of the imminent availability of immunosuppressive drugs. This was precisely in the midst of that black period that I described in Chapter 20, between the identical twins (1954) and the first successful drug immunosuppression (1962). All the livers we transplanted in these dogs were rejected at about 6 to 8 days.

Although we were also developing methods for transplanting the intact whole spleen, that work has now been forgotten because there is as yet no practical application. Immunologically, this was of interest because the spleen is itself an immunologically competent organ (i.e., it is an integral part of the body's immune system), and it mounted a brisk reaction of the grafted spleen against the new host, a phenomenon soon dubbed graft-versus-host disease. The transplant became a warlike invader rather than a mere stranger.

We could not demonstrate any beneficial immune phenomenon, such as antigen overload, from the transplanted liver and we were not yet aware of the especially favored transplantability of the liver, later shown to be the case in pigs by Roy Calne when he returned to England, and also suggested several years later by the work of Starzl in humans.

As told in Chapter 20, Roy Calne of England had come to work in our laboratories 2 or 3 years after we first began the liver transplant work, so he was well aware of what we were doing in liver transplantation and why we were studying it. He himself was working intently with Joe Murray on kidney transplantation, and it was not until he returned to Cambridge that he became one of the world's foremost experts in liver transplantation.

Although we were the first to report the operational details for removal of the entire liver, vascular shunts in place, and replacing it with a new liver in its normal position, we were not the first to consider transplanting the liver. Earlier, in 1953 or 1954, at about the time of the identical twin kidney transplant, C. Stuart Welch, Professor of Surgery at Tufts Medical School, was starting work on liver transplantation. Like us, he was experimenting on dogs, placing the liver in a new site in the abdomen, not in its normal position. For it to receive its normal anatomic double circulation of blood, it seemed best that the liver reside in its normal position. That was our endeavor. While Welch's work showed several other points that were helpful to us, Welch himself gave up the work after a year or two and moved away from Boston.

Although we had quite a team on the project, three surgeons became most importantly involved in the evolving work on liver transplantation. Two, Roy Calne and I had exchanged ideas at the Brigham/Harvard laboratories during Roy's stay (1960-1962), as just mentioned.

The third of this triumvirate, Thomas Starzl, was working on liver transplantation at Northwestern University in Chicago, later taking his studies to Denver and working intensively on the kidney. Two of the three, Starzl and Calne, both considerably younger than I, were to become prime exponents of clinical liver transplantation in its early years (1963 to 1975) before it emerged as a widely accepted treatment.

Our first brief paper on liver transplantation was published in 1959. The next year we described our work in detail before the annual meeting of the American Surgical Association. At that time Tom Starzl discussed our work in light of his own, and it was clear we were working in parallel. We enjoyed a congenial relationship, not one of rivalry, but rather openness so important for scientific advance in a new field.

In 1962 Alan Birtch joined me in the liver transplant work and took charge. He was a Johns Hopkins graduate who had finished his residency at the Brigham and had spent a year studying liver blood flow in the Department of Physiology with Professor A.C. Barger. Alan devoted himself to this field for several years, was the first to describe the obstruction of blood flow in rejection of the liver, and was one of those liver transplanters who suffered a severe case of hepatitis himself ("the liver's revenge") during his work, as described below.

From the Laboratory to the Operating Room

In 1963 we performed our first liver transplantation in a patient with a huge primary cancer of the liver. It was not successful; the patient died of pneumonia, at least partly traceable to the immunosuppressive drugs. The case was reported and illustrated in my book *Transplant: The Give and Take of Tissue Transplantation*, in 1974.

Tom Starzl performed his first human liver transplantation at about the same time as I did in 1963, but with a longer survival. Also in 1963, Roy Calne, now back in England, was starting his remarkable series of liver transplant operations. Within 2 or 3 years he reported his first human cases.

Roy Calne and Thomas Starzl were both to have a profound impact on the entire field of transplantation. Both are brilliant surgeons, teachers, and innovators, widely recognized throughout the world for their work. Both have received many awards, prizes, and honors, in their own countries and abroad. These two men, one in England and the other first in Chicago, then Denver, and later Pittsburgh, were to devote their entire professional careers to the development of transplantation. My life was enriched by close personal and scientific contacts with these two remarkable surgeons.

Roy Calne (now Sir Roy) was born in 1930 in Surrey. He attended Guy's Hospital Medical School in London and did his early surgical training there. After army service in Malaysia with the Gurkhas, he took a year at Oxford before coming to work with us in the summer of 1960. He returned to England in the late fall of 1961, just before that first successful immunosuppressed kidney transplant was carried out by Joseph Murray based on Calne's early work with 6-mp (see Chapter 20). Professor of Surgery at Cambridge University, he was the first to explore the use of a new drug, cyclosporine, for transplantation. He has been a central figure in the development of transplantation throughout the world.

Thomas Starzl was born in Le Mars, Iowa, in 1926. He attended Northwestern University where he obtained a Ph.D. in physiology in 1950 and an M.D. in 1952. After internship and a residency at Johns Hopkins, he worked in Florida and was then appointed to the faculty at Northwestern, becoming an assistant professor in 1961. While he was there, we began to correspond about our mutual interest in experimental liver transplantation. We first met in 1960 at the meeting of the American Surgical Association where I presented my paper, as mentioned above.

About 1960 Tom told me he would enjoy working in my department. While I would have been proud and pleased to add this young star to our group, it was perfectly clear to me that he needed to be at a university not only with strong backing from his chief, but with an empty slate in transplant science. My small laboratory was already overcrowded, and the Brigham was soon to have a large proportional share of patients with kidney failure on both Dr. Thorn's service and mine. We were doing as much experimental work in surgery, as much surgical transplantation, and as much dialysis as our small hospital and laboratory could possibly accommodate.

The surgical department of the University of Colorado at Denver was well known to me because my friend and Harvard Medical School classmate Henry Swan had been Professor and Department Head there for many years and helped to give this Rocky Mountain university, new to the councils of world surgery, a growing and secure reputation. I had been visiting professor there in 1958. Swan's work was in cardiac surgery. This was a perfect place for Tom Starzl to carry forward his work in transplantation under Swan's successor, Bill Waddell, a colleague from my MGH years.

In 1962 Tom Starzl moved from Chicago to the University of Colorado, where he pursued his work on transplantation of both kidney and liver with his usual energy and increasingly wide recognition. There he began his custom of teaching others the art and science of transplantation, as Joe Murray and the Brigham team had done before him. In 1972 he was made chairman of the Department of Surgery at the University of Colorado. Nine years later, in 1981, he was appointed Head of the Transplant Unit and Professor of Surgery at the University of Pittsburgh. He has become a pioneer in the use of a new drug for immunosuppression, known as FK506, and has recently (1992) published a book—*The Puzzle People*—telling the fascinating story of his life as a surgical scientist devoted to the development of organ transplantation.

Throughout much of his scientific career, Tom Starzl worked with Kendrick Porter of London, who carried out the pathological and microscopic examination of both experimental and clinical material from Starzl's work. This 4,500-mile collaboration, which lasted several decades, was in a sense a continuing link between Tom and our department, where Ken Porter had first started his transplant research in 1956.

Tom has contributed uniquely to transplantation science on a very broad base. He was one of the first to stress adding cortisone to azathioprine for treating rejection. Although we had used cortisone for this purpose as early as 1952, we did not report it as a separate drug regimen. Starzl also improved the use of cyclosporine in the same way, by adding cortisone. He has written several books that are widely used in the field of transplantation. By the magnitude of his enterprise in surgical care and the number of liver, kidney, bowel, and pancreas transplants he performed at Colorado and then at Pittsburgh, Starzl has become one of the leading transplant surgeons of his time. Several important physiologic facts have emerged from his study of liver transplantation, by which he has demonstrated genetic and enzymatic mechanisms underlying certain disorders of the liver. In some of these he has shown that transplantation is an effective method of treatment, even though other aspects of liver function may be normal. He has also demonstrated the migration of donor cells to other places in the recipient body, a new clue to transplant acceptance.

In those early days (1960 to 1970) liver transplantation moved slowly. Six years after the first clinical transplants a meeting was held in April 1969 in Cambridge, England, at which the first 91 patients were reported. Of these, only 10 were still living and only 3 had survived the operation for more than 12 months. The longest survivor at that time, a patient operated on by Starzl in Denver, lived for about 16 months. A year and a half later the total had increased to 133, and at that time the longest survival was 29 months (one of Calne's patients). A few years later I was asked to chair an international meeting on transplantation of the liver, examining the total record to date. While a half-dozen other centers were now carrying out the operation, Calne and Starzl had, between them, carried out over 90% of all the liver transplants in the world. Long-term survival was becoming much more frequent as the operation itself and the use of drug immunosuppression were both being perfected.

Beginning at that time (about 1975), liver transplantation came out of the research lab and underwent the same sort of expansion in use that kidney transplantation had shown about 10 years before. At the present time in most countries carrying out transplantation, liver and heart transplantation are second in frequency to that of the kidney, each involving about one-third as many operations as are done for kidney.

When I consider the tortured growth of science, the rivalries, ego trips, misunderstandings, backstabbings, fraud, misrepresentation, arguments over priority, and unhappiness that have marred so much of the story of scientists and science, I regard this period in early transplantation as a remarkably happy one. Only a few people were at work. They kept in touch, met together, bore good will toward one another, and together founded a new field of clinical and scientific activity.

Who Needs a New Liver?

Patients who need liver transplantation differ in important ways from those needing new kidneys. Chronic kidney failure is characteristically seen in teenagers or adults; only rarely are acute infections the cause. Cancer or other malignant tumors rarely warrant kidney transplantation. None of the kidney diseases is a result of self-indulgent lifestyles. Most of the diseases are chronic.

In sharp contrast, liver failure treatable by transplantation includes a large cohort of young children whose bile ducts fail to develop (biliary atresia); some of the greatest triumphs in liver transplantation have been in that childhood group. Chronic alcoholism is one of the commonest causes of fatal chronic liver disease. It was clear from the outset that no alcoholic should receive a lifesaving liver at the sacrifice of an alternative recipient unless a certifiably prolonged abstinence had been achieved. Acute fulminating fatal hepatitis, much to the surprise of all, can be treated by transplantation, with long-term survival. And livers with primary malignant tumors can be successfully replaced if the cancer is caught early. Late malignancy would almost never be an acceptable basis for transplantation because of the virtual certainty of spreading disease, visible or not.

The clinical experience of Alan Birch and myself with only four cases (two adults and two children) in 1963, 1964, and 1965 yielded no long-term success. We felt we should await the perfection of immunosuppression before proceeding further with liver transplantation. Our former student (Roy Calne) and our collaborator in Denver (Thomas Starzl) took up the work with greater success and in far greater numbers, as mentioned above, and by 1975 liver transplantation was gaining general acceptance. We had been active participants in the years of struggle (1957 to 1965) but had passed the torch to others during the early years of success (1965 to 1975). While I have been criticized for not going ahead with clinical liver transplantation, it was in good hands, and I have no regrets.

The Revenge of Immunosuppression

Much of this story about transplantation has been upbeat and optimistic. Fair enough, since it was an entirely new, rapidly growing, and increasingly successful way of treating sick people. But the picture is not always so rosy. Transplant operations (especially those of liver and heart) are still associated with significant mortality. For some patients the drugs simply did not keep immunity suppressed. For others, although the drug did its job at first, there was later a chronic rejection (seen especially in the kidney) that claimed the organ after several years. Kidney transplantation is associated with a 95% (or higher) survival rate at one year if living donors are used, with some diminution when cadaver donors are used. For liver and heart, this figure for early survivorship is only slightly lower.

In a dire sense, immunosuppression has also had its revenge. In Emerson's words in his essay *On Compensation*, "It would seem there is always this vindictive circumstance stealing in at us unawares... this backstroke, this kick of the gun, certifying that the law is fatal; that in nature nothing can be given, all things are sold."

From the earliest days of the use of azathioprine (Imuran) and now with cyclosporine and FK506, reducing immunity has led to the growth of malignant tumors in a small fraction of cases (about 10%). In one case a lymph-related tumor appeared at the exact site where antilymphocyte serum had been injected. Cancers of several types have appeared long after transplantation.

The simplest explanation of this emergence of tumors in patients under immunosuppression is that the normal immune system constantly exerts a sort of roving policing or surveillance, killing off tumor cells (that may be immunologically distinct from the host's own cells) when they arise. Then, when the policeman is suppressed or inhibited—when the cat's away—the tumors emerge. The longer the followup, the higher the incidence of tumors under immunosuppression. Israel Penn, a world expert on this problem, estimates that at 20 years after transplantation the incidence of malignant tumors will rise much higher. That is why we need a better method of achieving graft acceptance, some way of inducing tissue tolerance without toxicity and global loss of immunity.

There was one other unexpected aspect of liver transplantation. Sort of a diabolical justice. The liver's revenge. While working intensively on liver transplantation, Alan Birtch came down with a very severe case of hepatitis. Tom Starzl also contracted this disease, as did Roy

Calne. A nurse working on liver transplantation died of the disease. I had formerly been stricken with a severe case of hepatitis in 1946 and thought I was immune. During my liver transplantation days, I came down with the disease a second time, although a rather mild case. Several other liver transplanters contracted the disease. I do not know any explanation for this unexpected outbreak, this epidemiology. Did laboratory animals (dogs) carry this virus in the liver without showing the disease itself? That seems to be the most logical explanation.

No mere rhetoric can do justice to the role of patients and their families in the development of transplantation. Patients give so much of themselves and contribute so much to our understanding, often knowing their own gloomy prognosis. Understanding all the risks and travails of the course, they make their choice in hope and faith and always with the assurance of helping others should their own course falter or fail, as it so often did. In these crucial early years of our work (1951 to 1975) our patients were the real heroes.

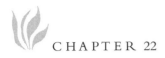

CHAPTER 22

Broadening Scope; New Problems; *Nonnumquam, Nocere Est Renovare*

Starting in the middle 1960s, a few years after the case of M.D., an increasing number of scientists, physicians, and surgeons began to explore the possibility of treating disease in other organs by transplantation. This work is still going on; new horizons for transplantation and new ways of transplanting human organs and tissue will be discovered for many years to come.

The Heart

The story of heart transplantation recapitulated that of kidney and liver transplantation. Success depended on suppression of the immune system with drugs, as was first done successfully in M.D. There was another similarity: at the beginning only a few people were working on heart transplantation, as had been the case with the kidney, in only one or two laboratories. They were getting started rather quietly as far as the rest of the world was concerned. Few physicians or surgeons—let alone the media and the public—knew of the work. As a generality, if you would look for what is coming next in science, do not read the papers. Go to a scientific meeting or visit a lab. This was true for kidney, liver, and heart, but there was a difference. The first kidney transplant was scarcely noticed in the papers. I am not even sure it was mentioned. The first human liver transplants were also neglected by the press, probably because reporters could not understand what people were talking about: transplanting the liver? How do you do that? What for? Where? Why? There was no frame of reference.

In heart transplantation the breakout from the laboratory to clinical reality made a splash that was heard around the world. Or rather, a typographical bang. Front-page headlines of newspapers appeared in type 2 or 3 inches high. Everyone knew where the heart was and what it did. While only a pump, it is rather central. As the ancients considered it the seat of the soul, so also most people still grant it some sort of special status in the hierarchy of internal organs. King. Or maybe Queen.

The major biological difference between the heart and the other organs that had already been transplanted (kidney, liver) lay in the fact that the heart consists almost entirely of muscle. It contains only a few specialized cells that do metabolic or glandular work in secreting hormones. It also contains an important nerve network—the conduction bundles—that coordinates its beat. While its muscle is a little different from the muscles that move our arms and legs, it is nonetheless muscle tissue. Because the heart is largely muscle, with less cellularity, there were some who thought it might be less antigenic. I was one who held that optimistic view. As it turned out, the heart can be rejected just like any other transplant and requires drugs to suppress immunity so it will remain secure and beating normally in its new host.

As was the case with both the kidney and the liver, three major figures in surgery and science were the prime movers. In heart transplantation they were Richard Lower and Norman Shumway (of Minneapolis and Stanford) and Christiaan Barnard of Capetown, South Africa. In addition, there was a fourth, a great friend and advocate of young people in surgical research: Owen Wangensteen of the University of Minnesota.

The work of these men on the experimental surgical transplantation of the heart started in Minneapolis in the late 1950s and early 1960s. Owen Wangensteen, a Minnesotan of Swedish extraction, was for almost 50 years the leader of surgical research in the Midwest. What he liked to call his "small agricultural college" rapidly grew to be a great power among American universities, especially in surgical research. During the years 1956 and 1957 the University of Minnesota housed several people who were to become stars in the field of cardiac surgery and cardiac transplantation. Curiously enough, Wangensteen's own interests lay in the gastrointestinal tract and ulcer disease. He never appeared to have much interest in heart surgery or transplantation. But his laboratory and the milieu of inquiry he fostered were at the heart (or at least the root) of the matter.

Norman Shumway received his medical degree from Vanderbilt University in Tennessee in 1949, then enrolled at the University of Minnesota where he entered the surgical Ph.D. program of Wangensteen, receiving his degree in 1956. Christiaan Barnard, a graduate of the University of Capetown, came to the University of Minnesota in 1956 as a student under Wangensteen, working with C. Walton Lillehei and Richard Varco, two Minnesota surgeons who were developing open-heart surgery. Barnard worked in Minnesota until 1958, when he took a surgical appointment back home at Capetown. Shumway's studies had to do with the effect of temperature on disturbed rhythms of the heartbeat, a topic of importance in open-heart surgery and later in heart transplantation because of the low temperatures required for preserving the heart while it is disconnected from the circulation. Shumway left Minnesota in 1957, soon moving to Stanford University for a notable career in heart transplantation.

Richard Lower was another Michigan transplanter (Hume was born in Muskegon, Shumway in Kalamazoo, Lower in Detroit). He had attended medical school at Cornell, with a surgical residency at the University of Washington in Seattle, whence, in 1957, he moved to Stanford and worked with Shumway. About 1959 they began to experiment with removing the heart and suturing it back again in the same animal. Richard Lower, working in Shumway's laboratory and assisted by Eugene Dong, then performed the first successful heart transplantation in a dog, in December 1959.

Shumway carried out his first successful human heart transplantation at Stanford on January 8, 1968. By that time Richard Lower was developing cardiac and thoracic surgery under David Hume at the Medical College of Virginia; Lower could soon demonstrate one of the longest survivors of heart transplantation.

Meanwhile, that other Minnesota graduate student, the South

African Christiaan Barnard, had pushed ahead a little bit faster and was able to scoop the world by carrying out the first clinical cardiac transplantation in Capetown on December 3, 1967. For those interested in dates, this was 13 years after the first identical twin kidney transplant, 5 years after the first immunosuppressed transplant (kidney), and 4 years after the first two human liver transplants.

Barnard's patient was a 53-year-old man, a diabetic with repeated heart attacks and now severe failure of both the right and left sides of his heart. The donor was a 24-year-old woman who had been struck by an automobile in an accident only about a mile from the hospital. Starting the operation in the middle of the night, Barnard completed the transplant, and the patient was back in bed the next morning. The threat of rejection was treated with azathioprine (patterned after the work of Murray, Calne, and Hitchings 5 years before) as well as cortisone and irradiation. The patient died on the 18th postoperative day from a combination of rejection and pneumonia, much as our first liver transplant patient had died 4 years before. Barnard carried out several more transplantations in the next year or two, achieving survival of 20 months in his third patient and over 12 years in his fifth patient. In his seventh patient a long-term survival approaching 20 years was realized, the kind of result all patients and transplanters seek.

While Barnard was thus the first, it was Shumway, working at Stanford, continuing his work at a slower and quieter but less erratic pace, who soon led the world both in numbers of hearts and in results. Twenty-three years later, in 1991, his department at Stanford could report 687 heart transplantations in 615 patients. Some required a second transplant when the first failed. The late survivorship was 81% at 5 years, and the longest survival was also about 20 years. Shumway's program took the lead in cardiac transplantation, much as those of Starzl and Calne had in liver transplantation and the programs of Murray, Starzl, and Calne had in kidney transplantation.

In discussing liver transplantation, I mentioned that there was no fallback position, since there was no artificial organ analogous to the artificial kidney. The artificial heart later showed signs of becoming useful in this role. It is a machine that accepts blood from the great veins running toward the heart (the venae cavae) and forcefully pumps it into the artery leaving the heart (the aorta). Blood clots tend to form in all mechanical devices, including this one. A major use for an artificial heart, as more practical versions have been developed, is to tide over a severely sick patient awaiting transplant. When the device is used for short periods as a bridge, the clotting tendency is less pernicious. On more prolonged use, clotting has been the principal agent of failure.

Chauvinism in Surgery

Cardiac transplantation was so spectacular both to physicians and to the public that two remarkable phenomena ensued, unprecedented in the history of science and surgery: national surgical chauvinism and an ego epidemic. Shortly after that first announcement by Christiaan Barnard, other nations considered it important to demonstrate that they, too, could do heart transplants. It was a matter of national pride. Several cardiac surgeons in several countries were anxious to jump on the bandwagon and demonstrate that their nation and its scientific resources could accomplish cardiac transplantation.

Laurie and I happened to be in London at the time of the first successful cardiac transplantation there. Considering the usual British soft-spoken undersell, we discovered that boasting and crass showmanship could be prominent even in Great Britain. The surgeons, in full operating regalia, appeared on the steps of one of the London teaching hospitals to the shouts of cheering crowds, bands playing "Britannia Rules the Waves" and "God Save the Queen" with the waving of flags, guardsmen in bearskin busbies hovering around on horseback. British reserve was cast into those waves that Britannia rules.

Closely linked to this national chauvinism was an ego epidemic, personal chauvinism in a sense. This took the form of the performance, in 1968, 1969, and 1970, of a large number of cardiac transplantations (about 50 or so) by surgeons who were masters of cardiac surgery but had no experience with either experimental or clinical transplantation. In fact, none of their hospitals had shown any interest whatsoever in transplantation while other humble toilers in the vineyard had been sweating away at it for 15 years. The results were disastrous. Mortality was unacceptable.

At first the newspapers, even some of those in the United States with a long tradition of scientific conservatism and responsible reporting, greeted all this with elation. Presumably a new era had arrived. One prominent surgeon declared that life expectancy for man would now rapidly move up to 150 years. Actually, there never was at any time, either then or now, any evidence whatsoever that transplantation of organs would prolong human life beyond its ordinary expected span. Quite the contrary, the name of the game in transplantation (as in most of surgery) is to improve the quality of life for a few threatened people during those short years allocated to them by a kindly providence. The public health impact of sporadic heroic treatments in any field will of course be near zero as judged by life expectancy data. The principal and daily mission of clinical care is the relief of suffering; only on rare occasions does it prolong lives in an aggregate or populational sense.

Even the press soon began to realize that something had gone dreadfully wrong during the ego epidemic of heart transplantation. There were articles in a few newspapers with strong bioscience reporters who suggested that, possibly, these transplant operations were being done by surgeons, by teams, who had no experience with the rest of the art and science of transplantation. Within 3 years the epidemic died where it began, while the work of Shumway proceeded steadily forward.

During the years of the first immunosuppressed kidney transplants (1959 and 1962), the early liver transplantations (1963 to 1966), and the first heart transplantations (1968 to 1973), great progress was being made in tissue typing, tissue groups, and immunogenetics as well as in the legal and ethical aspects of donor procurement. All these were to help progress in all sectors of transplantation science and practice.

The Lung

Transplantation of the lung presents a special problem: to be useful the lung requires the simultaneous circulation of both blood and air. The entire lung is in minute-by-minute contact with the outside world through inhaled air that permeates its every segment. This distribution of outside air must be balanced by the distribution and circulation of the blood, so that red blood cells can pick up oxygen from the air and exhaust their carbon dioxide. Air and blood must reach every little air pocket (alveolus) in the lung, and they must reach it together, at the very same instant. Once there, they are separated only by a thin and highly specialized membrane. Breathing a lot of air (ventilation) into the lung without good circulation accomplishes nothing. Pumping in a good flow of blood (perfusion) with no air to inflate that segment is also courting disaster. The ventilation-to-perfusion ratio (balance) is the key to lung function. A healthy ventilation-to-perfusion ratio is essential to success. Achieving this balance was a major problem in lung transplantation.

One of the first human lung transplants with at least a short period of survival was carried out by James Hardy and his associates in Jackson, Mississippi, in 1963. The patient had been suffering from emphysema (chronic lung insufficiency, often the result of heavy smoking) and survived for 18 days. Another early experience but with long-term survivorship was an operation done in Belgium by F. Derom at the University of Ghent in November 1968. The patient was suffering from silicosis, a form of lung scarring found among miners and industrial workers. He lived about a year. Both these patients underwent transplantation of a single lung. As I pointed out before, in surgery it sometimes pays off to take the bolder and seemingly more radical course. The inequality in perfusion and ventilation between the recently transplanted and the native (opposite) lung was often the source of trouble. If both lungs are transplanted at once, this inequality between the two sides is minimized. Healing of the bronchi (air passages) stitched or sutured together is also a problem, with failure bringing almost certain death. Joel Cooper of St. Louis has resolved this ingeniously by supporting the blood supply using a graft of peritoneum (from the abdomen).

In patients with severe chronic lung disease, the heart must work much harder. This applies particularly to the right ventricle of the heart, which in these patients must pump its blood through an obstructed circulation in the lung. Heart failure, especially right heart failure, is therefore commonplace in chronic lung disease such as emphysema. While the procedure of transplanting the heart and both lungs together seems an exercise in surgical heroics, in some cases it is the simplest choice. Considering the intricate circulation between the heart and lungs, which can be left undisturbed when both are transplanted together, the transplant is done with only a few blood-vessel suture lines. Despite its early severe difficulties, transplantation of the lungs has now emerged from this trouble-some period.

The Pancreas and the Endocrine Glands

Most cases of diabetes are traceable to inadequate or poorly con-trolled production of insulin from those little islet cells, first described by Langerhans, in the pancreas. The administration of insulin regulates the blood sugar but does not prevent other complications of diabetes, which often affect blood vessels, the eye, or the kidney. Because insulin admin-istration does not do the whole job, attempts to transplant the pancreas began in the early and mid 1960s.

Each organ transplanted presents its own special problems. Early efforts to transplant the pancreas failed owing to a special arrangement within this organ. The pancreas secretes highly corrosive enzymes that will digest protein and even the pancreas itself. These enzymes are se-creted into the upper intestine to digest food. To isolate the delicate insulin molecules from these destructive enzymes had been the problem 40 years before, when insulin itself was isolated. In nature the two are completely separated even though coming from the same organ: insulin goes directly into the bloodstream, and the enzymes go into the intestine to digest food.

In telling the story of transplantation in our time, I have men-tioned only a few names of pioneers and leaders. Some names have been essential to this history, and so it is with Richard Lillehei and John Najarian. Dick Lillehei, the younger of the two brilliant Minnesota broth-ers (his elder sibling had been a pioneer in open-heart operations), began working intensively on pancreas transplantation in the early 1960s. John Najarian, a native Californian and graduate of the University of California in 1948, was a key player and captain of a winning football team. He received his M.D. from the University of California and pursued his sur-gical residency and fellowship years there, becoming assistant professor and head of the transplant service in August 1964. In 1967, he was appointed Professor and Chairman at Minnesota, succeeding the remark-able Wangensteen mentioned above.

Najarian has focused on several special aspects of transplantation science, particularly the development of antisera (usually horse sera) against lymphocytes and thymocytes, the cells responsible for rejection. These are sometimes an aid in immunosuppression. When he arrived at Minnesota he found an active pancreas program already under way under Richard Lillehei and David Sutherland, who performed several of the first pancreas transplants. As of 1991, Najarian could report 1,200 kidney or kidney-pancreas transplants in diabetic patients. His department has become a center for the study and treatment of severe diabetes, often the childhood or juvenile type, especially in patients with failure of both kidneys and loss of their sight. The relief of these crippling complications has revolutionized the expectations of childhood diabetics and their physicians.

Somers Sturgis, Head of Gynecology in our Department of Surgery, attempted in the 1950s to transplant ovaries in a way that would preserve their internal secretion of hormones (estrogen and progesterone) and help make patients who lacked normal ovaries more truly female. He did this by placing the ovarian tissue in small envelopes (Millipore filters). In animals, some ovarian function was observed and it looked encouraging. However, there were no clinically successful ovarian transplants.

Certain patients suffering from deficient thyroid or parathyroid function would benefit immensely from transplantation of those endocrine glands. These—as well as pancreatic islets—were studied in our department by John Brooks. As Sturgis had with the ovary, Brooks used a Millipore filter to protect the tiny transplant. The idea here was to place the organ in a filter that would let the oxygen of the blood plasma in and let the hormones out but exclude the destructive immune lymphocytes responsible for much of tissue rejection. This approach never became clinically useful.

The Newest Field of Surgery and Science

The magnitude of this new field of science and surgery is indicated by the figures for transplantation in the United States. In 1989, there were 8,890 kidney, 2,160 liver, 1,673 heart, 413 pancreas, and 67 heart-lung transplants. There was continued growth in 1990: 9,600 kidney, 2,700 liver, 2,100 heart, 549 pancreas, 202 lung, and 50 heart-lung transplants. With donor availability as the limiting factor, these figures for transplant frequency seem to be attaining a plateau, as shown by the numbers for 1993: 9,551 kidney, 3,062 liver, 1,607 heart, 384 lung, and 658 pancreas or pancreas/kidney transplants. There have been 2,000 bone marrow transplants annually in recent years.

Estimating the total worldwide experience, we can use data gathered from the Worldwide Transplant Center Directory (using Terasaki's summary of May 1992). This showed a total of 241,048 kidney, 19,448 heart, 1,600 heart-lung, 1,184 lung, 41,764 bone marrow, 21,324 liver, 2,144 pancreas, and 2,854 kidney-pancreas transplants. While these are the best figures we have, there are gaps because of the failure in the early days to obtain data from Russia, China, and parts of central Europe. Thus, the impressive total endeavor in transplantation over the course of 40 years sought to relieve suffering and prolong life (or both) for about 360,000 patients, the great majority of whom were operated upon in the last 20 years, since 1975.

No matter what the numbers or the underlying science, no matter how arcane the methods or how hidden the secrets of the art, ultimate acceptance of organ removal and transplantation must rest entirely on one criterion: its effectiveness balanced against its risk, the latter in part a function of the extent of damage to the rest of the body by the disease in question. To be acceptable—and ethical—the benefits of a new procedure (once tested and adopted for general use) must far outweigh its risks.

Statistics—risk-benefit analysis—play a key role in the ultimate decision for transplantation whether the question be ethical, financial, or biological. What is the relative likelihood of success? Ironically, in transplantation, statistical values are the basis of ethics: is transplantation in this patient morally acceptable?

And yet statistics can never tell the whole story. For two reasons. First, early in the application of any new technology, whether it be space travel or heart transplantation, you cannot rely on statistics because there is not enough experience to provide a basis for statistical analysis. As new treatments arise, that special problem of insufficient numbers inevitably arrives for each. The numbers are too small. In most of transplantation, we are now emerging from that blurred area of uncertainty and anecdote. Second, statistics may be a false guide because the accumulation of a few brilliant results in experienced hands, of sick young people now made well, may blind the eye to the likelihood of failure at the extremes of age or in less experienced hands.

There is no way that a central agency of ethical judgments can make rules for what is ethical and acceptable for all patients in all centers. Flexibility and individual judgment must prevail for many years in any new field. The armchair ethicist devoid of personal experience or current knowledge has no way of assessing the advisability of new procedures. While we must beware the enthusiast who pushes his own operation or his favorite drug too hard, we must equally beware the detached Olympian. The opinion of an inexperienced ethicist may be ethically unacceptable.

From Primum Non Nocere *to* Nonnumquam, Nocere Est Renovare

Primum non nocere ("first do no harm") is an ancient maxim of Hippocrates (though not part of the Oath) that is more honored in the breach than in the observance. No one ever took it very seriously, because it is often necessary to do harm so that good may later result.

Consider cesarean section, the most ancient of surgical heroics. With the mother almost dead, the procedure of saving the baby by removing it surgically from the womb was the final stroke of doom for the mother, certainly at the time of Caesar and right up to the middle years of the last century. One of the most dangerous of injuries done in the name of treatment was intentional hemorrhage, or bloodletting. All too often this "venesection," "bleeding," or "leeching" failed in its mission; if large in volume, it added to the patient's burden. When carried to extremes (as it seems to have been in George Washington's final illness), little benefit accrues and major injury results.

Think of amputation for compound fractures, universal during the Civil War. Or removal of the eye for a small cancer of the retina. Or minor insults such as taking blood from one person to give to another. Radiation treatment, chemotherapy, and surgery all do some harm so that the patient may then heal and return to family and society.

"First do no harm" should be changed to "Sometimes we must

hurt if we wish to heal." Such a revised motto, enshrined in Latin, might go something like this: *Nonnumquam, nocere est renovare*—"Sometimes, to hurt is to heal."

Transplantation epitomizes the fact that we must do injury so that healing may follow. While much of modern medicine and surgery undertakes risks and causes damage in the hope of conferring later benefits, in most instances the risk is to the patient and not to another person. In transplantation, the procedure sometimes places two people at special risk for the benefit of one. In this sense the revised medical motto cited above acquires an added social dimension.

Waiting Lists; Drawing on Other Species (Xenotransplantation)

The mounting lists of patients awaiting transplantation in this country far outstrip the rather constant and constrained numbers of organs available and transplants accomplished. The Europeans are about five times more successful than we are in this national effort. Even if we were to increase our success rate in cadaver donor procurement to that level, we would still fail to meet the need.

Some numbers will illustrate the problem.

As of late 1994, a waiting list of almost 4,000 patients is being treated by transplantation of human cadaver livers at a rate of only about 175 to 250 per month. The number of additions to the waiting list is about equal to (or slightly more than) the number of transplants accomplished. With the liver, as with the heart, lethal disease treatable by transplantation waits for no one. Deaths on the waiting list occur at a rate of about 15% a month. Additions to the waiting list occur faster than the death rate. An analogous situation applies to the heart, with 3,000 on the waiting list. In the case of the kidney, the availability of dialysis mollifies the situation because many patients can be carried along on the artificial kidney, but almost 27,000 patients are waiting. While there is no doubt that a newly invigorated public drive for donors and for better public understanding of this need will help save lives, we will never come close to an acceptable rate of donation as based on cadaver resources alone.

These facts make it essential that we succeed in establishing the use of animals as donors, otherwise known as xenotransplantation (*xeno-*, by its Greek root, means stranger). It is not difficult to visualize animal farms where genetically pure, disease-free strains would be raised for this purpose. We raise animals and use them for our food, to obtain protein for our own use. Why not, with equivalent ethics, husband their growth to save lives with their organs? While zealots will press legislators to oppose the farming of donor animals, it is an essential next step for the United States. We use the pancreas of animals for insulin, pituitaries for growth hormone, bones for gelatin, and meat for meals. Why not use the heart to pump blood?

Far more of a hurdle than public education is the obstacle posed by the immune disparity between species. There have been six or eight heroic efforts at transplanting animal organs, carried out by teams of sophisticated surgeons and scientists. All have failed. The breakthrough is not yet here. There are portents of good things to come, such as the genetic engineering of molecules that bind or inactivate the harmful slings and arrows of the immune armory. But their clinical uses lie in the future.

It is important to stimulate, support, and encourage young scientists who are as single-minded in their assault on the immune barrier to animal organs as we were in arriving at immunosuppression to transplant within species. Some scientists now living will provide a solution—possibly one whose general shape we cannot even imagine now—for the vexing problem of xenotransplantation. The field of transplantation, cultivated by a few in the 1950s and yielding an immense harvest of welfare to the sick, now obstructed by lack of donors, will then take its next giant step. Not many years left in this century. Maybe the next.

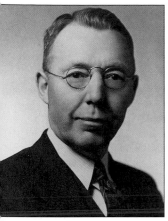

Leland S. McKittrick, surgeon of the Massachusetts General Hospital (MGH) and New England Deaconess (Palmer Memorial) Hospital. It was as McKittrick's assistant that FDM began surgical practice in 1943.

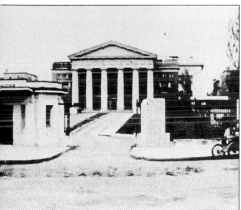

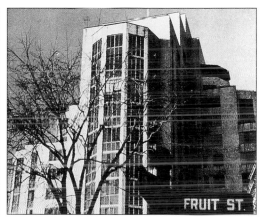

Entrance to the old Peter Bent Brigham Hospital (PBBH) as seen from Brigham Circle, about 1920.

The MGH at the time of FDM's internship. The large building (completed in 1939) was the George Robert White Building, which was given over entirely to surgery.

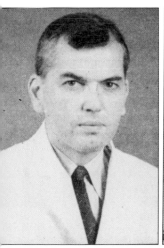

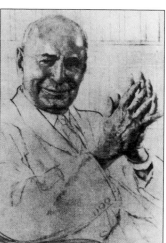

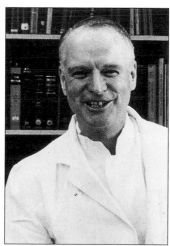

Three teachers at MGH who strongly influenced FDM's career plans (*left to right*): Fuller Albright, Director of the Metabolic Ward 4 in the Department of Medicine; Edward Delos Churchill, Homans Professor and Head of the Surgery Department; and Oliver Cope, Churchill's assistant and Director of the Department during Churchill's wartime absence.

Plate 9

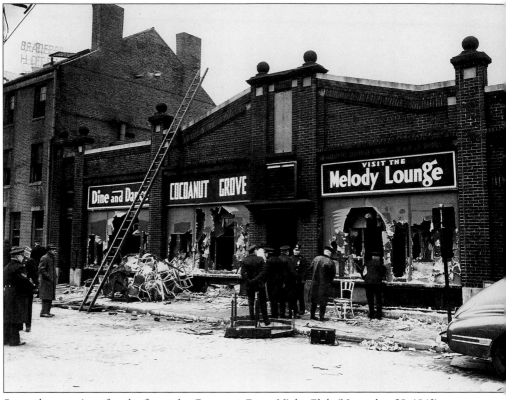

Scene the morning after the fire at the Cocoanut Grove Night Club (November 28, 1942).

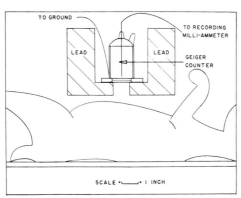

Drawing by FDM for one of his early articles on the use of radioactive dyes (1943) showing an anesthetized rabbit positioned under a Geiger counter. An abscess in the animal's belly could be detected when the tagged dye was injected intravenously.

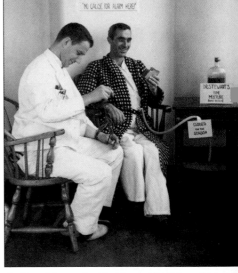

A Grand Rounds skit (about 1940) in which a patient joins in the fun as his feeding tube is finally removed. FDM, then a junior resident, confirms that the hated tube has in fact been withdrawn and is "closed for the season."

Plate 10

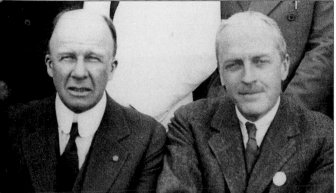

John Homans (*left*) and David Cheever (*right*). These two mainstays of Brigham surgery served on the staffs of Harvey Cushing, then Elliott Cutler, and finally FDM. They are shown here at about the time of their retirement, in 1951.

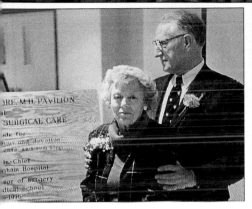

_aurie and FDM in 1981 at the dedication of the eventh floor of the new Brigham and Women's Iospital (BWH) tower. This floor included the 3artlett Unit (named after Laurie's father), the _aura B. Moore Unit, and the FDM Unit for Comprehensive Care.

J. Hartwell Harrison, Elliott Carr Cutler Professor of Surgery and Head of the Division of Urology, as a young man (about 1950). Harrison's work made safe kidney transplantation possible, because he was the surgeon for all living donors in the early cases.

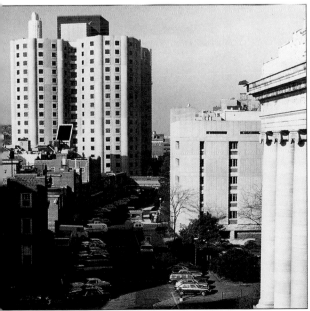

View up Shattuck Street about 1980. Harvard Medical School (HMS) main administration building on the near right. In the background is the newly completed tower of the BWH.

Plate 11

FDM playing the accordion for a Christmas party in the Surgical Office, about 1952. Holding the music is Mrs. Soma Weiss, widow of the beloved teacher of internal medicine for FDM's generation at HMS. To her right is George Thorn, singing along.

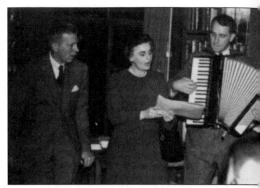

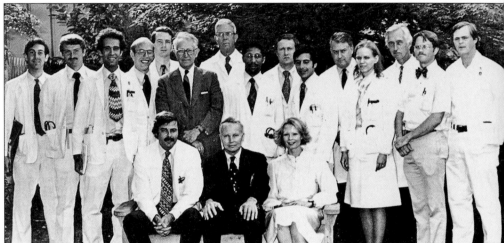

Members of the surgical staff in 1978, two years after John Mannick took over as department head: Seated on bench *(from left to right)* are George Linville, John Mannick, and Jeanne Petrek. Standing are *(front row)* Eric Shaeffer, FDM, Frank Smith, George Kacoyanis, Sigurd Guyton, Fred Mansfield, and Tom Hosea and *(back row)* Peter Einstein, Robert Beattie, Kurt Newman, Robert Olson, John Brooks, Clyde Lindquist, Nathan Couch, and Philip Drinker.

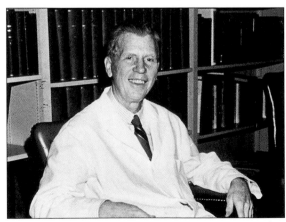

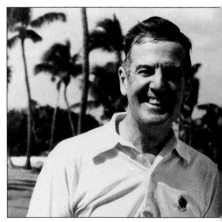

George Widmer Thorn, Hersey Professor of the Theory and Practice of Physic, about 1950. An inspiring colleague as Physician-in-Chief at the Brigham, Thorn was a seminal figure in the development of the artificial kidney, transplantation, and the treatment of adrenal disease.

F. Stanton Deland, attorney, Harvard Overseer, golfer, yachtsman, and long-time friend of FDM. Deland was the guiding genius in the four-hospital merger that led to the building of the new hospital.

Plate 12

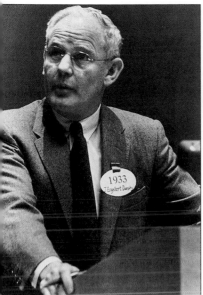

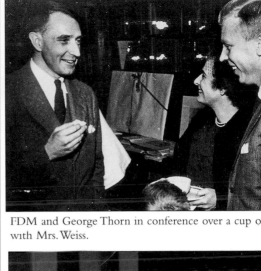

FDM and George Thorn in conference over a cup of coffee with Mrs. Weiss.

Englebert Dunphy, a graduate of the Cutler years at the Brigham, later a staff member with FDM, and then Professor and Head of the Departments of Surgery : Portland (Oregon) and San Francisco University of California).

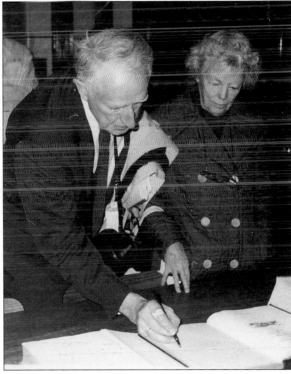

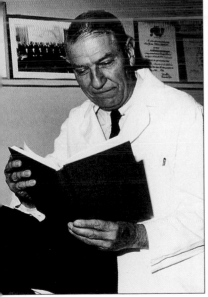

On a trip to Beijing, China, in 1981; FDM and Laura Moore at the Library of the Chinese National Academy of Sciences, autographing books by FDM that were ready and waiting for the author's arrival.

Gustave J. Dammin, Professor of Pathology, steadfast guide to the entire transplant program.

Plate 13

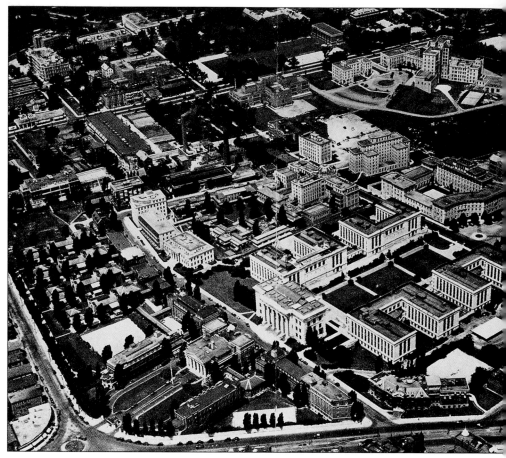

Here and on the opposite page are two aerial views, taken in 1934 and 1994, showing the Brigham Hospital and a portion of the Harvard Medical School, along with some of its nearby hospitals and laboratories. Brigham Circle can be seen at the lower left in both photos. The two Greek-pillared porticos of the Brigham (*bottom center*) and the Medical School (*just behind, to the right*) have remained unchanged. Francis Street stretches upward to the left; parallel to it and to the right is Shattuck Street.

In this 1934 view, the plantings around the four Brigham pavilions and the open spaces among the surrounding hospitals lend the scene an almost rural/suburban aspect. At the intersection of Shattuck Street and Huntington Avenue (*below right*) stands Huntington Memorial Hospital. Children's Hospital can be seen to the left of the Medical School, with Beth Israel Hospital above and to the right.

Plate 14

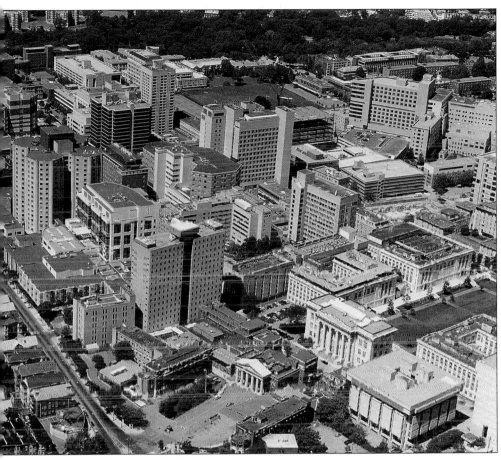

In this 1994 view the construction of the past 60 years becomes evident. The new tower of the Brigham includes the four hexagonal buildings (*center left*); below it is the Center for Women and Newborns and the two tall, rectangular towers of the Thorn Research Building, with the lower structures of the Ambulatory Care Center between them. Now, the intersection of Shattuck Street and Huntington Avenue has been taken over by the Countway Library of Medicine (*below right*). New construction at the Children's and Beth Israel Hospitals as well as the Dana-Farber Cancer Institute and the New England Deaconess Hospital has helped to convert the entire neighborhood into a huge medical center. The two Greek porticos remain as testimony to the classical architecture of the turn of the century, Harvard Medical School having been completed in 1906 and the Brigham in 1912.

Plate 15

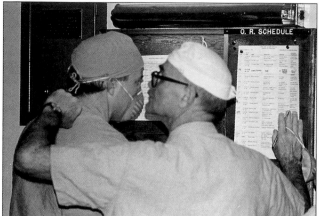

Characteristic scene in the PBBH operating room corridor. Roy Vandam, Professor and Head of the Department of Anaesthesia, may seem to be checking the operating list with one of the staff anesthetists, Patrick Bennett, but in point of fact he is looking at his watch to see if progress is on schedule.

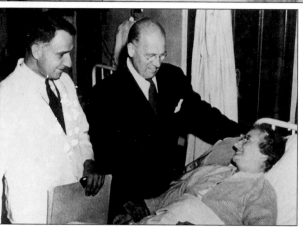

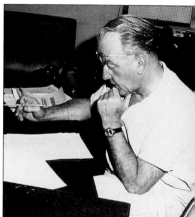

Visiting Professor Sir James Paterson Ross of London is at the bedside with FDM. Several students could gather for conversation with both the patient and the visitor. This patient was flattered by so distinguished a visitor from abroad. She and Sir James corresponded for some years after this visit.

Characteristic scene in the surgeons' room, about 1965. Dwight Harken is dictating operative notes after one of his operations on the heart for relief of mitral stenosis.

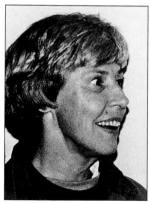

Sally Hurlbut, FDM's scrub nurse for many years and daughter of close friends Dr. and Mrs. Robert S. Hurlbut of Cambridge.

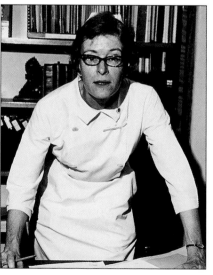

Marion Metcalf, extraordinary nurse who was Head of the Department of Nursing at the PBBH and subsequently in charge of all nursing for the four merged hospitals.

Plate 16

BOOK ❦ SEVEN

Heart Disease and Cancer

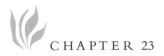

CHAPTER 23

Opening Its Valves and Then the Heart Itself

In the spring of 1941, as a junior surgical resident 2 years out of medical school, I scrubbed in on an operation at the MGH in which Edward Churchill removed the calcified pericardium (the envelope or sac surrounding the heart) in a young man with constrictive pericarditis. Pericarditis is a chronic disorder, sometimes due to tuberculosis, in which the pericardium becomes thickened, calcified, and stony hard. A pump such as the heart must be allowed to fill and swell before it can contract to eject its blood. The iron grip of constrictive pericarditis interferes with the heart's normal distensibility, impairs its filling, and therefore reduces its output of blood. The operation to remove that calcified sac (known as pericardiectomy) is a tricky one because the heart muscle beneath the stony sheath is very thin.

In those days the use of blood transfusion was limited, and there was no such thing as a pump-oxygenator to take over and maintain the circulation if the heart was torn or damaged during the operation. When the operation goes well, the heart, released from this death grip, can distend with blood and pump it out to the arteries. The patient can gradually resume normal activities but, depending upon the duration of the constriction and its effect on the heart muscle itself, can rarely indulge in more strenuous work. Churchill was a careful, precise operator, and his patient got along very well.

Churchill and Harken

Churchill was the first surgeon in the United States to perform pericardiectomy. Although a pioneer in cardiac surgery, his main interest was in lung surgery. He demonstrated that lobectomy (removal of one or more lobes of the lung) could be done safely, with a low mortality even in patients with chronic bronchial infection (bronchiectasis) or for lung cancer, and in certain cases of tuberculosis when the bronchial passages became narrowed.

Seven years after that operation of Dr. Churchill's, in the fall of 1948, I was recruiting new staff to bring our department at the Brigham up to strength. I asked Dwight E. Harken to head up thoracic surgery. A few months earlier I had left behind me the impressive strength of the MGH in thoracic surgery. Now at the Brigham I found a total vacuum in that field. No one on the staff was doing thoracic and cardiac operations regularly, attending the relevant meetings, or making an academic commitment in this area. Harken had already gained a reputation and had developed a bustling practice in thoracic surgery in the Boston area. He did his work largely at the Boston City and Mount Auburn Hospitals. In addition—and most unusual for the late 1940s—Harken was already becoming known as a cardiac surgeon. During the war he had removed 145 bullets and shell fragments from the hearts of wounded soldiers in 134 operations with no deaths. Several of these metallic objects lay free within one of the four major chambers of the heart. He removed them by opening the heart, a procedure he had probably performed more frequently and more successfully than anyone else in the world at that time.

Despite this impressive record as a cardiac surgeon and the fact that during the previous 6 months he had operated on two patients for disease of the heart valves, it was Dwight's skill in thoracic surgery (i.e., operations involving the lungs and chest) that led me to seek him out for our staff. We had many patients with lung disease who needed surgical care and many residents and students who needed instruction in this field. While he more than fulfilled our needs for a chief of thoracic surgery (and very promptly), Dwight Harken's main interests continued to be in the development of heart surgery.

The previous June (1948) Harken had carried out his first successful operation to relieve narrowing (stenosis) of the mitral valve, one of the four major valves of the heart. The name "mitral" was adopted by the early anatomists because the valve resembles the two portions of a bishop's miter, or hat. This valve is located in the channel between the left atrium (which receives blood from the lungs under low pressure) and the left ventricle (which pumps blood out through the aorta to the rest of the body under high pressure). When the mitral valve closes normally with each beat, as it should, blood can flow in one direction only, vital to proper function of the heart. Narrowing of the mitral valve is almost always produced by rheumatic heart disease in childhood.

While I was well aware of Harken's interests, neither he nor I could have foreseen the number of patients with mitral stenosis who would seek his help over the next few years. By 1955 he had operated on over 1,000 such patients, most of them at the Brigham, and had become universally regarded as one of the world's foremost cardiac surgeons. It was through my long acquaintance with these two men—Edward Churchill, my professor, and Dwight Harken, my staff member—that I came to have intimate contact with and continuing enthusiasm for cardiac surgery. I was never a cardiac surgeon myself.

Churchill and Harken stood in sharp contrast to each other and were of different generations (Harken in his middle 30s and Churchill in his 50s). While colleagues on the faculty and in the same field, they were never close personal collaborators. Both were middlewesterners, Churchill from Chenoa, Illinois, and Harken from Osceola, Iowa. Churchill was not given to talkativeness and at times could be somewhat withdrawn and austere, bearing a rather lofty if not Olympian demeanor. By contrast, Harken was informal, forward, red-haired, and appropriately flamboyant. He was given to speaking out boldly, lecturing frequently, and seeking to interest cardiologists in his work, as well as the students, residents, internists, and the many visitors who trailed behind him on rounds. While Harken admired Churchill's wisdom and skill, Churchill was at times rather critical, not only of Harken but of any plans for surgery within the chambers of the heart.

When I was ready to propose Harken's appointment to the Dean and to the Harvard Corporation, I needed the approval of Churchill and the two other senior professors (Gross at the Children's Hospital and Fine at the Beth Israel Hospital) to ensure an appropriate title. Churchill was down on mitral surgery. In this, as in one or two other judgments about the future of cardiac surgery, he was still swayed by the notion expressed by cardiologists at the turn of the century and in the 1920s that even if the narrowed valve were widened, rheumatic damage to the heart muscle itself in cases of mitral stenosis would prevent rehabilitation. He had been a young surgeon 20 years earlier when Elliott Cutler in Boston and Henry Souttar in London had attempted to open the narrowed mitral valve surgically and had failed. He was convinced that merely opening up the valve orifice would be in vain; the heart muscle would never recover. Churchill, my revered professor, a man of profound surgical and philosophical wisdom, appears now so clearly to have been in error in this judgment.

In contrast, Harken had the faith, the enthusiasm, and the ingrained optimism of the true pioneer. He was not worried about heart muscle damage because early in his work he showed that this concern was not borne out. Many of his patients—and I saw many of them with him—thrived beautifully after operation. Before the operation their skin was bluish and they had difficulty breathing because their lungs were filling with fluid. Their hands and feet, legs and arms were often shriveled up for lack of blood supply or swollen with edema; unable to work, they could not climb stairs and were often totally bedridden. After the operation, they could walk and exercise for the first time in years. As their hearts resumed more normal output of blood and provided nourishment to body cells, they pinked up and gained weight and could climb or even run up stairs. This was remarkable testimony to the buoyancy of the heart muscle as well as the human spirit. Mitral stenosis truly was a point defect, a focal, surgically accessible disorder, the repair of which rectifies many of the other bodily troubles it engenders. A narrowed mitral valve was just that: a logjam in the flow of blood through the heart. Open up the logjam, the river flows again. Cardiac output and health are restored.

The role of Edward Churchill in heart surgery was not confined to his pioneering operations on the lungs and pericardium nor to his skepticism about mitral valve surgery. His most notable contribution to cardiac surgery came about almost inadvertently, unbeknownst even to him at first. The story of the origin of the pump-oxygenator is a fascinating one. Although development of this machine moved forward with his departmental support, it never attracted his enthusiasm.

John Gibbon Comes to Boston

In June 1930, 10 years before that pericardiectomy, 15 years before Dwight Harken's early valve surgery, and only 6 years after Cutler's failed attempts to operate on the mitral valve, a young surgeon of Philadelphia came to the MGH to work as a research fellow with Churchill. John H. Gibbon, Jr., son of a famous Philadelphia surgeon, arrived to study surgery of the lungs. While working in the laboratory at the MGH, he met Miss Mary Hopkinson, one of Churchill's laboratory technicians. John and Maylie (as she came to be known) worked together throughout that first year, became engaged, were soon married, and continued to work together over several decades to accomplish one of the greatest engineering feats of this century.

In February 1931, Churchill assigned Gibbon the task of monitoring an extremely ill patient who had suffered several pulmonary emboli (clots that passed from the leg veins to the lungs). Gibbon's job was to sit with her and measure her pulse and blood pressure (vital signs) every few minutes to keep close track of her condition. Churchill's idea was that if she threw off another big embolus (manifested by a sudden deterioration in these vital signs, particularly a fall in blood pressure), he would open the artery leading from the heart to the lung for a few seconds to remove the obstructing clots, which would otherwise be fatal within minutes. In this particular case, her vital signs did deteriorate, a clot did come to the lungs, and she lay at death's door. Although the operation was attempted, the patient died (as did all others who underwent this operation until 30 years later, in the 1960s).

In assisting on this case, the young Gibbon had plenty of time to reflect and consider other, better ways of doing this operation. He began to develop the concept of a machine that could accept all the blood as it returned to the heart via the great veins (several quarts per minute), remove its burden of carbon dioxide, add oxygen, and then pump the oxygenated blood back into an artery under high pressure. If this could be done safely, even if for only 3 to 5 minutes, clots could be surgically

217

removed and patients might survive. His dream of an artificial heart and lung to tide over the critical period while the heart was open was to become a reality only because of the dogged persistence of Jack and Maylie Gibbon. It took 22 years. And then it opened up not only the heart but a whole new world of surgical care.

Gibbon and his new wife returned to Philadelphia to continue their joint project. Three years later, in 1934, they returned to the MGH and Churchill's department to spend another fellowship year working on their concept. While Gibbon was grateful to Churchill for providing facilities and support for this important work, it was clear from Gibbon's later tales that his boss always remained skeptical about the feasibility of an artificial pump-oxygenator as a temporary substitute for the heart and lung. Churchill was not alone in this skepticism. Undaunted, the Gibbons carried on and in 1937 published an article describing their work at the MGH, entitled "Artificial Maintenance of the Circulation during Experimental Occlusion of the Pulmonary Artery."

Twenty years later, just months before the pump-oxygenator was first used successfully, a respected physiologist stated that a pump-oxygenator substitute for the heart and lungs would never be possible because all that pumping agitation and friction would destroy the red blood cells. As is so often the case with science, the aging expert was a naysayer and the youthful enthusiast proved him wrong.

Before telling the rest of the Gibbons' story, we should look back at some of the other things that were going on in cardiac surgery at that time. Some of these remarkable developments were occurring close by, at the Children's Hospital in Boston and on our own service at the Brigham, while others were to take place in Baltimore at Johns Hopkins. All were destined to change heart surgery and, later, be improved themselves as a result of the pump-oxygenator.

Opening the Mitral Valve and Closing the Patent Ductus

Several scholars of heart disease had predicted around the time of World War I that there were two point lesions in heart disease that invited surgical repair: narrowing of the mitral valve (described above) and persistence of the open (or patent) ductus arteriosus. The ductus is a large artery that is open in the fetus when circulation of blood to the lungs is unnecessary because the mother's blood supplies oxygen to the infant. While still in the uterus the fetus has no need for lungs and has no air to breathe anyway. The ductus bypasses the lung. Immediately after birth, as the infant cries and takes its first breath this blood vessel starts to close. But if the ductus fails to close and remains open, heart failure gradually ensues, followed by infection and death.

While a few visionaries such as Elliott Cutler recognized these surgical possibilities, the usual pronouncements (more frequently heard) were those of conservative surgical sages with negative opinions who believed it was not only impossible but even perhaps sacrilegious to operate on the human heart. Never mind the needs of patients or the attractiveness of subjecting these ideas to scientific scrutiny in the lab. It just never could be done. Nor should it be tried. God did not have that intent, they preached. Maybe someone should have reminded them that God had also been quoted as being opposed to relieving the pain of childbirth, almost 100 years before.

In 1924-1925 Elliott Cutler, then a junior faculty member at Harvard working at the Brigham under Harvey Cushing, was inspired to try to widen the opening of the narrowed mitral valve in patients with rheumatic heart disease. He carried out six such operations on patients dying of mitral stenosis. In most cases he used a long punch-hole instrument (he called it a valvulotome) that could be introduced through the thick wall of the left ventricle and advanced blindly (by feel) up to the mitral valve. Once there, it would be used to punch a hole in the valve to relieve the obstruction and let the blood flow through more easily. At the time of the first operation he performed, his special instrument was not yet ready, so he used a long narrow scalpel to pry open the adherent leaflets of the stenotic valve. This one patient was somewhat improved and lived over a year. Later patients, in whom the punch-instrument was used, died soon after the operation. Possibly his new punch-instrument was more damaging than the scalpel. While Cutler clearly perceived the potential damaging effect of the valvulotome, he did not see a possible significance in the survival of his first patient, in whom it was not used.

In 1925, Henry Souttar of London carried out an operation with the same purpose on a 19-year-old girl and was knighted for his work.

He approached the problem differently. He inserted his finger into the thin-walled auricle (or atrium) of the heart, placing sutures as a purse-string around the finger in the heart wall, and cinching them up tightly to prevent a leak. Then, feeling for the valve with his "entrapped" fingertip, he could dilate or even break apart the leaflets of the narrowed valve. His patient improved and lived for 5 years. Thus, of the seven patients who underwent mitral valve operations in the 1920s, one lived for over a year (Cutler's first patient) and one lived for 5 years (Souttar's). While these two operations could hardly be considered total failures, that idea some-how got rooted in the literature and in the mind of Dr. Churchill, who always referred to them as failures. Little or no attention was paid to the fact that the two survivors were patients in whom the narrowed leaflets were pried open and no valvular tissue was removed or severed.

In 1938, 13 years after Cutler's attempts at mitral valve surgery, two efforts were made at the same time and in the same city—Boston—to close the patent ductus. One was by John Strieder aided by a cardiac physiologist, Ashton Graybiel, at the Boston City Hospital. While their first operation appeared to go well initially, they could not tie off the ductus completely as they had hoped. The patient died a few days later of acute gastric dilatation, a disorder that today would be readily diagnosed and successfully treated.

The other effort to close the ductus was by Robert Gross, a junior member of the Harvard surgical faculty (working at both the Children's Hospital and the Brigham), and his collaborating cardiologist, John Hubbard. Together they developed a plan to ligate (i.e., tie off) the open ductus. In August 1938, evidently ignorant of the work being carried out by Strieder only a few miles away, Gross successfully ligated the patent ductus in a child. Several more such patients were successfully treated within a few months.

Some weeks after one of Gross's first attempts at ductus ligation, the child died of sudden massive hemorrhage when the ligature cut its way through the delicate wall of the artery. Gross swore that he would never again simply tie the ductus. Instead, using an elegant technique that required great skill, he would divide it completely and close the two short ends with sutures. As a student I watched one of these operations and, like all who saw them, was immensely impressed with the skill, dexterity, and gentleness with which Gross handled this large, thin-walled blood vessel, which was carrying a large volume of blood at high pressure. Word of his success immediately earned Gross a well-deserved reputation and an international following. He had demonstrated that the heart and its nearby great vessels were not sacrosanct at all and could be repaired surgically. Following these operations on the blood vessels near the heart, it became clear that the heart itself would soon be opened with success. The surgical world was ready, but as the war approached and then intervened, it was not clear just how, when, or for what condition this advance would take place.

Just before the war Alfred Blalock at Johns Hopkins, along with his cardiologist colleague Helen Taussig (an expert in congenital heart disease), devised an operation to reroute (shunt) the blood in certain types of babies who were born with a severe heart deformity and whose skin was blue (cyanotic) from lack of oxygen. Total repair of this complex defect would not be attempted for another 10 years, but Blalock's operation on the great vessels near the heart offered remarkable relief and new hope for patients with heart disease, especially children with congenital heart deformities, and gave them many good years of life.

Following the war, Dwight Harken returned from England fresh from the experience of his surgical successes in treating heart wounds. Immediately he took up his principal interest: surgery of the mitral valve. On June 9, 1948, 5 months before I asked him to join our staff at the Brigham, he performed his first mitral operation. After joining our staff he did several more. Of the first six patients, two lived flourishing lives after the operation and were relieved of their heart failure. To Harken's surprise, it was discovered that 4 days prior to his first mitral valve repair, Charles Bailey of Philadelphia had carried out a similar operation. Bailey's first two patients died, but the third lived for 23 years. As was the case with Gross and Strieder, here were two surgeons arriving at the same historic point at almost the same moment. Without getting into the epistemology of such coincidences, I should point out that such convergent evolution is a commonplace in science. When the time is ripe, more than one person is likely to pick the fruit. Credit should go to both because controversy over priority is damaging to the reputation of both parties and to the public's respect for science and scientists.

After Harken's mitral stenosis operations, four of his first six and six of his first 10 patients died. As he told the story, he became discouraged, went home, and told Mrs. Harken that he was through with cardiac surgery. Hearing of this, his medical collaborator, Laurence Ellis, visited Harken at home and convinced him to carry on. How right Ellis turned out to be! Of the next 15 patients operated upon for mitral stenosis, 14 lived. Soon the world of cardiology learned of this success, and matters developed rapidly, just as they had with the ductus operation. In 1964 Harken and Ellis reported a series of 1,571 such patients. In the group with medium-grade disability, the mortality was only 0.6%; in those most severely crippled, the operation was understandably more hazardous and was associated with a 17% mortality. Rehabilitation to normal living for patients with mitral stenosis had never been attainable before. Even the most conservative cardiologists who had cautiously withheld operation from their patients finally came to realize that by accepting this risk they might offer the possibility of a new life to many. One of the first cardiologists to demonstrate by physiologic measurement the drastic improvement in heart function in these patients was Lewis Dexter, who became another of Harken's close collaborators.

Harken widened the valve as Souttar had, with his own index finger (able to feel and sense the valve anatomy) inside the heart. There was no cut made that removed tissue from the valves themselves.

Most of the patients with mitral stenosis were operated on at the Brigham, with Harken working as a member of our staff, teaching students and residents. Leroy Vandam was in charge of anesthesia. As mentioned above, I had asked Vandam, who had been at the University of Pennsylvania, to come and join our department in 1954. He picked up the anesthetic care of the cardiac surgical patients at that time and standardized their anesthesia with a minimum of risk, as he had likewise done for transplantation. Lewis Dexter ran the Cath Lab for study of these patients. Several of the Brigham cardiologists, including Samuel Levine, Bernard Lown, Richard Gorlin, and James Dalen, worked with Harken in this increasingly massive undertaking. With their support, medical conservatism gradually yielded to the seeming radicalism of surgical procedures for valvular disease—operations now accepted everywhere as routine and, once mitral stenosis is established, the sooner the better.

At our weekly staff meetings (described in Chapters 10 and 12) we discussed all deaths and complications. There were many deaths from mitral stenosis surgery to discuss in those early days (1948 to 1955). Sometimes the residents became restless and discouraged. They met with me privately to urge that we discontinue mitral surgery for a few months. Yet even the most skeptical of our students and residents were attentive as Dwight Harken, who was always frank, open, and self-critical in his account of each case, told what had happened and why, as well as how he hoped to improve the operation. It seemed clear to me that the results were improving rapidly and that case selection was one of the keys to mortality. We should never yield to the temptation to take on only the easy cases because they pose a lesser risk. Some of our early cases were the most neglected, high-risk ones. I later encountered a similar period of gloom among our younger staff during the early, dark days of transplantation, under immunosuppression. In both instances, we accepted plenty of the tough cases (especially at the beginning, when the "bad old" cases were still out there) as well as the easy ones. As time went on, more of the patients were those with a shorter, more recent illness and lower risk for operative fatality. Morbidity and mortality rates were discouraging at the beginning, but the gloom soon lifted with many brilliant successes and the certain knowledge that the failures were never buried in the record room or hidden in the pathology department. They were always analyzed and discussed openly by Harken and the residents. This openness led us rapidly out of the dark days.

The enigma of selecting patients for a dangerous new operation in lethal disease pertains both to new surgery and to new drugs that might be useful in desperate situations. It is tempting for the pioneer, in order to keep mortality low, to confine early trials to those patients at lowest risk (those who need the new treatment least). But always there is the pressure to offer the treatment mercifully to desperately ill patients who seek help and want the favor, the gift, of a try. They would rather die during the operation than go without trying. Harken operated in many of the most urgent and risky cases. That he succeeded as often as he did in those early days of developing the new concept of operating on the inside of the heart is a tribute not only to his skill but also to the steady improvement in all aspects of surgical care.

Soon the heart was to be opened much more safely. Before carrying that story further, we must catch up with the Gibbons in Philadelphia, as well as some remarkable surgical innovators in Minneapolis.

John Gibbon Opens the Heart

On May 6, 1953, John Gibbon repaired a congenital defect in the heart of an 18-year-old girl. This was an interatrial septal defect, a hole in the septum or membrane separating the two upper (low-pressure) chambers of the heart, the atria or auricles. Jack, with Maylie's assistance, used a pump-oxygenator for the first time in a human being. With the help of this device—his new machine—he could open the heart and sew up the hole while the new device pumped and oxygenated all the blood and kept the patient alive. Once the heart was closed and resumed its beat, the machine could be disconnected. This was just 22 years after he sat at the MGH measuring the vital signs of that patient suffering from repeated pulmonary emboli.

Many of us who were friends of Jack Gibbon knew of his work in some detail and of his resolute pursuit of a single objective. Despite being subjected to a good deal of kidding about its impossibility, he persisted, from time to time publishing articles or speaking at meetings to relate his progress.

On one occasion our small travel club of surgeons was meeting in Philadelphia. One of the high points of the meeting was to be a visit to the Gibbons' laboratory to see how the Great Machine was coming along. I remember the day well. We trooped in, 10 or 15 of us, and were asked to take off our shoes and put on rubber boots. This quaint custom is standard practice in most operating rooms in Great Britain, as if they were so accustomed to torrents of blood (as in eighteenth-century amputations) that they had never modernized their footwear as American surgeons had.

We were then ushered into the operating room of the Gibbons' laboratory. At that time the pump-oxygenator was approximately the size of a grand piano. A small cat, asleep to one side, was the object of all this attention. The cat was connected to the machine by two transparent blood-filled plastic tubes, one deep dark red (venous, deoxygenated, going to the machine) and one bright pink (arterial, oxygenated, returning blood to the cat). The contrast in size between the small cat and the huge machine aroused considerable amusement among the audience. The bulk of the machine was not required for pumping but rather for adding oxygen to the cat's blood and removing the carbon dioxide. As Gibbon had often described to his colleagues, this function of gas exchange had always presented the main difficulty.

Watching this complicated procedure, concentrating mostly on the cat, whose heart was about to be completely isolated from its circulation, opened, and then closed, we began to sense that we were not walking on a dry floor. We looked down. We were standing in an inch of blood.

"Oh... I'm sorry," said Gibbon. "The confounded thing has sprung a leak again."

There followed several noteworthy events. First, our small audience could not help but be impressed by such good humor in the face of embarrassment in front of a critical group of old friends. Second, Mrs. Gibbon, with characteristic presence of mind, quickly spliced the leaky tubing. And third, the experiment was successful in that the cat's heart was isolated from its circulation, even if for only about 45 seconds while it was quickly opened and closed, and the animal recovered uneventfully. At that time the Gibbons' objective was 30 minutes of successful machine perfusion with the heart open. Within another year or two, perfusions of such durations were to be achieved in human patients.

With the successful operation in May 1953 and a few more like it, Gibbon retired from the operative field of cardiac surgery. He modestly stated that he was not a heart surgeon. His main interest was in surgery of the lungs. He felt there were other men better prepared as cardiac specialists to pick up where he had left off. Among them was John Kirklin of the Mayo Clinic, one of the first to put the Gibbon machine to extensive use. His first successful operation was in March 1955. Four of his first eight patients survived. All were children with congenital heart disease who were terminally ill and about to die before he operated on them. Now they were made well.

225

Other Ways: Toronto and Minneapolis

Other surgeons concerned with this matter of isolating and opening the heart while pumping the blood around by some other means were also models of ingenuity and innovation. In 1950 William Bigelow of Toronto had reported cooling a patient to about 20°C (hypothermia) so he could reduce the brain's demand for oxygen and thus ensure its survival and incidentally the survival of kidney and liver (and in fact, the whole patient), even though he was opening the heart and stopping all function for several minutes. Henry Swan, our classmate at medical school, and later professor at the University of Colorado, was also using hypothermia when operating on children with heart defects. In 1952 F.J. Lewis of Minneapolis further improved methods for the use of hypothermia.

Meanwhile other Minneapolitans were studying the most spectacular and possibly the most imaginative of methods for patient support during repair of the heart. C. Walton Lillehei, Richard Varco, and their team developed a method by which the blood vessels of a sick child were temporarily connected to those of its parent to allow the parent's heart and lungs to function as a pump-oxygenator for the sick child. By conducting blood from the child's vein to the parent and then returning it from the parent back to the child's arteries fully oxygenated, it was possible to isolate the child's heart, open it up, and repair it. Their first successful case using this cross-circulation technique was in 1954. In all, they carried out 45 such operations, with a 63% survival. All the patients, mostly children, were desperately ill and dying. This was a heroic, difficult, and complicated procedure, involving risk to the well donor (the parent whose heart was doing the pumping). In 1955 Richard DeWall joined them and devised a new kind of bubble oxygenator that was soon used along with the Gibbon pump to replace the awkward, cumbersome, and risky cross-circulation method.

Catheters in New Places

With the ability to open the heart safely came a new era of hope for blue babies and for adults in heart failure or with cardiac pain. Progress this far, and surely no further, could not have come about without a way to achieve more accurate diagnosis from within the heart.

In 1929 Werner Forssman, a surgical intern planning a career in urology, bravely introduced a long, thin tube (otherwise known as a catheter and usually used to empty the urinary bladder) into one of his own large veins that lie in front of the elbow. He threaded the catheter up the vein and around the bend at his shoulder. He kept on pushing until he knew, based on the length that had disappeared into his vein, that the catheter must have gone down into his heart. So he walked down the hall to the x-ray department and asked them to take a picture. There it was. The tip of the catheter sitting in the right atrium. So much of science is so simple! At least, it always seems that way in retrospect. Maybe, as in this case, it is having the idea in the first place: a tribute to the complexity of the human mind.

By means of catheterization, in which the lowly catheter was applied to the heart (as opposed to that more humble organ to which it was accustomed), cardiac surgeons could be more certain of doing the right thing.

André Cournand and Dickinson Richards of New York took up this work of cardiac catheterization in about 1945, followed shortly by our own Lewis Dexter. When you take blood straight out of the chambers of the heart and measure its pressure, oxygenation, and carbon dioxide content, you can also use the catheter to inject a dye and measure the heart's output of blood. You can inject fluid that shows up on the x-ray and see the pattern (anatomy) of blood flow. Within a short time it became possible to pass the catheter up an artery (rather than a vein) to take blood samples directly from the high-pressure (left) side of the heart and to examine the aorta, that huge, high-pressure conduit that conducts blood from the left heart to the rest of the body. In 1956 Cournand, Richards, and Forssman were awarded the Nobel Prize for this work. Ten years later it was by this procedure, used by Mason Sones of Cleveland, that coronary artery disease could be accurately seen and then repaired.

It is a source of consternation that Nobel recognition was never awarded to Gross, Gibbon, Harken, Lillehei, Blalock, Kirklin, Rob, DeBakey, or any other of our surgical colleagues who were pioneers in making stunning discoveries in the care of cardiovascular disease. Somehow, it took transplantation to wake up the Nobel Committee to what had been going on in surgery.

The Clicking Dogs

Dwight Harken also experimented with ways of fixing the aortic valve, the high-pressure one-way valve at the output channel of the left ventricle. This required a stiffer valve, for which a ball valve seemed well suited. His work with ball valves was based on the prior success of a young Brigham surgical resident, Charles Hufnagel, in perfecting ball valves for placement in major arteries. Hufnagel did this work in the dog, that sacred laboratory animal most suitable for much of the research that has resulted in so many advances in surgery and helped relieve the suffering of so many people. When it came to the development of transplantation and cardiac surgery, surely the dog was man's best friend. Thereby hangs the tale of a few wagging tails.

In the 1950s Charles Hufnagel was working to perfect a ball valve that could be used within the heart. To study these devices he placed them in the aorta in a large series of dogs in our laboratories at the Harvard Medical School. When he accepted a job as professor at Georgetown University, he asked me if he could take these dogs with him to Washington. Of course I agreed, because these dogs were extremely valuable, priceless. There were no others like them anywhere in the world. Also, they had become pets of the laboratory team. Their long-term followup over the course of years would be necessary to determine the extent of wear and tear on the ball valve.

So he loaded all his dogs into a small trailer to drive them from Boston to Washington. When he reached northeastern Connecticut, he needed to make a pit stop at a filling station. As Hufnagel disappeared into the rest room, the attendant heard a dog barking in the trailer and thought an animal probably wanted out to irrigate a local tree. So, thinking there might be one or two dogs inside, he opened the trailer door. About 25 dogs bounded out, barking and sniffing and wagging their tails delightedly. This is a part of Connecticut along the road about halfway between New York and Boston that is largely uninhabited, quite a wild place for this canine diaspora. Yapping with joy at their release from the noisy trailer, the dogs disappeared into the hills of Connecticut.

This would have been a terrible loss to science and cardiology had it not been for the ingenuity of Hufnagel, the dismay of the filling station attendant, and the willingness of the local dogcatchers to cooperate in an unusual medical adventure. All the dog officers were given stethoscopes and were instructed to hold down any dog they caught, stray or otherwise, and listen to its chest. One of the dogs had returned to the trailer, and the dogcatchers were all given a chance to listen to what a ball valve sounded like, clicking back and forth in the chest with every heart beat. Unmistakable. If the dog clicked, keep it.

It wasn't long (about a week) before all the dogs were rounded up from the forests of northeastern Connecticut and sent on their way to Hufnagel's laboratory at Georgetown University. This work, these valves, and his study of these dogs in inventing a new device have given him a secure place in surgical history.

Sticking With It

The tenacity of scientists in sticking with a problem until it is solved has often been described in this book. Prime examples were Hufnagel with his ball valves and the Gibbons spending 22 years to take the idea of a pump-oxygenator from theory to reality. But possibly the finest example of such tenacity is the work of Dwight Harken, who stayed with the problem of intracardiac surgery over the course of half a century, from his wartime work until his death in 1993. In his illustrious career, Harken also developed an artificial mitral valve as well as a way of correcting an abnormal heart rhythm by means of a new pacemaker that would take over only when the heart needed it (the demand pacemaker).

Dwight resigned from our department in 1969, the year of his 60th birthday, and was succeeded by his assistant, John J. Collins, a former Brigham resident. With a surgical team large in comparison with Harken's one-man team back in 1948, Collins has operated upon a great many cardiac patients of all types, including transplants, and has achieved one of the lowest mortality rates in the country. As Harken's successor, he has mounted a remarkably successful program in cardiac surgery and transplantation.

All physicians, surgeons, and patients who are caught up in the web of heart disease owe a debt of gratitude to that hard-working Iowan. Dwight Harken died in Cambridge on August 27, 1993, as this chapter was being prepared. And now his son, Alden Harken, graduate of Western Reserve Medical School and of the Brigham surgical residency, carries on his father's tradition of teaching and innovation in surgery as Professor and Head of the Department of Surgery at the University of Colorado in Denver.

Although formidable physiologic and medical problems are encountered in both cardiac surgery and transplantation, these two new fields would not have been brought to practical reality had it not been for the surgical laboratories in the universities of the United States. After the events of these past 50 years, surgical research need not apologize to the rest of biomedical science. Often frowned upon by those whose work is at the bench of basic science, American university laboratories of surgery (in both Canada and the United States) have brought that same quality of science from the bench to the operating room via the laboratory.

By any measure—most particularly the number of people cared for and the number of physicians and surgeons caring for them—cardiac surgery is the largest new field of surgery to have developed in the half century since World War II. As a result of their care by surgeons, thousands of people are relieved of cardiac pain, their lives sometimes prolonged; some patients with heart attacks (acute myocardial infarction) have lifesaving operations on the coronary arteries during the acute phase of that disease. Possibly most important and meaningful for society as a whole is the fact that many children, ranging from newborns to teens, can be given a whole new life now that the cardiac defects with which they were born can be repaired. The gain is in quantity of life for some and quality of life for all such patients.

Surgery of the heart is also the field in which surgeons have most clearly entered the previously sacred precincts of nonoperating physicians: the internist, the pediatrician, the cardiologist. The advent of cardiac surgery has given these physicians a new series of decisions to make and new avenues of hope for their patients. And even as some of the cardiac surgery is giving way to simpler, less invasive, often x-ray-guided treat-ment (e.g., balloon angioplasty, aneurysm repair), it was the new plateau reached by surgical scientists just before and after World War II that made further advance possible.

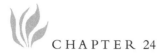

CHAPTER 24

Adoptive Immunotherapy of Cancer

From that first patient of mine who died after a breast operation in 1942 (Chapter 10), up to and after my retirement in 1981, I was concerned daily with cancer. General surgeons, the breed of which I was an example, are the people who take care of cancers of the breast, thyroid, stomach, colon, liver, and pancreas. The solid tumors. Cancer of the breast leads the list, being (along with lung cancer) one of the leading causes of death in American white women over the age of 50. Breast cancer is sensitive to many influences. It is a tumor that can often be cured if removed early, and one that continues to be the subject of intense research not only because of its prevalence, but also because of its responsiveness to chemical and hormonal changes. And yet, like most of the solid tumors, once it recurs after operation, cure is almost never achieved ("never say never").

Starting in the 1960s breast cancer became the main subject of my clinical research. Despite repeated optimistic press announcements and alleged breakthroughs, it was continuously borne in on me that the solid tumors, such as those of the breast, represent the best examples of curability by early surgical removal but also our most dreadful failures once the tumors return. Then, in the 1980s, one of my former residents, Steven Rosenberg, began to achieve success with his lifelong ambition: the treatment of cancer by increasing the patient's own powers of immunity sufficiently to throw off, or reject, the tumor. This concept, that the body's defense against a cancer could be enhanced by having the patient adopt some genetically strengthened immune cells (often the patient's own cells, reinfused) is, in his terminology, adoptive immunotherapy.

It is the purpose of this chapter to tell the story of our years working to improve the care of cancer of the breast, limiting the extent of initial surgery; of the problems posed by advanced breast cancer and by other solid tumors; and of the new hope for cure of some solid tumors arising from Steve's adoptive immunotherapy. But first, some definitions.

Bad Actors: The Solid Tumors

The word tumor literally means "swelling" and is indicated by the Latin suffix -*oma* (as in carcinoma, sarcoma, lymphoma). If, under the microscope, that swelling consists of rapidly duplicating cells, it is called a "neoplasm," meaning "new tissue growth." Some (but not all) neoplasms are malignant, which means they tend to spread to other organs and, if left to their own devices, will kill their host (the patient). Thus, all cancers are tumors, but not all tumors are cancers. The word "cancer" is derived from the Greek and Latin terms for crab, because of the crablike growth of some of these cancers, noted even by the most ancient physicians, the more precise term being "carcinoma" (crab-tumor). The crab is the astronomical symbol for the Tropic of Cancer. In this chapter we are using the broad term "solid tumor" to include a large but special group of cancers.

The group of solid tumors includes most of the familiar cancers. They have several characteristics in common. For one thing, they start as small cellular growths—lumps—localized to one microscopic place. The malignant process often seems to start in a single cell or in two or three neighboring cells probably subjected to the same influences and possibly communicating with each other chemically. As the solid tumors grow in size, some cells (the malignant tumor cells) begin to migrate elsewhere (metastasize), where they form additional solid masses of tumor that may be as tiny as half a pinhead or as big as an orange. Most cancer cures today are achieved by total surgical removal of very early solid tumors. Most solid tumors are amenable to early surgical removal. Thus the solid tumors are the surgical tumors.

Four of the commonest cancers in the United States are solid tumors: cancers of the lung, breast, large intestine (colon), and skin. The group of solid tumors also includes cancer of prostate, uterus, pancreas, ovary, testicle, kidney, liver, thyroid, esophagus, stomach, tongue, and bone. If the cancer originates in the liver, it is considered a primary (rather than metastatic) solid tumor of the liver (hepatoma). Cancer of the skin may be of the skin-colored type, usually a hollowed-out ulcer (squamous cell carcinoma, caused in some cases by exposure to the ultraviolet rays of the sun), or it may be a jet-black mole-like tumor (malignant melanoma). Basal cell skin cancer (also related to sun exposure) is generally a harmless small lump. A biopsy, or removal with microscopic examination, is essential for differentiating these three very different types of skin cancers. Most brain tumors are also classified as solid tumors.

By contrast, there are the nonsolid tumors. These affect the blood and lymphatic systems and bone marrow and include the leukemias (cancer of the leukocytes or white cells), lymphomas (arising in the lymph nodes or lymphocytes), and some rare cancers of the bone marrow elements. Although these tumors are not usually amenable to early surgical removal, many are sensitive to radiation and to chemotherapy (treatment with drugs and chemicals). In fact, some of the best results of radiation and chemotherapy are achieved in these tumors.

Since World War II, an international effort has been devoted to improving the dismal outlook of patients with advanced solid tumors: those in whom, after that first hopeful removal, the tumor has returned or metastasized. Our failure here has always been the bad news.

The good news is that coming over the horizon during the past decade is an entirely new form of treatment based on stimulation of the patients' own lymphocytes (immune cells) to improve their immune capability. These cells have been stimulated to multiply and to reject advanced cancer, wherever it is, completely and permanently. While only a start, and still imperfect, this approach is so drastically different from our old ways and has so clearly demonstrated encouraging results in a few patients that it must be included as a part of any story of cancer surgery in the last half of the twentieth century.

Radicals and Conservatives

During this half century, there have been persistent efforts to expand the scope of the initial surgical removal of the original tumor by extending the primary operation and removing more nearby lymph nodes and even normal tissues on the grounds that they might contain cancer cells.

In Latin, the word *radix* means root. A radish is a root. Things that dig at the roots are radical. A radical operation attempts to dig out and remove all the tumor at its very roots. To save something is to conserve it. Conservative operations conserve or spare more of the patient's normal tissue. These clinical meanings are important, particularly as they stand in contrast to the usual political or social meanings of these words. In medical discussions we should stick with the medical meanings. Thus, radical is not always new or destructive and conservative is not always old and safe.

Around the turn of this century, advances in surgery, especially the increased use of blood transfusions, made it possible to develop more radical operations for early cancers. In the case of breast cancer, the prototype was radical mastectomy, developed by William S. Halsted at Johns Hopkins around 1890. Similar extensions of surgery were developed in other countries and for other cancers. For breast and other types of cancer (colon, prostate, and uterus all being examples), the more radical operation was at first a great improvement over the crude efforts to remove cancers by conservative limited excision, which often led to disastrous spread. In the world of 75 to 100 years ago, radical operations were a breakthrough, curing patients who previously had no hope of cure. Although we are moving away from them now, let us give them credit for the very real improvement they conferred over what went before.

Then, near the time of World War II, there occurred two simultaneous but divergent departures from the accepted surgical approaches of the time: one further to extend and the other drastically to constrain the removal of early solid tumors. Not only have many surgeons of our generation participated in these changing surgical modes and methods, but we have also been keenly aware of the public accounts of these changes as reported in papers and magazines and on television. I cannot blame the public for being totally confused. It sounds almost as though one surgeon or one medical school was advocating a new procedure on the basis of local pride or prestige, staking out turf, while others found fault. In point of fact these more radical departures were always undertaken for a specific reason, to be justified by increased survival of patients having such operations, on the basis of 5-, 10-, or 20-year followup and as contrasted with other procedures. At their worst, these conflicts over how much to undertake at the first operation have been a war of words and a battle of personalities; at their best, they are a war of numbers, a vast battlefield of statistics. And if we are talking about 5-year survivals, do not forget that it will always take at least 5 years—and more realistically, 8 or 10 years—to gather such data for a large number of patients. Attempts to extend the radical operation for breast cancer were undertaken, particularly by Jerome Urban in New York and Owen Wangensteen in Minnesota.

At that same time (approximately 1945 to 1960), other surgeons began a move in the opposite direction, advocating only limited removal of small, highly localized, early and favorable (i.e., not aggressive) tumors. Those interested in this more conservative approach pointed out that if the tumor is found to be local, well defined, and unlikely to recur, local surgery should suffice and nothing further needs to be done. In such cases radical mastectomy is an unnecessarily extensive operation. I was of this school. On the presumption that some tumor cells were likely to be left behind, we often combined restricted local removal with radiation therapy, as did McWhirter of Scotland, one of the earliest and most vocal advocates of surgical restraint immediately after World War II.

Curiously, advocates on both sides of this controversy agreed that less is better if the tumor is local, not aggressive, and noninvasive. A big if. Starting about 1960—a little later than many, but sooner than most—I abandoned radical mastectomy save in a few special instances, as mentioned above. I favored using the simple mastectomy, in which the breast alone is removed and the lymph nodes under the arm are sampled to see whether or not radiotherapy or chemotherapy should be given. The woman no longer has a breast. But she has a better likelihood of 5-year survival than if the lump alone is removed. Many patients of mine who were in their middle 40s or 50s, who had borne and nursed their children, and whose husbands did not require the cosmetic/erotic symbolism of an intact breast, said to me, "Dr. Moore, take off my breast if it is necessary. What I want is to be alive to see my teenage children graduate from college." Besides removing the local tumor, we removed some lymph nodes to examine them under the microscope and find out whether or not the tumor was truly local, favorable, and noninvasive. A vocal feminist claque grew up around this problem, loudly proclaiming any removal of the breast to be brutal and unnecessary mutilation. Few patients agreed with such a polarized view.

One is left with a clear sensation of forward movement away from the automatic, unthinking application of the Halsted radical mastectomy. And a reaffirmation of the faith that patients should seek a doctor whose honesty and experience they trust, one who will not pressure patients into doing his (or her) own thing. If the doctor is a radiotherapist, for example, we hope the opinion of a surgeon will be sought, and vice versa. If a team exists in the modern configuration of a tumor clinic, all voices must be heard.

The Free Interval and Advanced Disease

Once the first deed is done—that is, the primary treatment (usually surgery, often with radiation and sometimes with chemotherapy) is complete—and all known or visible disease has been removed or treated, the patient enters the free interval. "Cure" means that the free interval will last 5 or 10 years or for the rest of the patient's life. In essence, cure means that the patient will die of something other than cancer.

If the free interval comes to an end much too soon, after a month or even a decade, because the tumor has returned either at the same place (local recurrence) or elsewhere (metastases), we then encounter nature's obstacle, a wilderness of the unknown. It is important to realize that biomedical science deals with such a wilderness at every frontier. In recurrent cancer this is a wilderness with many points of entry but no clear trail to the clearing on the far side. The stark reality is that almost all patients who enter this wilderness with advanced disease will die. We are unable to guide them through.

Here is where our own efforts in breast cancer were expended most intensively over a period of almost 30 years. Certain hormones stimulate the growth of breast cancer. Removal of the glands secreting those hormones was often helpful. We carried out many total adrenalectomies to remove one source of the stimulated estrogen or female hormone. Working with Donald Matson, we removed the pituitary (hypophysectomy) to eliminate all endocrine influences. We used cortisone in conjunction with chemotherapy, employing various types of drugs and chemical substances. Some of our most successful cases were those in which the ovaries and then the adrenals were removed and, even before the patient came out of anesthesia, high-dose chemotherapy was started. Surprisingly, a few of those patients are still alive and well after 20 years. In these trials we were working with new combinations of old methods and trying with some success to give our patients a few good months or years.

Maybe the most important thing I did during these years was to encourage wide collaboration within our hospital. We never instituted treatment of advanced or recurrent cancer without seeking the opinion of those who had skill and experience in other forms of treatment: radiation, drugs, or hormones.

Steve Rosenberg Makes Lymphocytes Multiply and Work Harder

It was against this background of frustration with the ineffective treatment of advanced cancer that we hailed the first reports by Steven Rosenberg of his use of genetic manipulation to treat late cancer as a ray of hope.

In 1962 Crick, Watson, and Wilkins were awarded the Nobel Prize for discovering the precise arrangement whereby an array of chemical substances—nucleic acids, the genetic material—is transmitted with exact accuracy from parent to offspring. They had done this work about 10 years previously. Those precise sequences were shown to encode the choice of amino acids for protein synthesis on minuscule assembly machines (ribosomes) in each cell. These molecular sequences, programming the synthesis of proteins, exist in large molecules of deoxyribonucleic acid, or DNA. DNA contains all the genes of the person, and the gene-encoded control of protein synthesis governs the character of everything of which we are composed, from the most subtle enzyme reactions to the color of our eyes and hair, the shape of our heads, and the way we walk, talk, and think. And why we resemble our parents. Discovery of the genetic code and its mode of transmission changed all of biology, and now—long predicted and hopefully anticipated—it is finally bringing new hope in the treatment of cancer.

In 1985 Rosenberg reported some of his first results with the application of genetics in the treatment of cancer using the patients' own lymphocytes and compounds made by genetically engineered bacteria. For the first time in history, doctors heard reports of patients who had been near death with recurrent masses of a solid tumor but who were now alive and well, no visible tumor anywhere, after their own lymphocytes were stimulated to become better tumor killers and then given back to the patient.

The principle he set forth was to borrow some of the patient's lymphocytes, identify those particularly prone to kill cancer cells, grow them rapidly outside the patient's body by using a cell stimulant called interleukin-2 (IL-2), and then inject them back into the patient, maintaining their growth stimulus with more IL-2. He had been working with certain very recalcitrant solid tumors, especially malignant melanoma and cancer of the kidney. Some of the early results were encouraging. A few were spectacular.

Crick and his coworkers were neither the first nor the last to win the Nobel Prize for elucidating the chemical compounds within the cell that pass along genetic traits to offspring. And Rosenberg was not the first—and surely will not be the last—to treat cancer by changing the patient's immunity, an idea that goes back many decades. Other attempts to alter the patient's immunity in cancer have involved some immunologic stimulus, such as the toxins used by Bradley Coley in the 1920s, the tubercle bacillus, or another bacterium called *Corynebacterium parvum*. Contrasted with these efforts, Rosenberg's work is unique because it involves, not a toxin, but rather the patient's own immune cells. After the cells were reintroduced, there was a remarkably favorable response in many patients. About 10% were completely rid of their cancer, some maintaining this tumor-free status after treatment was stopped. Rosenberg was the first to bring such a method to reality.

Steven Rosenberg was born in New York City in 1940. After

attending the Bronx High School of Science, he graduated from college at Johns Hopkins in Baltimore and completed medical school there in 1963. He then began a surgical internship in our department at the Brigham. Three years into his clinical work he took time off to do postgraduate study for the Ph.D. degree in biophysics at Harvard. Between 1968 and 1974 Steve completed his senior and chief residency in surgery at the Brigham and the West Roxbury Veterans Administration Hospital. Again he took time out for a year of study with John David at the Harvard Medical School in the field of molecular immunology, which focuses on the chemical weapons that immune cells use to kill invading cancer cells. He then spent 2 years in postgraduate study of immunology at the National Institutes of Health (NIH). There has always been a joke over the fact that surgical residencies at the Johns Hopkins seem to last longer than they do at the Harvard hospitals. Steve's residency in our department, lasting almost 11 years, probably set some sort of record. Steve says, "It took that long for Dr. Moore to approve me as a surgeon." Since he was, from the start, clearly an able operative and clinical surgeon, his comment refers modestly to the fact that he took time off during his residency years to earn his doctorate and to become an expert in protein structure and immunology.

Upon completing his surgical residency at the Brigham, Steve was made Chief of Surgery at the National Cancer Institute (NCI) as well as Professor of Surgery at both the Uniformed Services University and George Washington University.

The Care of Lieutenant L.G.

In 1978 Steve Rosenberg began to study the production of a growth factor for T lymphocytes. This substance was later identified as a lymphokine (or lymph-cell stimulator) known as IL-2, mentioned above. Genetic modification of a bacterium was used to synthesize this human-type cell stimulator in large amounts—an early example of genetic engineering. He then showed that mouse lymphocytes multiplied a thousand-fold or more when grown in a tissue culture along with IL-2. Thus stimulated, some of those cells attacked fresh tumor cells, and he called these "lymphokine-activated killer" (LAK) cells. After several years of experimentation in animals, he was ready to introduce LAK cells in the treatment of human cancer.

The story of one of his early successes tells the tale better than I could. This story appears in Steve's recent book about his research, *The Transformed Cell*. I am indebted to him for permitting me to retell this story here and for contributing additional details.

Lieutenant L.G. first came under Rosenberg's care at the NIH in 1983 at the age of 33. A naval officer doing many energetic and challenging jobs usually carried out by men, she was a doer, an achiever, a matter-of-fact person accustomed to accomplishment, with a considerable personal investment of skill and effort. As we shall see, these habits of work and lifestyle explain, at least in part, her tenacity in weathering the prolonged, uncomfortable, and stressful treatment that lay ahead.

A few years before L.G. came to Rosenberg, a black skin mole behind her right shoulder had started to look different and become more active. When there is a change in the way a black mole feels or appears or if it develops a red border, the person should consult a doctor without delay. Being a naval officer, she was taken care of at the Bethesda Naval Hospital. Biopsy revealed a malignant melanoma (the dangerous black cancer of the skin). While the lymph nodes draining the area appeared normal under the microscope, the melanoma was thick and invasive. Melanoma is one of the tumors where, under the microscope, one can make a pretty good guess as to whether it is a rather harmless tumor or a dangerous one. This one was the dangerous kind. After removal of the melanoma she entered her disease-free interval, full of hope and confi dence.

Early in 1983 she was transferred to a position in Guam as lieutenant commander and flag secretary, working with the admiral's staff. Within a few weeks she began to notice some hard lumps under her skin. The Navy doctor biopsied one of these and discovered that it was the same malignant melanoma. Her disease had returned and metastasized. As we have seen in breast cancer, so also in melanoma, this occurrence has always spelled the beginning of the end.

Like so many patients in this ominous fix, she was willing to try anything reasonably likely to ensure her survival. She underwent some experimental clinical treatments at several naval hospitals, but without success. One of her physicians mentioned Steve's beginning work at the NIH, so she went to Bethesda to explore this possibility. On her arrival she was found to have many round lumps of tumor in her lungs and hundreds of lumps under her skin. Her sense of participation and determination to get the job done was expressed in her main fear (as she described it) on entering this complicated new treatment: that she might not measure up to the doctor's expectations.

She began her new treatment under Steve's care in November 1984. To begin with, some blood was drawn, the lymphocytes were separated, and killer cells were isolated and stimulated to grow by using the genetically engineered IL-2. On November 29, 3.4 billion killer cells grown from her own lymphocytes were infused back into her bloodstream. This treatment made her ill, an illness made worse by repeated infusion of more IL-2 used to stimulate the LAK cells even further. Although IL-2 alone is toxic and makes patients sick, its bad effects usually wear off completely.

This intensive cycle of treatment continued for 6 days, at which time the dose of IL-2 was further increased. Now Lt. L.G. became extremely ill with nausea, vomiting, and muscle weakness. Despite this, she wanted to go ahead, to continue with the treatment to stimulate the killer cells. On December 10 she received a seventh infusion of her own lymphoid cells and two more doses of IL-2.

Despite her resulting illness and some worrisome signs, and with her full approval, Rosenberg and his team persisted. While she seemed to be tolerating the treatment a little bit better, she had a severe crisis a few days later. She was not breathing adequately. Her life was clearly threatened by the treatment itself. She developed pulmonary edema (water accumulating in her lungs) and appeared to be on the brink of total respiratory arrest. As an emergency procedure, she was intubated, oxygen was administered with assisted respiration, and she was given drugs to hasten excretion of water and salt, which helped to unload all that excess fluid. Not only had she been through a severe crisis resulting from an absolutely maximum push of IL-2/LAK treatment, but in fact she had received more IL-2 and killer cells than had any other patient up to that time.

As she climbed out of this crisis, she showed emotional scars from her terrifying experience. At first, her tumors showed no change. But there was one hopeful sign. The day she was returned to her regular ward from the intensive care unit, biopsy of the tumor showed focal necrosis of tumor cells under the microscope, a pathologist's term meaning that some of these cells were dying. In due course she was discharged from the hospital, her status insecure, and her outcome uncertain.

About 2 weeks later, she came back for her first follow-up appointment. She was feeling much better. Maybe this was the best sign of all. Another biopsy was done and the pathologist now saw "the appearance...of tumor cell ghosts consistent with [the] previously diagnosed malignant melanoma.... Lymphocytes were seen.... No viable (i.e., living) tumor is identified." As you might guess, cell ghosts are the shadowy remnants of dead cells as seen under the microscope. While this was a remarkable phenomenon and one rarely seen before in such widespread malignant melanoma, there were some worrisome developments. In some of the metastatic areas of tumor spread (especially her lungs), the tumors were not getting smaller. This was puzzling and discouraging. With such a new treatment, no one could predict what lay ahead.

A month later (March 20, 1985) the patient returned again for follow-up and immediately told Steve, "My tumors are going away!" Many of the tumors she could feel under her skin were shrinking and disappearing. Again there was a biopsy. All the tumor cells were dead. Before treatment, x-rays had shown a great many tumors; now there was none visible anywhere or discernible by x-ray, CAT scan, or MRI. Her cancer had completely disappeared. Here was the dream of every cancer patient, every family, every cancer researcher for the past century, coming true.

Typical of her indomitable spirit, she was now applying for return to active duty in the Navy. Since none of the navy physicians had ever seen a patient who was dying of malignant melanoma get well and go back to work, she had a bit of trouble with her petition. In fact, it required action from the Secretary of the Navy, who promoted her to Commander.

Without going into some of the exciting details of the later career of this naval officer, so devoted to her national service responsibilities, I will add that L.G. has remained well and completely free of tumor. Seven years after her treatment (at about the time Rosenberg was writing his book about this work) and when he was helping me describe her case here, she was perfectly well. She has remained well now for 9 years.

How could anyone fail to see a bright light of hope in the gloom of the cancer problem in such a patient as this and the many others like her in Rosenberg's studies at the NCI. "One swallow does not a summer make" and one case does not make a series. But there have been many instances in these 50 years when one case made a splash whose ripple spread very far: Gross' first ductus closure, Harken's first mitral valve repair, Murray's first kidney transplant, and now one of Rosenberg's first IL-2/LAK patients.

Not all Steve's patients do this well. About 35% show tumor shrinkage, 10% show complete disappearance of tumor, and 5% remain free of tumor after treatment is stopped. That is why he and the many others who are following his lead are trying to improve this approach to immune treatment.

Favorable responses to the treatment of late cancer have been gauged by reductions in the size of the tumors, in symptoms, or in the adverse physiologic effects of the tumor. The frequency of this response is then expressed as a rate or percentage of treated patients who respond. In considering positive responses to adoptive immunotherapy such as those of Lt. L.G., we are encountering an entirely new phenomenon: an early response that is not a mere shrinkage indicating borderline, arguable improvement, but one that involves complete destruction and disappearance of the tumor. While the statistical cure rate is still low, it is significant that such responses occur at all.

Because of the work of Rosenberg and others involved in genetic manipulation, the treatment of advanced cancer has taken a new shape and will never be the same again. These patients and this work have demonstrated a new way out of the wilderness. The detailed procedures in use at this moment are surely not the best, the safest, nor the last word. Progress thrives on constant change. Malignant melanoma and cancer of the kidney have been the most responsive to adoptive immunotherapy; trials have now begun in cancers of the breast, bowel, and lung.

We owe a debt not only to Steven Rosenberg, but also to French Anderson, Vincent DeVita (recently director of the NCI), and their many collaborators. They are a part of our national scientific establishment at the NIH, supported by a nation of taxpayers. If ever there was a national effort, this is it. Many other cancer centers both here and abroad have taken up Steve's work, sometimes modifying it in an effort to improve the results.

Who will be helped? Only a few of us in the older generation. Many of our children. Some sort of immune treatment will be a commonplace for our grandchildren's generation as they reach the cancer age. Were they to develop advanced cancer from one of the common solid tumors, they will enjoy the option of immunotherapy based on genetic engineering, a new and more hopeful treatment that might return them to a normal life.

BOOK EIGHT

Surgery Abroad and Back Home

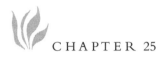

CHAPTER 25

Korea

(1951)

In the summer of 1951 at the request of the Surgeon General of the Army, I took a trip to Korea to consult with Army surgeons analyzing the patterns of wounds and illness. Two special problems were designated for particular attention: blood banking and blood transfusion, with their threat of potassium toxicity, and epidemic hemorrhagic fever (EHF). Visits therefore included the forward hospitals, the mobile army surgical hospital (MASH) units, and the base hospitals in both Korea and Japan.

One occasion I recall vividly. We were flying at about 2,500 feet in an army L-5, a two-seater artillery spotting plane. About the size of a Piper Cub but very sturdy. All khaki-colored, army style. The pilot was a young officer, flying us north across the Chinese lines. Our own front lines, dimly seen as trenches on a ridgetop, lay out there, behind us. The scene was one of dense forest, hills, and low mountains to all horizons, reminiscent of Vermont or New Hampshire.

There was some artillery crossfire. The pilot had said we would be flying through the flight pattern or trajectory of our own big guns. He seemed unperturbed. I tried to be. A sudden noiseless whoosh went by us and jostled the plane. It was not so much a noise as a small tornado, a very sudden and intense compression of the air and of our eardrums. A moment later we heard the explosive sound, again not so much a bang as a sudden rush of noise. That was the gun behind us shooting off the shell that had whooshed by us. Soon we climbed out of this artillery trajectory pattern. While the pilot was unmoved by this safe deliverance from the geometry of gunfire, it seemed to me to be progress, at the very least.

The pilot pointed out the Chinese lines below. We could see some trenches and an occasional tent. Then, just behind them, some white shell-bursts. Not just the white of smoke or fire, but snow-white. Like cotton. "Phosphorus shells," the pilot volunteered.

The medical department of the U.S. Army cared for casualties of the enemy, both Chinese and North Koreans as well as Turks (on our side) and other U.N. troops, including Aussies in our MASH. I had seen some Chinese who had been wounded by phosphorus bursts. Phosphorus wounds were an unsolved problem. The little bits of highly reactive phosphorus continued to burn deep in the wound and burrowed into muscle, bone, or arteries for hours or days. A fiery, burning-burrowing pain. Also a continuous hazard to survival. Nothing you could do about it. Phosphorus shells do no more troop damage than ordinary shells. They are weapons of terror. But isn't that true of all weapons?

There was no antiaircraft fire. If there had been, we would not have stayed up there for long. The only hazard to our spotting plane was rifle fire from below. The MiG was an early Russian jet that the Chinese had modeled after the German Messerschmitts of World War II. It would have made short shrift of us. The United States did not have jets at that stage of the Korean War. None near us, at any rate. While the Chinese occasionally flew over the lines with a few MiGs, our air power remained completely dominant. That is why we could conduct helicopter evacuations successfully and take a leisurely trip with a low-flying artillery spotting plane.

We didn't see much sign of human activity that I could recognize or interpret. It was all under camouflage. After the pilot talked to the artillery fire control people, we turned back. Upon landing we inspected the fuselage and wings and found a few small bullet holes. "The infantry always shoot at us," the pilot said, in passing. I was driven back to the MASH, a short distance away, in a jeep.

I had witnessed an unusual view—for a doctor—of the violence of midcentury. Over the Chinese lines, watching our artillery bursts.

People I could not see, dying violent deaths. Thirty years later, when I visited our friends in China and welcomed some Chinese visitors to our hospital and our home, I did not talk about the Chinese lines or the Chinese winter offensive that drove MacArthur and our troops back with such suffering, or the casualties on both sides.

One of the most peculiar aspects of the wars of this century has been the quick and total reversal of social and nationalistic antagonisms. Think of the Germans. Two terrible wars. Now our allies. The Russians: friends, allies, then enemies, then friends again. The Italians. The Japanese. The Chinese. Over a few decades, each has made the transition from hated ogres (caricatured in cartoons as ghastly enemies) to friends, or vice versa. Although wars of implacable hatred between the French and the Germans have cost millions of lives since 1870, these two nations are now trying to form a combined army.

Helping Out at a MASH

During my brief visit to Korea there was no major attack on either side. Just constant skirmishing and those night patrols, conducted by both sides. The "no-man's-land" was strewn with mines, swept by machine-gun fire. On several occasions, survivors of these night patrols were brought to the MASH by helicopter (chopper) early the next morning. Just after sunrise. I made the acquaintance of several of these wounded men, helping them when they first came in, seeing them through their operation and wound debridement, through setting of their fractures, and following them until a week or so later when they could be sent back to Japan. By chance, when I was visiting one of the base hospitals in Japan, I saw several of them there again.

For a surgeon who had not been exposed to the care of the wounded in World War II, these night patrols certainly presented a terrifying aspect. A few men, often volunteering for the task, would go forward under cover of darkness and try to feel out the disposition of the enemy. The enemy was well aware that such patrols were coming, as indeed we were of theirs. So land mines were set. Among the worst of these were the Chinese shoe-box mines, informally put together, with a trigger mechanism and explosive charge plus many small pieces of metal in a container about the size and shape of a shoe box. When a soldier stepped on one, it was impelled upward by the first charge and then exploded the second charge at about the level of the soldier's pelvis, producing terrible wounds of the upper thigh, buttocks, rectum, and genitalia. Many of the amputations that we had to perform were rather high in the thigh because of these shoe-box land mines.

The wry humor of the GIs is notable. One of the statements, oft repeated, even as someone was being brought back by chopper from one of those night patrols, and all the intensive care team were at the ready (warned by radio), "This is the only war we got, so we better make the most of it."

The Threat of Potassium Toxicity

The blood-banking method for the care of the wounded in the early years of the Korean War was based on "theater banking." That is, the collection of blood from soldiers nearby. Edward Churchill had initiated this method while serving as chief surgeon in the Mediterranean theater during World War II. Universal donor blood kept at icebox temperature for up to 10 days and in some cases 20 days was then transfused without cross-matching in the advanced battalion aid stations. Because of helicopter evacuation of casualties, these forward surgeons (and even those farther back in the MASH units) received casualties who would have been found dead on the battlefield in any prior war. Massive transfusions were urgently needed. These were men with bullet wounds of the great vessels of the abdomen along the spine (aorta or vena cava), enormous wounds of the liver, and penetrating wounds of the upper part of the heart or lungs. The throat. The brain. Blood was used in vast amounts. Transfusion reactions were rare. Although we suspected that some cases of renal failure might have resulted from undetected blood-group incompatibility, this was never proven.

The surgical services at the various MASH units were concerned with potassium toxicity from this over-age icebox blood. This topic was one that we had studied intensively for the Army about 8 years before, during World War II. When blood is stored over long periods of time, the high concentration of potassium inside red cells begins to leak out into the plasma, where it does not belong. Normally there is a 30:1 ratio of potassium concentration between cells (high) and plasma (low). Leak of this potassium from cells to plasma is a chemical sign that some of the stored red cells are no longer viable. They have started to live out their life span in the icebox and are now dying. If a bottle of banked blood is kept too long, this leaking potassium can build up to dangerously high concentrations in the plasma, making the transfused blood toxic to the recipient. If a severely wounded soldier was also threatened by kidney failure, this blood-bank plasma potassium could be especially dangerous. To prevent this hazard it was essential to monitor the icebox storage time. After 7 to 10 days, unused blood was henceforth to be removed from storage and spun down to separate the red cells so that low-potassium plasma could be salvaged for transfusion in patients with wounds and burns.

Although the artificial kidney had been developed at the time of World War II, it was not used during that war. In fact, it was only later that Willem Kolff emigrated from the Netherlands to the United States and distributed the artificial kidneys he had made to physicians who might improve them by using more sophisticated engineering. As described in Chapter 19, one of these designs was sent to George Thorn at the Brigham, where it was quickly improved into a usable washing device to remove toxins from the blood of patients whose kidneys were off duty either temporarily or permanently.

Four or 5 years later, by the time of the Korean War, things had progressed significantly, and the Army possessed several of these artificial kidneys, all of them in the hands of expert young officers well schooled in the chemistry and care of renal failure. Many patients who developed renal failure after severe wounds were being dialyzed, and some of them, whose kidneys otherwise would have failed, were pulling through to complete recovery.

Epidemic Hemorrhagic Fever

Americans and United Nations troops in Korea, including particularly the Turks, Australians, and New Zealanders, suffered extensively from a devastating disease never before seen by our infectious disease specialists. This was epidemic hemorrhagic fever (EHF). Although EHF occasionally afflicted natives of the Far East, little was known about it. For a time the predominant explanation for its high incidence (and high mortality) among newly arrived U.N. troops was lack of immunity. Soon it was discovered that some Korean troops had the disease, as did the Chinese north of the 38th parallel. Supposedly they had been exposed for years but now became sick. Why now?

As it turned out, EHF was not a matter of the patients' disordered immunity but rather of the personal habits of ground squirrels that lived in burrows. It took some sleuthing to discover the animal reservoir that kept this disease going. When a battalion reached the site of a planned encampment, bulldozers would scrape the topsoil away to clear an area for pitching tents. This de-surfacing exposed the squirrels' underground burrows. Terrified by this turn of events, the little beasts scurried off to seek safety, leaving traces of urine and feces. It was this offal and excreta of squirrels that spread the virus of this disease, so rampant among troops. Since the Korean War, EHF has died back to the rarity it once was. But now, 40 years later, we are learning that the hantavirus and the disease it causes in the American Southwest is a similar (if not the same) virus and similarly spread by the excreta of gophers and ground squirrels.

During the period I was in Korea there was a severe outbreak of EHF; many men came down with this disease and died. The reason I was particularly asked to help treat these patients was that, although they were suffering an infection, their response resembled the response to a severe burn. As in a burn injury, EHF caused huge amounts of fluid (edema) to collect in the tissues in front of the spine, from the upper part of the chest all the way down to the pelvis. The concentration of red cells rose while blood volume fell; patients went into shock and often died of renal failure. In more senses than one, they were burned by the virus.

Those of us studying this disease came to the obvious conclusion that, just as for a severe burn, the first step was to give the patient enough plasma and fluid to keep his blood flowing, restore a normal blood volume, and avoid renal failure. Delivered promptly in adequate (often huge) amounts, this fluid infusion (including plenty of plasma) worked like magic and put the patients back into good shape. Even without antibiotics to fight this microorganism, the men were better than able to fight the infection and survive. The second and major need was for an antibiotic that would control the microorganism producing this disease. This need was never met.

We looked into several of these problems, particularly at one MASH unit, where an active and productive surgical research team was working under the guidance of John Howard, a surgeon of Philadelphia. Howard and his group did a superb job of studying these patients and translating the results of their research into improvements in clinical care all across the front. For me, it was a privilege to work with John and help in whatever way I could.

The Wounded and Their Surgeons

The front at that time included regions known as Punchbowl and Heartbreak Ridge. These battlefields consisted of steep escarpments with the front line precisely on top, facing the enemy's front line on the opposite ridge. The forward battalion aid stations were situated just behind the front lines along the slopes of these ridges. The second line of hospitals—some of them MASH units, others a little bit smaller than a MASH—were not far behind. All were close to the combat areas. Such proximity to immediate care translated into low mortality from wounds. A situation not always possible in war.

If there were wounded awaiting care, a helicopter could land on the small pad at the front line itself. The Chinese and North Koreans gave those choppers about 2 minutes to alight, pick up one or two wounded, and take off before they resumed shelling of the area. This local custom of military medical chivalry brought severe yet still salvageable wounds to the MASH soon after injury. If there were Chinese or North Korean soldiers wounded from a patrol the previous night, we took care of them also. The gunners knew that.

The battalion aid stations were mere hutments or caves surrounded by sandbags, often on a steep slope, and subject to enemy artillery fire. Probably most of these shells had been lobbed toward the front line, but being a little bit long, they came down just behind it and lit on the steep slope in the region of the battalion aid stations. The wounds cared for in these aid stations were in many cases less severe than those selected for the immediate helicopter ride.

It was at the battalion aid stations that my belief was reinforced—as if such reinforcement would ever be necessary—that the soundest medical education consists of good basic physiology, anatomy, biochemistry, and pathology. In the words of A. Baird Hastings, our teacher of biochemistry, "The most practical thing in the world is sound basic research." To this, add "and teaching." The young doctors in those battalion aid stations had just finished their internships and many had no interest in a career in surgery. Yet there they were, faced with some of the most urgent surgical problems you could imagine. They were not treating casualties by rote but rather by superior intelligence. These young doctors could think on their feet, applying their knowledge of physiology, anatomy, and biochemistry and often improvising brilliant solutions to seemingly insoluble problems. They obtained battery-powered electrocardiograms for those with wounds around the heart or lungs, seeking the most accurate evaluation possible as to what organs were injured and deciding whether or not an immediate operation was required. Although these young medical officers transfused a lot of blood, they didn't waste the precious stuff. They examined their patients in great detail and made precise diagnoses of the nature and extent of their wounds. For the most part, those battalion aid stations did not have x-ray machines, although one or two had small ones that could operate on portable generators. If major surgery was required (as in a belly wound, for example), the patient was promptly shuttled back to the MASH by jeep or chopper.

Occasionally, among those young doctors, I would encounter one of our medical students of a year or two before who had taken my courses and sometimes quoted some aspect of our studies in improving the care of burned or wounded patients. That certainly was a thrill for me.

The Case of a Severely Wounded Soldier

One of my memorable patients (because of the coincidence of long follow-up) was a large, handsome, athletically built young black soldier. This soldier had been wounded by a shell or mine fragment entering the right upper quadrant of his abdomen, the chunk of steel emerging through his chest in back. One need not have studied human anatomy to realize that such a wound as this might involve liver, diaphragm, lung, and pleural cavity. Being a shell fragment rather than a bullet, it was destructive. Slow. Irregular. Wobbling. Not like the clean wound of a high-velocity bullet.

Because he was wounded at night, he was brought to a battalion aid station rather than being taken immediately by chopper to a MASH. I happened to be there at the time, and I helped a young lieutenant start transfusions and get the patient stabilized. At dawn we called a chopper to take him back to the MASH. Choppers could not fly unless the ground was continuously visible. That meant no flights at night or in thick fog.

An hour or two later I went back to that MASH and assisted a young major in the operation. The upper part of the patient's liver was badly shredded. Fortunately, no major bleeding persisted or else he would have died at the aid station. The right lower lobe of his lung was also severely torn. We knew we were going to have plenty of trouble with this combined injury. Dirt, shreds of uniform, and dead tissue were cleaned away, removed, debrided. One lobe of his lung had to be removed along with a portion of his liver. The diaphragm was sutured, some drains were placed, including a drain into his common bile duct, and the wound was closed loosely to prevent trapped infection, always a threat in dirty war wounds.

Within a few days, that which we had feared became evident. A bronchobiliary fistula developed, a situation rarely encountered in civilian surgery. This is an abnormal opening (fistula) connecting the biliary tract (which normally conducts clear brown bile into the gastrointestinal tract) with the bronchial tree (the system of airways leading down into the lung). In no way could his body form the necessary scar tissue fast enough to close off this opening made by the traveling shell fragment. From time to time he would cough up bile, and it would also emerge from the drainage tracts. Because of our drains, this bile leak was not fatal. Maybe not fatal, but extremely unpleasant.

As soon as it was possible, we reoperated, closing off the bronchobiliary opening by interposing some healthy tissue. We then re-expanded the remaining lung and tucked the liver back where it belonged. Chancy, dangerous surgery so soon after a major wound. He seemed to do quite well, although the large gash remained in his upper abdomen and back.

By coincidence, a couple of weeks later I saw this same soldier while I was making rounds at a base hospital in Japan where the wounded were taken before being sent back home, the most blessed event that could happen to them. He was doing well. He recognized me, put out his hand, and said, "Thanks." I asked him about his plane rides, when he was going home, and where home was. Soon. Detroit. He smiled warmly at the thought. I had a good look at his dressing and his healing wound. The bronchobiliary fistula was closed and dry. Our repair had held. He was beginning to heal up, and soon he would be back home.

One of the many good things that the Army Medical Corps did was to see to it that men who were evacuated to the States were taken to major hospitals near their homes and folks. I can imagine the joy and cheering and good times when this husky soldier, now thin and wan but still handsome, arrived in Detroit. The wonders of surgical convalescence, the help surgeons give, the support of people you love and need. Getting better. And getting people well.

Japan, and Home

Back in Japan, visiting MacArthur's headquarters (I never got to meet the general himself) and our base hospitals, the scene was one of planned organization, rigid discipline. The advance northward into China, the counterattack by the Chinese, and the winter retreat leading finally to the peace talks all occurred after my visit and somewhat to the east of the area where I had been working.

With World War II in the more distant past and the bitter, agonizing national pain over Vietnam yet to come, this interim war in Korea has been caught in between and somewhat forgotten by history. Yet by its sheer magnitude in terms of American casualties and commitment, as well as the terrible destruction wrought by artillery and bombs, the Korean War was big enough and bad enough to occupy the full attention of this country for several anxious years. With new tensions in Korea, that war may be coming back into historical focus. In any event, its surgical lessons have never been forgotten.

I was away from this country only briefly (2 months). This was nothing compared with the experience of many friends who spent 3 to 5 years in the service during World War II. But even this short visit gave me a glimpse of the surgical problems peculiar to the military and a more realistic view of the human suffering of war. Suffering borne with stoicism and sometimes even humor. I gained a great deal of respect for our average American GI and his young surgeon.

Every war and each battle is fought in a different cultural and physical environment. The nature of the political engagement itself, the weapons used, and the natural environment determine the surgical and medical needs. But the reaction of men under fire, the unrelieved stress of lethal threat, and the plight of the severely wounded have remained unchanged over the centuries. Now, as always, the mercy of prompt surgical care and expert nursing is the only balm for wartime suffering.

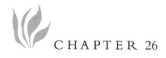

CHAPTER 26

Ibn Saud: Caring for the Royal Family of Arabia

(1961)

Now and then most everyone has a dream that turns out to be an uncannily accurate and detailed prophecy of things to come. Extrasensory perception? A space-time warp?

On a certain Wednesday night in November 1961, I had a vivid dream about being in an oriental court with a robed and burnoosed king. His court was elaborate, Persian rugs under tents. Primitive regal splendor, but at the same time brutal and ominous. In a desert. A detailed picture. I thought nothing of it save for a lingering question: "Why now?" I told Laurie about it and went about my usual day. Breakfast. Off to the hospital.

That afternoon we were in the midst of our weekly Thursday afternoon student seminar, meeting with some fourth-year students who were presenting informal papers for discussion and criticism. About half-way through the seminar, around 4:30 PM, I heard the telephone ring in the outer office. Not unusual. But then Doris Lewis, my secretary, interrupted the class and asked me to pick up the phone. Highly unusual. She had a funny look in her eye. I knew it was important. It was the U.S. State Department asking if I could leave that afternoon for Saudi Arabia to attend their ailing king, Abdul Aziz, Ibn Saud. He was sick and his doctors had sent for me.

This event would change my life for a while and my view of the

260

Arab world and the Moslem religion for a long time. Six months earlier I had been a guest at the American University of Beirut in Lebanon, attending the Middle East Medical Assembly, where I had given several papers on a variety of surgical topics. There I had met an American surgeon, William Taylor, who had come from his job in Dhahran, Saudi Arabia. He was a full-time physician for the Arabian-American Oil Company (ARAMCO), the principal agent for export of Arabian oil to Europe and the United States. The relationship of Saudi Arabia to ARAMCO, and through that corporative intermediary to the United States, was very close.

When I met Taylor at the medical assembly, we did not discuss Saudi Arabia, ARAMCO, the trans-Arabian pipeline (TAPCO), or the royal family of Saudi Arabia, but instead talked about some of the projects I had been working on and some of the medical problems he had to cope with in Arabia. When the king became ill, the decision to call me was in response to Bill Taylor's suggestion.

Flying to Arabia was an experience in itself. Although I had visited several out-of-the-way places in the world, including a few primitive Third World countries, I had never visited one under the iron hand of a rich, despotic royal dynasty. When we reached Saudi Arabia, it was night. From the high-flying plane all we could see were hundreds of fires from the towering exhaust pipes of the oil rigs. These fires were not oil wells burning (as we saw after the desert war with Iraq in 1991), but rather the constant burning off of the flow of natural gas that was emitted in huge amounts from rigs on the big dome near Dhahran. This can be seen in some American refineries and oil fields, but not over such a large area, extending to both horizons. A great deal of energy was being wasted on the cold desert air.

Shortly after my arrival I was taken to see the king. He was practically blind (not totally blind, because he could see a bit around the edges of his cataracts). He had a problem with recurring pain in his chest and abdomen. In addition, he had developed a ventral (abdominal) hernia and a groin hernia lower down. Because of his pain (unrelated to the hernias), medical specialists (from England) had already recorded several electrocardiograms. In their opinion, the king had not suffered a heart attack.

The king, with his blindness, undiagnosed chronic abdominal

pain, and more than a suggestion of severe liver disease, certainly could not be cared for adequately in Arabia, even in the shiny new hospital that ARAMCO had built in Dhahran for its American employees, where Bill Taylor had been in charge. It was clear to me that the king should come to Boston.

Making a plan for the king required not only the usual examinations, x-rays, and consultations, but also a meeting with the king's brother, Faisal, who was then the ranking prince and presumed successor to the throne. I remained in Dhahran for less than a week while the royal retinue got organized. I was given a brief tour down the Persian Gulf coast to Qatar, one of the coastal Emirates, to catch a glimpse of the culture of the Arabian peninsula. The eye-seeking black flies on the faces of infants. The peasants and commoners who were not only poverty-stricken but living in primitive and disease-ridden conditions, literally on the sand. The people were several centuries out of phase with their royalty, who sped by in Cadillacs, dust flying.

To bring the king to Boston, ARAMCO hired a large jet that could accommodate about 100 people. They filled it not only with the king and his immediate retinue, but also with his chief of state (an intelligent, highly educated Arabian aristocrat who was an expert on Middle Eastern history), various sheiks and hangers-on, and four of his favorite concubines. I rode with the crew in the cockpit of this huge plane. We landed at Naples to refuel. Coming in at night, airport runway ahead, a royal retinue behind, it was certainly a moment to wonder at the experiences a lifetime in surgery can bring.

The Royal Retinue

Of all the king's retinue two persons were especially notable. One was the announcer. He was a large black man, a royal slave from the Horn of Africa, about 7 feet tall. His bare chest was crossed with bandoliers filled with ammunition, running from shoulder to hip, and he carried a loaded automatic rifle. His job was to tell everyone what was going on. Back in the camel days, radio was not available to do the job. Hence the announcer.

The other remarkable person was a small, rotund schemer and

specialist on insider influence, sinister in both appearance and reality, known as Sheikh Id (pronounced "share-eed"). He was always fully burnoosed, bejeweled headband in place. Id was crucial to the maintenance of the king as an institution. His closest personal confidant. There is no truly analogous person in our government; the closest parallel might be a few of the president's White House advisors, some of whom in the last 20 years have turned out to be equally adept as schemers, plotters, and influence-peddlers.

There was no simple way to get rid of Sheikh Id. Nothing whatsoever could be done about him, even by the ARAMCO executive who was a specialist on the royal family and stayed with us throughout the entire episode. Sheikh Id was the ultimate power behind the throne, although he was usually found in front of it.

The king had 55 daughters and 45 sons, or so it was said, a low batting average, considering the value placed on male offspring in the Moslem world. He was falling behind the 0.500 mark. Nonetheless, many of these princes and princesses were upset by Sheikh Id and his manipulations around their father, without his or their approval. I never became party to any of this intrigue. That would have been even more unhealthy than what I was already doing.

About 4 years later we noticed in the paper that there had been a suspicious accident on a flight from Saudi Arabia to Switzerland. The plane appeared to have been sabotaged. The crash occurred in the Alps. Not much was found. Well planned. One of the passengers listed was a certain Sheikh Id. The newspaper just listed the names; the press didn't know about Id. Possibly somebody had decided to eliminate him. Too bad this had to take so many others with him. Whatever his ultimate fate, we just had to put up with Id as best we could.

A Diplomatic Welcome

Our hospital administrator, William Hassan, of Lebanese descent, did a superb job during all the pomp and splendor of the royal visit. He spoke Arabic naturally and fluently. The choice top floor of the private wing of the Brigham was given over to the royal family. The head nurse there, Miss Bunevith, was not only an excellent nurse but also a diplomat.

She took care of the Arabian entourage with great talent, finding places for both Id and the announcer. While by current standards such might be regarded as a misuse of hospital beds, it is not every day one is called upon to attend royalty.

I had always been a little skeptical of formally garbed state department types wearing spats and double-breasted vests. Black fedoras. On the second day of the king's stay, one such functionary came to visit the king, preceded by suitable fanfare from the announcer. He had brought the king a gift from President Kennedy, who also sent a bunch of roses daily.

Arabic is a difficult language. Few Westerners have mastered it. Lots of nouns. For example, the words for white horse, black horse, brown horse, and chestnut horse are each different nouns. I ushered our impressive diplomat into the royal presence and introduced him to the king via the announcer and an interpreter. We had sidetracked Id for the moment. Our state department dignitary sat down beside the king. I remained there for a moment, wondering what would transpire when an elegantly clad state department official visited the king of a desert empire, sick in bed. Our diplomat immediately began conversing in fluent Arabic. The king broke out in a broad smile. He was immensely pleased and delighted. There and then I dropped my prejudice about pretentious state department types.

At a medical meeting about that time, one of my friends asked, "But Franny, what did you do with the concubines?" Answer, "The nurses' home, of course." Our student nurses took good care of the harem, gave them plenty to eat, and showed them where to spend their fortunes on clothing even though clothing was often stated by detractors to be unnecessary for their principal function. They were pleasant women who did not conform to the *Playboy* image of the slim, suave, largely nude inhabitants of a harem. More like plump peasants well draped in voluminous silk dresses with long sweeping skirts.

Caring for the King

The king's blindness (due to cataracts, with only a trace of trachoma) was reversed by our ophthalmological surgeon, Trygve

Gundersen. Once the king's eyesight was restored, he fired all his concubines.

The surgical procedures on the king were fairly simple ones. I explored his abdomen, hoping to find the source of his pain, and repaired his hernias. It became evident that he suffered from severe cirrhosis of the liver. Devout Muslims are never supposed to touch alcohol. Although cirrhosis can be produced by substances other than alcohol, it is nevertheless a common cause in the Arab world.

We took x-ray pictures of the king and in each we found bullets. Several of them in various places. These were the low-velocity missiles of muskets used in the many battles and small wars in which he had fought alongside his father, liberating and uniting the peoples of the Arabian peninsula after World War I, following the demise of the oppressive Ottoman Empire.

It soon became apparent that medical help for the royal family of Saud would not be confined to the king but would be extended to most of his retinue and relatives (many of whom arrived later) and would be provided by many members of the Brigham staff; the public health and tropical medicine experts at Harvard, including the School of Public Health; and even the pediatric staff at Children's Hospital. The king sent for several princes and princesses (some of them children), ministers, and palace guards in need of medical help. One of the elegant, sophisticated, educated, and beautiful young princesses (many of whom had been sent to Paris for their education) had an ominous bone cancer from which she later died.

Arabian Days...

During their visit, our Arabian guests provided some diverting moments.

Coincidentally, the president of the Boston Red Sox baseball club, Thomas Yawkey, a distinguished and respected sports figure, was a patient in the hospital on the floor below the king, and he asked if he could pay a call on His Royal Highness. We ushered him into the royal presence with both Sheikh Id and the announcer in attendance. He made a short polite speech with good humor and friendly jokes expressing the hope that the king might come to a Red Sox game before he returned to Arabia. After what had obviously involved considerable thought and planning, Mr. Yawkey presented the king with a brand new baseball autographed by the entire Red Sox team, including Ted Williams.

After a polite acknowledgment, smiles, and bows by the attendants and leisurely coffee all around, (and of course an announcement by the announcer), the king examined the baseball carefully, staring at it, feeling it, turning it over in his hand. Then he held it up to the light and said slowly and clearly (via his interpreter): "What does one do with this object?" Before anyone could reply, he asked for a pen, autographed the ball with his scrawl, scarcely more legible than an X, and returned it with a broad and contented smile to an astonished Mr. Yawkey. There are some situations that you just can't do anything about.

Pouring midmorning coffee involved a bit of ceremony. An expert servant (always male, often a tall black slave) took a long-snouted, burnished-silver coffee pot and held it up with one arm, as high as he could. In his other hand he held, as low as he could, a small beautifully gilded coffee cup. Then he poured a long, thin stream of steaming hot coffee from the pot to the cup. Not a drop was spilled. No comment. No praise. Try it sometime. But not over your wife's best carpet. To qualify for this exercise, the coffee must be boiling hot.

The ARAMCO executive told us that the Arabian royalty prized as slaves the tall, handsome African people from the Horn of Africa just across the Strait of Hormuz. The women were retained as wives or concubines. The men performed many tasks, were often honored, and in time had their own slaves: slaves' slaves. Whatever the nature of this abject captivity or enlightened bondage (we never knew which), we did not learn any more about it and were advised not to inquire.

The king enjoyed giving away wristwatches. He had hundreds of gold Swiss watches with his picture on the watch face. These he distributed liberally, starting with the airplane crew. All members of my family received one. He also gave us a beautiful silken flowing robe, along with a burnoose (a jeweled headband) and a gold-plated belt and dagger. Some of my children used this costume to good advantage in school plays.

... *and Nights*

At one point during the king's stay, Laurie and I gave a dinner for the Saudi Secretary of State and invited several scholars of Middle Eastern history from Harvard and other universities, some from as far away as U.C. Berkeley. The Secretary of State spoke fluent English and was an elegant conversationalist. He was a remarkable resource on Arabian and all of Middle Eastern history, much of it still unwritten. Our former teacher and professor at the MGH, Edward Churchill, had spent a good deal of time in the Middle East at the American University of Beirut and was pleased to meet the Saudi secretary at our dinner.

Finally, after several months, the king and his retinue made ready to return to Arabia, with a stopover in Florida. Before they left Boston, ARAMCO arranged a huge banquet at the Copley Plaza Hotel in Boston. Laurie and a few other wives were invited. Although Laurie had not yet met the king, we had entertained several of his retinue at that dinner for the secretary of state.

Many of our most eminent senior staff in medicine and cardiology were Jewish. They had consulted on and helped care for the royal family without complaining about the partiality being shown the royal retinue; these staff members were invited to the banquet and came. I was proud of our staff for their cooperation and backing. It was a rather quiet time in Arab-Jewish relations. In fact, at the time of my previous visit to Lebanon, there were even Jewish students at the American University of Beirut and Jewish doctors at the Middle East Medical Assembly. Never, since.

After the banquet at the Copley, the king and his group went to Florida and rented a large villa in Palm Beach. Trygve and Harriet Gundersen and Laurie and I were invited down there to visit. We had dinner with the king. It is very difficult for us in our culture to realize how absolutely unprecedented it was for two women to be guests at dinner with the Arabian king.

Our sedate dinner was an event. The king was dressed in his Arabian robes with his crown headband inlaid with jewels (our guess was rubies, diamonds, and pearls) and a gold-plated dagger in his belt. His lower legs were bare, as were his feet. In this unfamiliar environment of mixed company, strangers at that, he kept nervously adjusting his robe to cover his lower legs, much like a woman sitting in a chair with too short a skirt who self-consciously keeps trying to pull it down to lengthen it, but to no avail.

We attempted to converse with him through an interpreter but the interchange was sparse. We gained some solace from the knowledge that we, and especially our female companions, were experiencing something of the utmost rarity: an informal coeducational dinner with the king of Arabia. His discourse was polite and gentlemanly, and he seemed to enjoy his unusual company very graciously.

After he returned to Arabia, the king survived for a short time, his condition essentially unchanged. He died (in 1964), presumably of a heart attack, and his brother Faisal took over.

Faisal, and a Transient Hope of Liberalization

I had met Prince (later King) Faisal the evening before our departure from Arabia on the king's chartered plane. This meeting was a colorful event. At night, with covert-secrecy-security precautions, I was driven over the open desert in a large, black stretch Cadillac to Prince Faisal's portable palace, a large, tented structure designed to accommodate him during his journey from Riyadh to Dhahran because of his brother's ill health. I entered the huge, compartmented tent, where magnificent Arabian carpets were spread directly over sand, as the floor. On entering, I first passed between two upright burning, smoking, knotted logs of the type we associate with medieval castles. Then a trumpet sounded. Escorted by another prince, with our interpreter immediately behind me, I walked between two rows of huge black men dressed only in breechclouts, ammunition bandoliers crossed over their chests, shiny golden swords crossed over my head, and entered the throne room where sat Prince Faisal. A graduate of Princeton, he said in perfect English: "Welcome, Dr. Moore. Won't you tell me about His Royal Highness?"

Prince Faisal, though not as visible as Sheikh Id, had much more to say about what transpired on the international scene. Sheikh Id was strictly local. Faisal was in striking contrast to most of the other Arabian men we saw. Not only was he educated at an Ivy League college, but he was also married to an American lady and was monogamous. When his wife became queen, she introduced education for women, founded a women's university, and began to make some long overdue changes in Arabian society. At that time, partly because of Faisal, women were not always required to wear a chador. A few years later, with King Faisal's Queen in charge, the liberation of Arabian women was well under way. Faisal instituted economic and legal reforms. Then the inevitable occurred. Faisal was assassinated. In Arabia, primogeniture is not the custom. Rule (and/or wealth) often passes to a brother or cousin. With such huge families there are lots of choices. Another brother succeeded to the throne.

Although I have not followed the matter closely, I have learned from more recent visitors that Arabia—now 20 years after Faisal, and possibly dominated by Iran— has again reverted to a fundamentalist Moslem posture, the women being shielded and chadored. The immense injustices of their society have become further entrenched. These customs are seen as injustices not only in women's eyes, but also in the eyes of many of the younger generation of Arabian men and women, especially those who have visited the West. Under Ibn Saud there was a beginning liberalization (rather slow and mostly by default) that was given new impetus and support by Faisal (intentional and well planned but brief). But now has come the retreat to severe social and political, and strict religious, fundamentalism.

Images remain of the sadness of a proud old society, its ruling dynasty unable to cope with the wealth and temptations thrust upon it by a fluke of geology: the Dhahran oil dome. Images too of a sick, primitive, unsophisticated but kindly king overtaken by history.

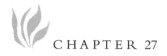

CHAPTER 27

The Midnight to Washington: National Responsibilities

octors and medical scientists fall into that large class of people whose expert knowledge is considered useful to government. This group wends its way to the banks of the Potomac on repeated occasions. In my early days this trip was made via the midnight train to Washington. My ties have been with the Army, the National Research Council, the National Academy of Sciences, the National Institutes of Health (NIH), the Uniformed Services University of the Health Sciences, and the National Aeronautics and Space Administration (NASA). In case that seems like a long and pretentious list, I should remind the reader that I have been at it since 1942 (about 53 years).

The Surgeon General's Committee

In 1952, after my return from Korea as a consultant to the Army, I reported my findings to the Surgeon General. Consequently, he asked me to visit army research units both in this country and abroad to review their research and their role in teaching army medical officers. On the basis of this work, I was asked by the Surgeon General to chair a new committee on the metabolic care of wounds and burns. Part of the job of our committee was to visit such hospital units to review their studies and plans. We journeyed to army medical research units in San Francisco,

Denver, and San Antonio, and to army-sponsored burn units, such as that in Charleston, South Carolina.

The largest unit for the care of burns in the United States was the Army Surgical Research Institute at the Brooke Army Medical Center in San Antonio. This unit developed rapidly during the 1950s and still remains the treatment center where severely burned service personnel are flown from all over the world. As one of the foremost burn units in the world, it has produced many remarkable advances in burn care. Surgeons who later took leadership positions in civilian burn units had studied there, including John Moncrief, Curtis Artz, Everett Evans, Bruce McMillan, Basil Pruitt, and Douglas Wilmore.

Early in its history, the San Antonio Burn Unit was the scene of a disaster when the whole unit was overwhelmed by a bacterium called *Pseudomonas aeruginosa*. Although this organism rarely causes disease in otherwise healthy people, it can be both invasive and destructive in a debilitated and severely ill burned patient. Once this germ becomes established in a hospital, it is difficult to banish completely because it resides in dust on the floor and walls as well as on bedding, utensils, and even drinking-water vessels unless these articles are all heat sterilized. *Pseudomonas* adheres to the person and clothing of physicians and nurses unless they are extremely careful.

Those in charge of the San Antonio Burn Unit and our consultant committee were slow to recognize that this severe, localized, self-perpetuating epidemic was due to an especially virulent strain of the bacterium and that patients, personnel, walls, and floors were harboring it. Once confronted, this epidemic was overcome by heroic methods of isolation and the restoration of structural and total environmental cleanliness. This burn unit was not the only one to suffer the blight of uncontrolled *Pseudomonas* infection. Several others elsewhere in the country developed the same plague and could be cleansed only by equally heroic measures. Our own burn unit at the Brigham was threatened, but fortunately we were able to eradicate the contamination in time to prevent the infection from reaching epidemic proportions. The San Antonio contamination had given us a warning.

As a consultant to the Surgeon General, I was also asked to witness, for the first (and only) time in my life, what I considered to be unethical experiments on human beings. Several members of our committee and one or two from other consultant groups were singled out to go on a secret mission. We were not told much about it and had to go through a loyalty-security-psychological clearance process even more rigorous than that ordinarily expected for army consultants. After this we were flown to a secret base, the exact location of which we never learned, where antipersonnel gases were being tested on volunteers from among our own GIs.

These nerve gases were not the quickly lethal ones being developed by the armies of many nations at that time. Such deadly poisons could be tested on animals for both offensive and defensive purposes. Instead, these were psychoactive gases that disorient people so they are unable to understand or obey commands, unable to determine direction or purpose. These gases depersonalize troops. Scramble their brains. Knowing what I did about drugs and anesthetics, I realized that in testing such dangerous gases there would be the problem of dose variability, especially since the gases were inhaled. Some of these volunteers could inhale large doses by pure chance with possibly severe or permanent brain damage. And as for the concept of volunteers, this was analogous to the ethical problem of doing experiments on prisoners. Who wouldn't volunteer if it got you out of prison? These young men got a lot of special perks as well as early discharge from the service in exchange for acting as guinea pigs to test nerve gases, or rather antipersonnel measures.

I was shocked by this. We were told, "An enemy will use it on us so we must know how to protect ourselves and counteract its effects." This argument is hard to fight. After the flight back to Washington, I slinked home to Boston, shaken and humiliated. I had seen something I was powerless to stop or control and realized it was only a small bit of what might be going on. On many other occasions I had seen the results of bullets and explosives (including nuclear blasts) tested on animals. I was accustomed to the realities of military research. But this was different.

Later on, some of these volunteers exhibited delayed emotional problems and self-destructive behavior. It was hard to know what was cause or effect. I never knew the answer. I suspected that in this instance the medical establishment—stressed by Korea and Vietnam and motivated by an urgent need for defense—had crossed a clear ethical boundary.

Later, too, as I was to learn over the course of several decades, our government has been especially vulnerable to accusations of careless disregard in the handling of the hazards of radiation injury and causes of suspected or real injury. As an institution, our government is prone to cover up or gloss over allegations that discredit either individuals or institutions such as the Army, Navy, NIH, Atomic Energy Commission, or any other large agency. If these matters of potential embarrassment pertain to bodily or psychological damage affecting troops or the public, or miners of uranium, or those living near nuclear plants or test sites, or workers with nuclear material, or patients in a government-sponsored radiation experiment, otherwise sensible officials become pathologically protective. Those "psycho" gases, and radiation exposure in nuclear plants and bomb testing were prime examples. "Truth is the first casualty of war"—but also of certain peacetime activities. Otherwise upright servants of the people become liars or tell their subordinates to lie.

Where there has been harm, or the suspicion of harm, beware a government spokesman or news release. Government agencies will admit a billion-dollar deficit or a billion-dollar cost overrun on an aircraft carrier. But when a person may have been hurt or killed, the reflex of government is to cover it up. If it is radiation that is the root cause of harm to people, even less will be said. There is a blind spot here about which I have become increasingly alarmed and apprehensive. A consultant such as myself, secure in his or her civilian position, must speak out about untruths or errors he perceives. Whether his perception be right or wrong in the eyes of history, if he does not speak out about this, who can?

Another duty of our committee of the Army Medical Corps was to review research proposals for funding. A tension, sometimes bitter, arises between animal researchers and the antivivisectionists. Usually I side with the researchers, but there were exceptions. An example was embodied in one proposal from a prominent medical school that was reviewed on several occasions. Because we were uncertain about the methods being used, I visited the laboratories. I considered those particular experiments on burned animals to be unnecessarily and unacceptably cruel and painful. The animals were not kept under anesthesia. A long and painful healing process often ended in death. How would such arcane and convoluted research help the care of burned people? I was no antivivisectionist and had done many animal experiments, but based on my reservations here we had the unpleasant duty of cutting off funding for that research completely. I made some bitter enemies; later they came to understand. This decision was decades before raids on labs by antivivisectionists and front-page stories from insiders about unacceptable conditions in animal experimentation.

On another occasion we visited a laboratory directed by a prominent surgeon, working under contract from the armed services, only to find that the work described in the proposals was not being carried out at all. Nowadays this breech would be considered science fraud and would probably attract the attention of the Congress. But at that time we were feeling our way with the review process. We took away the research grant. The "midnight to Washington" sometimes could impose an impressive burden.

NIH Surgery Study Section

Looking back on years of work with the NIH brings to mind a different yet typical experience.

The scene now changes to a neat office building on the campus of the NIH in Bethesda, a few miles north of the district line and across the street from the National Naval Medical Center and the Uniformed Services University of the Health Sciences. A group of 15 or 20 of us, mostly surgeons, would be sitting in a conference room there. With us would be one or two administrators and an executive secretary. At each place at the large table would be a neat pad flanked by several sharpened pencils. Also at each place would be a huge pile of research grants to discuss, copies of which we had already received. Coffee and danish on the sideboard. This scene was repeated hundreds of times every year: a consultant committee to some agency of the government—such as the NIH—meeting to vote on the acceptability for government funding of proposals from research labs all over this country and in Europe. We were determining make-or-break decisions on 100 or 150 research grant proposals seeking support, several millions of taxpayer dollars, for research on surgical topics in the medical schools of the United States and in a few universities abroad.

For me, this scene became a habit about 1956, a time when the NIH university grants programs were expanding rapidly. Specifically, it was the moment of opportunity for our government to support further development and perfection of pump-oxygenators for open-heart surgery as described in Chapter 23. I was working my 3-year stint as chairman of the NIH Surgery Study Section (1958 to 1961).

During World War II, financial support for research on the surgical care of the wounded was channeled through the Office of Scientific Research and Development (OSRD), a collaborative enterprise undertaken under the direction of the National Research Council (NRC), which is, in turn, an operating arm of the National Academy of Sciences (NAS). NAS was founded by Abraham Lincoln at the time of the Civil War precisely for such purposes: to put the scientific brains of the country to work for the common good.

In 1946 at the close of World War II, the OSRD function of channeling federal money to university laboratories was transferred to the NIH. Although OSRD funding for biomedical research during World War II seemed to be as generous as would befit a nation at war, it was but a pittance compared with the budgets soon to be voted annually by the Congress for university research through the NIH. At the peak of NIH funding, outlays for research—i.e., the total voted each year by the Congress for the support of medical research—was often in excess even of that requested by the administration. We were at the threshold of a heyday that persisted through the 1960s and 1970s before a tendency to scale back the annual increases became evident in the 1980s. By the standards of any other nation we are still very liberal in our public support of research.

The Surgery Study Section supported NIH funding for the majority of research undertaken to perfect the extracorporeal pump-oxygenator. This device was essential to the development of the field of open-heart surgery, yet its use now is so routine that it is rarely mentioned as an integral part of heart surgery. We arranged and funded the first international conference on extracorporeal pump oxygenation, bringing together surgeons, physicians, physiologists, biochemists, and mechanical engineers from all over the world to exchange data and ideas and help bring this device to its present state of perfection. It was this piece of machinery that made open-heart surgery possible and has been essential to the performance of heart transplantation.

The Uniformed Services University of the Health Sciences (USUHS)

A scene from the opening ceremonies of the USUHS on August 25, 1977, will display some of the Washington that we enjoyed. It was a brisk and windy day, bright sun with a few scudding puffball clouds. Laurie and I were sitting with a small group of men and women (most attired in the uniforms of the several services) in the imposing grove of tall and handsome pine trees in the low hills directly southeast of the U. S. Naval Medical Center in Bethesda, Maryland. Behind us was a large brick building, still in the final stages of construction. A naval band was blaring away, too loud and too close. We were there to celebrate the admission of the first class of medical students to the USUHS, the first full-time regular medical school since the American Revolution to be operated entirely by the federal government. It was a remarkable moment. There were speeches. David Packard, formerly Deputy Secretary of Defense, was the chairman of the Board of Regents. The board also included the surgeons general of the three armed services, as well as those of the Public Health Service and the Army Nurse Corps. Members of that board, together with spouses, joined in the celebration. Mr. Packard's address was one of pride at the accomplishment of building the new university. The President of the University, Anthony R. Curreri, a surgeon of our generation and Professor of Surgery at the University of Wisconsin, also spoke. Jay Sanford was the dean; Norman Rich was the first Professor of Surgery.

During World War I some medical courses had been given at the Walter Reed Army Medical Center to apprise the medical officers of the conditions they would face in France when treating men wounded in trench warfare. Sixty years before, during the Civil War, and again for a short time in the 1890s there had been a semblance of an army medical school in Washington. Walter Reed had been dean.

During World War II the need for medical personnel became more urgent. Medical officers of the Army and Navy (at that time there was no separate air force) would be better able to accomplish their mission with special training. New sorts of wounds needed new treatments: new conditions of war in desert or tropics, new diseases, and tropical parasites, as well as old diseases typical of overcrowded conditions and poor sanitation.

The government therefore recognized the need to provide an educational setting and postgraduate training for physicians in all the uniformed services (Army, Navy, Air Force, Coast Guard, and Public Health Service). This school was to be under the Department of Defense, also a creation of the postwar years. But it was not until the middle of the Vietnam War that a bill to establish such a medical school finally became law. Congressman F. Edward Hébert of Louisiana was the most vocal and persistent of advocates, so the medical school bears his name. His bill to establish the school had been signed into law by President Nixon in September 1972. A Board of Regents was established in May 1973 by presidential appointment, and an entirely new program of medical education for the armed services was gradually brought to life. I was appointed to the board in 1976 by President Ford.

The original idea was to provide specialized training to meet the needs of the military for physicians and surgeons, medical technicians, corpsmen, and nurses. At that time about 6 million servicemen and dependents scattered all over the world were cared for by the physicians, nurses, and hospitals of the armed services. While it was clear that our new medical school could never provide all the doctors needed for such an immense defense establishment, it could supply at least a few medical leaders committed to a career in uniform.

Now we were gathered to celebrate the admission of our first small class of 32 students—to be the class of 1981—and to dedicate the newly completed building. This was the initial proud step of that federal medical school. Later, when that first class graduated, Lewis Thomas—a leading interpreter of medical science—gave the commencement address. The second class had 62 students and by 1985 classes had increased in size to over 150 men and women, as mandated by the 1972 statute.

The mounting cost of medical education makes it hard if not impossible for many would-be students (and their parents) to afford it. Tuition was on the rise, but in most cases it was still far less than the true cost of educating the student. There were never enough scholarships and fellowships to take care of everybody. The financial arrangements for medical students at USUHS were (and still remain) unique. Each student is an officer in his or her service of choice, holding the rank of second lieutenant or ensign, and is paid an officer's salary—a good way to get around the problem of tuition. As you can imagine, the school has many applicants and is able to select an outstanding class.

Clinical courses (for example, in medicine, surgery, pediatrics, or obstetrics) are taught in the Army, Navy, and Air Force hospitals around Washington and around the country, as well as those in the Pacific and in Europe. The Clinical Center at the NIH is also available for teaching fourth-year courses. The students can elect courses in service hospitals hundreds or thousands of miles away.

Even before their first academic courses begin, the students receive field indoctrination in their particular branch of the armed services. If the Army, they might spend those first few weeks working with a tank, infantry, or artillery battalion. If the Navy, their first indoctrination might be in submarines. Most of the students choosing the Air Force option would already be flyers, but now they would be flying with other pilots in a variety of planes.

As befits the intense activities of a service career, physical fitness was always a part of the student mystique at USUHS. Dean Sanford exemplified this aspect of a service-related lifestyle and led mountain-climbing expeditions on the local Potomac precipices. The students were an orderly group. "Regimented," some critics would carp. That was not our impression. Hair was cut to conform to the dress code. Handsome young men and women well dressed and neat in their uniforms make an appealing sight whether the appeal is humanistic, patriotic, or just plain aesthetic. At commencement, as the students marched to their places, you were reminded of the order and discipline associated with West Point, Annapolis, or Colorado Springs. Quite a contrast to the costume so prevalent among college students of the 1960s and 1970s: untrimmed beard, long hair and headband, sandals, and sloppy jeans (including a guitar).

Periodically, the USUHS has come under fire from the Congress because it seems an expensive luxury to train medical officers specifically to care for the millions of people in uniform or their dependents when there is no way—beyond obligatory service for a minimum of 8 years—to ensure that they will stay on the job. The cessation of the Cold War and the consequent dissipation of the Soviet threat are likely to erode Congressional support for this medical school. Whether or not the intent of the Congress in establishing the USUHS will in the long run be considered valid depends entirely on the number of graduate physicians who remain in the armed services for significant periods of time beyond their obligation. All these young men and women are potentially leaders in military medical care and organization. If most of them leave the service, the investment is lost. It was our hope that they would remain on duty for a significant service career before giving it up to the temptations of private practice. Although we have only 20 years to go on, initial data from our graduates suggest that the investment is paying off as planned. Visits to army and navy hospitals have reinforced my feeling that this tiny fraction of the huge defense budget was well spent.

For almost two decades the USUHS has been a part of my professional life. Appointment to this board arose from my prior service with the Army Medical Corps as a consultant in Korea and with army research sponsorship, which began 25 years earlier.

NASA

As my responsibilities at the NIH began to wind down about 1968, I was asked to become a consultant to one of the Life Sciences Advisory Committees to NASA. The space agency first asked me to join an advisory committee in 1968 when NASA was first focusing on the physiological effects of prolonged space flight. This was on the eve of the Apollo program, one of the greatest feats of manned space flight, the moon walks.

Bentley Glass, physician, physiologist, and leading scientist of the State University of New York at Stony Brook, was asked to chair this NASA Advisory Group in the Life Sciences. He invited me to be a member of that group because of my knowledge of body composition (described in Chapters 13 and 14).

Under conditions of prolonged weightlessness, the human body undergoes massive changes in body composition. There is loss of muscle mass, blood volume (both red cells and plasma are reduced), cardiac output, and skeletal mass. There is loss (by inactivity) of the blood-vessel reflexes that support our circulation in the upright posture and prevent the pooling of venous blood in our legs. These changes in space are almost entirely due to weightlessness, to lack of gravitational force for the body to resist. Nothing causes loss of muscle like inactivity: think of the size of the muscles in a paralyzed leg or a leg long immobilized in a plaster cast. Travel in a space vehicle is a form of inactivity that affects all the muscles of the body except the heart and diaphragm.

We are accustomed to life in a gravitational ambience of about 1.0 G, the gravitational force as measured on Earth at sea level. Even when we are sitting in a chair, the muscles of the back and neck are keeping us upright, and the arms may be at work. Even in bed, the tone of some muscles is maintained at a resting level, not totally relaxed. In space at 0.0 G (or, more accurately, at microgravity—about 0.001 G), such automatic antigravity exercise is no longer required, and the heart does not need to pump blood uphill to the head. Everything is "on the level." An athlete getting ready for the season gets in condition by exercise known as "conditioning." On prolonged space flight the opposite effect is seen, a state rightly called "deconditioning."

Since measurements of this phenomenon were very much a part of our studies of body composition, we were able to help with advice on how to prevent this deconditioning in space by having the astronauts exercise against spring-loaded resistance devices. You can't lift weights for exercise when a 10-pound weight can be raised from the floor like a Ping-Pong ball.

Since 1968 I have continued as member of a series of NASA advisory committees in the biomedical sciences, finally ending up as a member of the Committee of the National Academy of Sciences on the Space Station. As we collaborate with the Russian Space Agency in our new space station effort, maintenance of physical conditioning over prolonged periods of travel in space, literally space-dwelling, will be a major research target of the entire effort.

A far more severe threat to astronauts in the high orbits of interplanetary flights is their exposure to space radiation. The orbits of all manned flights thus far, except those to the Moon, have been at altitudes of 150 to 300 miles, beneath the radioprotective shield of the magnetosphere. This is called low Earth orbit, or LEO. Once emerging from the protective zone of LEO (as on a trip to the Moon and Mars, for example), the spaceship and everyone in it is exposed to severe irradiation from cosmic rays and solar flare emissions. This will be a major hazard on any future interplanetary voyages and has been the main focus of my work on the NASA committees in recent years. In March 1992 I published a review of the available data on this matter entitled "Radiation burdens for humans on prolonged exomagnetospheric voyages." This is probably the last scientific paper I will ever publish and closes out a bibliography that began with "Studies with Radioactive Di-azo Dyes" in 1943 (described in Chapter 13).

Getting There, Awake or Asleep

For decades the best way to get to these meetings was to ride via the midnight train from Boston to Washington. The sleeper. Breakfast could be taken in the diner or at Union Station. And then off by taxi to the meeting on Constitution Avenue.

Nowadays, the first plane to D.C. usually leaves Boston around 6:00 or 6:30 AM. I could usually get breakfast aboard the plane (rather sparse), go to the meeting, check in at a hotel late in the day—or stay with a friend—and then after another day or two in the nation's capital, turn around and come home again. See patients, sort the mail, and wonder if spending that much time away was worthwhile.

Looking back, it seems that 50 years ago all this government consulting was somehow more leisurely and joyous than it is today. Less hassle and less political. More the feeling of a community of scientists joining in patriotic service. Under President Nixon, even appointments to NIH advisory councils became politicized for the first time. Some of the joy of public service disappeared.

The picture on a morning plane to Washington these days (especially the first plane on Monday) is such a sight, such a genre phenomenon, as to invite more artwork and satire than it has received. All the passengers are men (very few women, children, or families). They are clad in charcoal-grey suits, almost a uniform; earnest, sometimes joshing with each other but usually quite serious. As soon as tray tables can be lowered, they take out their pencils, papers, and calculators. All have leather briefcases or little valet cases. And laptop computers.

Some are going to Washington to sit with committees to some branch of government. Others are seeking government contracts, pleading cases, or lobbying. They have risen early. Their helpful wives have dished out some coffee and maybe toast. Soon they fall asleep over their tray tables, their work and computers laid out before them. A few minutes after takeoff they are roused for a small second breakfast. Back to napping. Then the announcement of the imminent landing. Stuff the work into the briefcase. Slam the laptop closed. Up go the tables. On go the seatbelts. Then the docking. All stand up. As the door of the plane is opened the men at the head of the line start to rock back and forth from side to side; they are beginning to walk out. They rush to a taxi (sometimes to an impressive limousine, the driver in uniform) and off to their jobs.

In its most comfortable period, during the years between 1950 and 1970 or so, travel on the airlines was almost as pleasant for the traveler as the trains had been 10 or 15 years earlier. It was not difficult to get reservations. In the early days at the East Boston Airport (not yet called Logan International) you could park your car right outside the entrance to the airline terminal. You walked across a little gravel parking lot and maybe a macadam roadway, checked your bags, walked outdoors on the tarmac (a British term borrowed by the Americans) to get to the plane, and then climbed a few steps to the downward-slanting tail section. Coming back on that same airline, it was a cinch. If it was raining, well that was just too bad. Back in 1940 I remember seeing a visionary picture of an airplane loading dock in a *Popular Mechanics* magazine. We wondered then how long it would be before we could actually walk from a terminal into an airplane without going outdoors and upstairs (in the rain). Soon, most of the planes had a third (forward) landing wheel, so they sat in a horizontal position on the ground. When new, this was in striking contrast to the DC-3 and its contemporaries, which rested in a tail-down sag until going fast enough to raise the tail off the ground. Level planes and loading docks helped air travel reach its apotheosis of comfort, about 1975 to 1980.

In the early 1950s, some of the regular commercial passenger aircraft began to provide sleeping berths. On one particular occasion, I was coming back to Boston from Seattle on a night plane. It was a four-engine prop plane with a big round belly, sometimes called a pregnant C-54. The opportunity of sleeping on a berth rather than propped up in a seat looked pretty attractive. The trip was being paid for by a medical society in Seattle. The trip would take 9 or 10 hours. Plenty of time for sleep.

With the props grinding away only a few feet from my ears as a kind of a constant soporific drone, I slept quite soundly. In the morning, I struggled into my clothes (much as in the old-time Pullman upper berth) and tentatively stuck out a foot, still bare. Then with my shirt on, but wearing pajama pants, I swung down to the floor into the aisle. At that moment I was facing toward the cockpit, since I had been sleeping in the most forward of the berths.

Behind me I suddenly heard laughing and was greeted by a nice round of applause, which shook me up a bit. When I turned around I could see that my matin arousal was being monitored by the rest of the passengers, who were seated in an orderly fashion, two by two, on each side of the aisle extending back 10 or 15 rows to the rear of the plane. They greeted my descent from the upper berth as sort of a theatrical performance. My audience totalled about 45 people. Looking at these admirers, I suddenly appreciated my shortcomings. My hair was tousled, my pants unbuttoned, I had no shoes and was padding toward the lavatory a few steps away, razor and toothbrush in hand. Fortunately for me, the lavatory was unoccupied and I could hide in there until I looked a bit more presentable. I then went back to where my berth had been, only to find that there was no place to sit. I was confronted, not with a genial black Pullman porter, but with a rather prim stewardess. This was a period when the appointment of a stewardess involved some overtone of nursing skills. She was thought of not merely as a passenger-handler, but as having some healing or nursing arts in her repertoire. Female pulchritude was still sought in such employment, not yet being regarded as sexist. Because the stewardess had already put the upper berth away and was still tussling with various things on the seats, it was quite difficult for me to extricate my pants, shoes, and socks. When I went back toward the lavatory to retreat again, somebody had beaten me to it. Occupied. Locked. By now the audience response had reached high levels of laughter, and I wondered if someone like Bob Hope might have done this better than I did. I never hired a berth again. Soon, they ceased to exist.

Looking Back

For doctors who made this trip for so many years, it was most often on a mission as a consultant or committee member. After a couple of days, we would return home laden with reports and briefings that were never read as carefully as we intended. We were anxious to get home for sleep in our own bed with our own spouse, and the next day, back to a different sort of reality: the operating room, students, and rounds. I felt great sympathy for my friends who lived on the West Coast. For them, this task involved, at a minimum, a 2- or 3-day trip. But that did give them lots of time to read!

Looking back on it all I still derive some small satisfaction from realizing that these journeys and government consultations are a part of the citizen's burden. Patriotism, if you will. The tangible reward is zero. The hours lost from your own work are, over the course of years, beyond measure. There ain't no glory in it. Few people even know where you have been or why you were away. You give a lot of your own time, of your reserve energy.

In return you receive a lot: you learn about how our government really works and about the medical, surgical, biochemical, and research details of problems we face. You gain respect for the many hard-working, conscientious, knowledgeable, and underpaid men and women who, together, constitute our government. Individually, none of these is responsible for its egregious excesses or abysmal failures. These are more often traceable to upper-level zealotry, selfishness (i.e., pork barrel), or outright stupidity. Our coworkers, even as high ranking as generals and admirals, were the toilers in the vineyard, not the dictators of policy.

Professors profess. They profess to know. Our government needs some of what they know. That is why you get started on that midnight to Washington. For me, this occurred in 1942, and it has never stopped. It is still going on, more than 50 years later. I have no regrets.

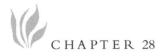

CHAPTER 28

Autres Chirurgiens,
Autres Moeurs

I f you are a teacher, it is part of your job to get out of your rut and see
how others are doing things, what steps are being taken at the fron-
tiers of your science or art, and bring those ideas home. Most certainly this inquisitiveness is important in surgery, where there is a tendency to enshrine even minor local traditions as sacrosanct. Better go see
other surgeons and other customs in other places. *Autres chirurgiens....*

One way of achieving such an interchange was the custom of
inviting visiting professors to our own institution to share their expertise.
The Brigham under Cushing had begun this "Pro Tem" tradition, meaning the "Visiting Surgeon-in-Chief Pro Tempore." In the old days, the
Pro Tem was invited to come and stay for a couple of weeks. Pretty
wearing for all concerned. Then the visit was cut down to less than a
week.

Cushing invited many luminaries to visit, including the Russian
neurophysiologist Ivan Pavlov and his British counterpart Sir Charles
Sherrington. And Sir William Osler. Following in this tradition, we
enjoyed being host to many distinguished visitors from abroad. Sir James
Learmonth was one of the first. He had been a Scots Jock (i.e., a Scots
GI) in World War I, was Professor of Surgery at Edinburgh, and was
knighted after operating on King George VI. Then we had Sir Arthur
Porritt, later Governor-General of New Zealand and thereafter one of the

first surgical lords. There was Sir Gordon Gordon-Taylor, one of the colorful older generation of London surgeons, as well as the younger generation of brilliant Britons as typified by Charles Rob, who later migrated to Rochester, NewYork, and then Washington, D.C. The visit of James Paterson Ross was described in Chapter 18. And Ivan Johnston of Newcastle. From France we welcomed André Monsaingeon from the University of Paris, from Australia John Ludbrook, and from New Zealand Michael Woodruff. From western Canada Rocke Robertson of Vancouver, later Professor of Surgery and then Vice-Chancellor of McGill University in Montreal. We invited visitors from all over the United States, including some of the senior men who were the very symbols of surgical change during and after the war, including Alfred Blalock of Johns Hopkins and Owen Wangensteen of Minnesota. In a reciprocal fashion, I was invited as visiting professor to many universities in this country and abroad.

While a little learning from abroad is a good thing, the tendency of American professors to spend a lot of time traveling can be pernicious. There was a joke about a friend of mine in Colorado who spent so much time on planes that he was called the "TWA Professor of Surgery." I tried to hold my own travels in check, but not always with success. At first I traveled solo to Washington, to meetings, societies, other colleges and universities. Later on (after our children had left for college) I told anybody who wanted to have me around that they should ask Laurie to come too. Worked fine. We circled the globe together. One of the pleasures of the academic life.

Britain

My first major trip as visiting professor was to the University of London in 1950. They also asked me to teach in Edinburgh, so this was a big trip for us. Laurie came. And then we went to Paris and Italy. On this trip we made personal and family friendships that have lasted all these years.

This was my introduction to the pomp and panoply of the Royal College of Surgeons. The atmosphere of the upper echelons of surgery in London had to be seen to be believed. At home I drove an old broken-down Pontiac station wagon into the unpaved Brigham parking lot, where I often got stuck in the mud or in a snowdrift. In London at that time, leadership mandated a Rolls-Royce (or a Bentley) and a chauffeur. Most of the ruling class of surgeons were also important potentates in national organizations and many were, sooner or later, knighted. About 30 years later a group of us Yankees were in London to visit with the four surgeons who were members of the House of Lords, so our traveling group had a chance to have a tea party with the surgical lords in the House of Lords and witness some of their quaint customs.

That first visit was only 5 years after the war and the hospitals were still pretty well broken down. There had simply not been time (or funds) to start reconstruction after the bombing and the fires. The National Health Service (NHS) was established in 1948, still brand new. It was possible for practicing surgeons and teachers in the universities to have only a fraction of their week occupied by NHS activity, so there was still free time for practice, research, and teaching. There was a virtual absence of organized departmental surgical research as we knew it and of research on large animals. Antivivisectionists in Britain had won their battle at the turn of the century. The familiar American animal laboratory where research and teaching could be carried out on dogs, cats, pigs, sheep, cattle, or monkeys simply did not exist. Only one animal research laboratory existed in London, and it was conducted under strict licensing arrangements by the Royal College of Surgeons. This was the Buckston Browne Research Farm, where Roy Calne did his epic experiments on kidney transplants in dogs using 6-mp (described in Chapter 20).

Among other things, it was this restriction that prompted so many young British surgeons to come to America. Over 50 young men from the United Kingdom worked with us at one time or another, many of them later assuming leadership positions at home.

In some ways the clinical traditions of British surgery, of operations and surgical care, contrast with ours. British surgeons are apt to pride themselves on speedy operations. They are more impulsive, possibly less prone to search out the root cause of error, seemingly less rigorous in aseptic technique, more authoritative. And the residents are more in awe of their seniors than they are here. Yet the two traditions are remarkably similar in basic surgical philosophy, and the cross-fertilization (dating back centuries) has been very intense since 1945. If I or my family should be taken ill and require major surgery elsewhere, I would accept Canada or Great Britain interchangeably as the best. If I found myself in some of the other nations on this Earth, I would flee in terror (if still able to run).

The most illustrious figure in the history of British surgery was Joseph, Lord Lister. By the peregrinations of his career, he could claim three cities as home: London, Glasgow, and Edinburgh. In turn, all three cities claim and celebrate Lister as their most famous son. Lister was the successor, in the mid-nineteenth century, of that paterfamilias of all surgical research, the Scots-born Londoner John Hunter, who lived and worked a century before. Laurie and I attended the Lister celebration in Glasgow in 1965, where I received an honorary degree, along with my long-time friend and associate, Bert Dunphy, former Brighamite, then Professor of Surgery at the University of California at San Francisco.

To visit Guy's Hospital and see the cornerstone bearing the date A.D. 914 is a lesson in humility. The oldest of our hospitals in the United States are only now about to celebrate their 200th anniversaries. Our traditions in surgery and academia trace more strongly back to the British Isles than to any other antecedents, although the British tradition was heir to some strong influences from both France (in the early part of the nineteenth century) and Germany (in the middle and latter parts of the nineteenth century).

France

Our first official visit to French surgery occurred in the early 1950s. André Monsaingeon, who had come to work with us at the MGH in the late 1940s, was now back in Paris as Professor of Surgery at the University of Paris, at l'Hôpital Paul Brousse, south of the city. Traditions of medicine and surgery, teaching and research, are very different in France. As an example, some of the French medical schools will admit as many as 1,000 students to the first-year class. The entrance examinations are very generalized; the student's name, age, or sex are not specified. Each has a number. From this huge egalitarian class (which would be impossibly expensive in this country), only a few are selected to go on to the second year. That initial intake of students is really an elaborate screening process to select those who should be permitted to advance.

The French Academy has an old tradition dating back to the great French teachers, such as Professor Louis, and the early surgeons epitomized by Dupuytren and Napoleon's surgeon, Larrey. One of the established traditions of this academy is that those who attend a meeting proceed to sip their cognac or drink their coffee and carry on conversations while the speaker is also speaking. This is very distracting to us Americans. I was asked to give a speech about some of our work in surgery. After I staggered through some fractured French that must have been acutely painful to the fine-tuned ear of the audience, André, who knew all about this work, took over and delivered the rest of my address, using my lantern slides. Yet even upon hearing his elegant French, the audience continued to eat, drink, and converse. This studied indifference might be a bit upsetting to the unwary. I assumed they were bored to death. Wrong. When it was all over, they asked a lot of questions, clearly demonstrating that not only had they listened to the lecture, but they had actually read some of my papers!

While London dominates much of British culture, it gets a lot of competition from Oxford and Cambridge. The Scots, with their university medical schools and hospitals, will never admit to any dominance by London at any time, in any connection, or even as competition. In France, Paris so completely dominates the intellectual and scientific life of the country that to the casual visitor it is hard to understand where the rest of the country fits in.

In the United States, the position of professor in a field such as medicine, pediatrics, or surgery is not celebrated except by those associated with academia and often times by few of those. In Britain, the professor is ranked in a sort of midposition. But in France and Germany, Monsieur le Professeur occupies a position of great eminence, and some of them have egos to match. We went to a formal dinner in Paris given by one of the most prominent surgeons in France. While I was busy trying to understand cocktail-hour French and possibly construct a few acceptable sentences, Laurie was quietly observing the decor. She later told me that there were six portraits and no fewer than 15 busts of our host in his apartment (abutting La Place de l'Etoile and l'Arc de Triomphe).

Scandinavia

All three of the Scandinavian countries have a tradition of pleasant human relationships, fine surgery, and trenchant science. Yet the three great countries are quite distinct.

Sweden is by far the largest (about equal to Denmark and Norway combined). The Karolinska Institute in Stockholm is the dominant biomedical research institution of Scandinavia and for a time received almost as much financial support from the National Institutes of Health as did many major universities in the United States. It is the source and scene of the Nobel ceremony. On its 150th anniversary I was invited to the Karolinska as the representative of American surgery and was asked to speak on behalf of the visitors from abroad.

The Danes are filled with good humor, good science, and a remarkably liberal tradition despite the terrible Nazi occupation. Professor Husfeldt was at that time the leader of Danish surgery. He had been active in the anti-Nazi resistance during the war, narrowly escaping with his life, and had supervised the passage to safety of thousands of German Jews through an underground transport system. He was widely recognized and revered for this role. I was flattered to be made an Honorary Fellow of the Royal College of Surgeons in London in 1967 at the same meeting where that honor was also conferred on Husfeldt.

Several Danish scholars came to work with us, including Bent Friis-Hansen in pediatrics, Knud Olesen in cardiology, and Helge Faber in endocrinology. The Danish residency system in surgery had such an inflexible pattern of promotion that it was not easy for them to get away to study abroad.

Norway is the smallest of the Scandinavian countries in population, has the longest coastline, and suffered the saddest and most brutal repressive occupation by the Nazis during the war. Carl Semb was Professor of Surgery in Oslo and a great sailor. His wife was a little bit overweight. They both joked over the fact that this was why he put her on the windward rail in his sailing dinghy and they won lots of races. Egil

Amundsen, a relative of the great polar explorer, was a frequent visitor to our department and to the Department of Physiology. At one point I was asked to be visiting professor at the University of Tromsö, the only medical school in the world north of the Arctic Circle. We took a boat up the west coast of Norway and spent a delightful week in Tromsö. It is dark there about 6 months of the year and is regarded as a hardship post. Many of the faculty rotate to the south to Bergen or Oslo to bask in a little sunshine from time to time. For those of us who live in lower latitudes, it may seem surprising to go to Bergen or Oslo for a southern sunshine holiday. But such is Tromsö.

At the time of one of our visits to Norway, our friend Fisher Howe, then a member of the State Department, was chargé d'affaires at the U.S. Embassy in Oslo. He asked me to speak there on the subject of the role of the U.S. government in American medicine. Most Europeans are critical of the United States for not having a broader system of health-care coverage for the population. I pointed out that we did have several programs. One covered about 6 million people (the armed forces, dependents, and retirees) and another, 28 million people (the Veterans Administration). The total is considerably more than the entire population of Scandinavia! But of course, despite this evidence of our size, I agreed with their basic point: we do not provide coverage of all our people for the financial burden of illness.

Germany

Our visits to Germany were mainly to Heidelberg and Munich. We never did get to Berlin. Professor Fritz Linder of Heidelberg had become a close friend of many American surgeons. He was made an Honorary Fellow of the Royal College of Surgeons in London at the same time I was. No German had been elected to honorary membership since before World War I. Feelings ran deep considering the thousands upon thousands of British soldiers who lost their lives fighting the Germans in two wars, not to mention the tonnage of bombs so recently dropped on London. So it came as quite a wrench (and the cause of some rather touchy speech-making) when Fritz Linder was offered this honor. He typified the new and warm relationship among West German science, western Europe, and the United States that slowly emerged two decades after World War II.

Visiting Munich in the 1980s, I recalled my first visit there 50 years before as a college student (in 1934). That was Hitler's first year. We were in Munich at the time of the Brownshirt rebellion when General Roehm and his followers sought to topple Hitler and his Blackshirts. After some maneuvering but not much gunfire, Hitler won. When they confronted each other near Munich, Hitler handed Roehm a loaded revolver. Roehm could have shot Hitler or himself. He shot himself. In his book on life as a Nazi bureaucrat, Albert Speer stated that this was the moment when he realized that Hitler was a criminal, yet Speer was trapped and remained in the Nazi government almost to the very end.

The Munich of our first postwar visit (1953) had been reduced to rubble by the Eighth Air Force. Even the place where the Nazi guard had an eternal flame burning to commemorate Hitler's first publicly violent demonstration (known as the beer-hall putsch) had long since disappeared. And with it the two uniformed, heel-clicking, goose-stepping Nazi Blackshirt guards with fixed bayonets, who guarded it when I was there as a college student.

While in Munich we took the opportunity to visit the famous library. One of the great anatomy books of all time is the *Fabrica* of Andreas Vesalius, published in 1543. Vesalius was Professor of Surgery in Padua. The illustrations of Vesalius' dissections were drawn by an artist (Jan Calkar) who was a pupil of Titian. These woodcuts persisted for 400 years. In the 1930s the New York Academy of Sciences had borrowed them, dusted them off, and reprinted a whole new edition using special acid-free paper and modern ink. Those precious woodcuts were then returned to the library in Munich. Some time in early 1945 that library was destroyed by an Eighth Air Force raid. During our visit we went to the library to learn what we could about the fate of the Vesalius woodcuts. The librarian was acutely aware of this tragedy and told us that the plates were probably deep under ground, buried in the rubble, if they had not been consumed by flames.

Greece and the Eastern Mediterranean

Though we visited Greece two or three times, we made only one major trip to the Middle East, in 1961. This was at the invitation of the United States Information Agency to teach and lecture in several countries. We visited Greece, Turkey, Lebanon, Syria, and Egypt. It was at the time of Nasser, when Egypt and Syria were united in a fragile political union: the United Arab Republic. There was a reasonable state of peace in the Middle East. We could drive without incident from Lebanon to Damascus across the Golan Heights. Jewish students attended the American University of Beirut. Neither before nor since has there been such a period of peace in the Middle East. It was on this visit that we met William Taylor, the ARAMCO physician in Dhahran whose friendship led to my visit to Arabia and Ibn Saud's visit to Boston (Chapter 26).

In the Arab world, autopsies are virtually unheard of. It seems immoral to introduce transplantation or cardiac surgery into a country where autopsy is forbidden and the surgeon cannot root out the causes of error or death. If an operation about which little is known is carried out and the patient dies, an autopsy is ethically mandated. If there is no way for the surgeon to find out what went wrong, it would not be ethically acceptable to perform the procedure in another patient. And yet in the Arab world, they do just that. They seem to get away with it. But at what cost? Surgical research as we know it is absolutely nonexistent in those countries. We often worry about the inappropriateness of introducing our advanced technology in developing countries. But how about teaching our science where there is no ethical or scientific standard of morality to give it validity? Some of the least developed countries are most anxious to establish transplantation or cardiac surgery. Whether or not they *should* do it, they surely will. Like so much technology transfer, teaching this type of surgery in such cultures is superficial and ineffective. It is like selling aircraft to people who don't know how to maintain them or presenting an ocean-going yacht to someone who has never piloted a sailboat. Only more dangerous. Problems of cultural difference run deep, and for the first time I began to feel them keenly. Why teach transplantation or heart surgery if the first 175 patients die and there are no autopsies? And no one cares?

We did not visit Israel until much later (1970) when we attended a large transplant meeting where I was to describe our early studies on liver transplantation. Israel stands like an island in the Middle East, an island of Western culture. In Israel, surgical research, teaching, publications, societies, and autopsies are all either part of the Western and American tradition or closely allied to it. While we can be proud of this important outpost in that part of the world, we must learn to respect the differences, of which there are many.

Down Under

For any traveler in medicine or science, the two island continents of Australia and New Zealand occupy a special place. Their scientific traditions have a historical basis in both Great Britain and the United States. The common language and a common spirit of congeniality, humor, athletics, and sports—and ethics—binds these nations strongly to ours. I was visiting professor at the University of Dunedin in New Zealand and later in Melbourne, Australia.

While we were in Australia, our host (Ross Sheil, formerly of our staff) decided to take us sailing in Sydney Harbor. Sydney has a large, beautiful, and protected harbor, completely landlocked. We went out in a little tender from the Royal Yacht Squadron, and there moored in front of us were two large sloops. One was immediately recognizable as *Gretel*, the Aussie 12-meter competitor for the America's Cup. Right next to it, almost as impressive, was an 8-meter sloop. Our host said, "Franny, which one of these do you think we are going to sail?" I replied, "I have no idea, but either one of them would be a first for me." We boarded the 8-meter. They immediately gave me the tiller. Up went the sails. Out came the cocktails and hors d'oeuvres, and we set off through Sydney Harbor, Australian style. I had to ask people about the buoyage system and try to avoid running into battleships, freighters, and ferries. There was a good breeze, and we moved along briskly. We had no power on board. Finally we came to an isolated beach, sort of a city park, maintained for yachtsmen. Here I "shot" a small buoy. I was proud of my skill (or luck) in being able to do this with reasonable success considering the strangeness (to me) of this large yacht. We then rowed ashore for a picnic on the beach. Surrounded by surgeons of Australia and New Zealand, some of whom had trained at the Brigham, many in charge of transplantation in their own local units, we had a great time. There was a kookaburra bird, which looks something like a kingfisher but about six times as large, screaming in one of the nearby trees. With the best of ornithologic intentions I held up a little piece of ham. The kookaburra came swooping down, snatched the ham, and flew off. The surgeons immediately jumped on me and said I should never have done that, because I was more apt to lose a finger than the ham.

In New Zealand I enjoyed the company of Gus Frankel, the professor at Dunedin, and through him spotted a young surgeon, Murray Brennan, who seemed willing enough when I suggested he might come to Boston to work with us. He came, married a beautiful American surgeon (one of our interns), raised a large family, and soon became Head of Surgery at the Memorial Sloan-Kettering Cancer Center in New York. Quite an import!

India

In India I was struck by the amusing but confusing admixture of British and American traditions. According to British tradition, all would-be surgeons had to go to London and pass the examinations of the Royal College of Surgeons. Merely to sit for these examinations was quite an honor. One heard about surgeons whose credentials included the phrase "Royal College of Surgeons, England—failed." Unlike the British College, the American board system of examinations follows the completion of the residency and, because of these prerequisites, is as good as closed to people coming from abroad. Nonetheless, many Indian surgeons have done fine work in various departments in this country, including ours, in both clinical work and research.

Many of the Indian population had been undernourished for many years, and I was struck by how small the people were compared with the average size of American patients. Often the disease process is far advanced by the time the surgeon is called in. Here is where one sees primary cancer of the breast that has spread all over the patient's breast and chest, like a great crab, as the ancients perceived in naming it cancer.

Hernias, which in this country are usually the size of a grape or, at their largest, an egg, here often descend into the scrotum and can reach the size of a football.

The professor of surgery at Banaras, Narsing Udupa, had worked with us for several years. He asked me to be visiting professor there. Laurie and I had a wonderful adventure. Banaras is also called Varanasi because it is situated along the west bank of the Ganges, bordered by the Vara and the Nasi Rivers. It is the only city in the world where the smog and foggy conditions are due to the accumulated smoke of saffron cloth and human bodies being burned in the ghats on the west bank of the Ganges. I noticed that the intensive care units of several of the hospitals conveniently situated on the sacred west bank of the Ganges, near the ghats. Not a topic you would bring up over tea.

Southeast Asia

Our visit to Thailand was part of the same journey as that to India and included Bangkok as well as Chiang Mai, where the professor of surgery was Okas Balankura, who had worked with us for a couple of years. Up at Chiang Mai the weather was clear and cool, since it is higher—in the mountains—and far removed from the stifling sea-level tropical humidity of Bangkok.

They have many unique problems in Thailand, one of which is tetanus (lockjaw). Tetanus is so rare in the United States that many American surgeons have never seen a case. In the rural parts of Thailand there were many unlicensed folk-nurses or self-styled physicians with no education or training. They did not understand cleanliness or sterilization. For all diseases they administered antibiotics by intramuscular injection with a long needle. A large fee was charged. Penetrating deep into muscle, these long needles were the ideal way to introduce an anerobic infection such as tetanus. On one ward I saw 12 patients with tetanus. Some cases were rather mild, but in one or two the disease was very severe, and prolonged periods of general anesthesia had been required to prevent lethal convulsions. We were told that, with time, most of these patients recovered.

China

In 1982, I was invited to visit China and was asked to bring three other members of my staff. While I could be relied upon to lecture on metabolic care, nutrition, and liver transplantation, the Chinese also wanted someone to teach about kidney transplantation, another who would cover intensive care, and a third, blood-vessel surgery. All these were new aspects of Chinese surgery. They had done their first kidney transplant only 3 years before, in 1979. The Chinese were beginning to encounter arteriosclerotic blood-vessel disease, that is, hardening of the arteries, so common for generations in the United States and Western Europe. No one knows quite why this disease was appearing in China for the first time at this period. The Chinese were beginning to need intensive care units and were becoming interested in the biochemical and physiological aspects of surgical care. To our surprise, one of our hosts, Professor Tseng Hsien-chiu, told me frankly that the government was difficult to deal with. I was a little surprised that he could state this so frankly. He said, "Building an intensive care unit in China is like trying to grow roses in concrete." However, he had managed to build a small unit in Beijing that was well equipped and provided good care for the few patients it could accommodate.

When we first arrived in Beijing we were ushered into the main library of the University of the National Academy of Medical Sciences. During colonial days this had been called Peking Union Medical College. Then it was given a communist title of the People's Republic. Shortly after we were there, the old name was restored, a historic reversal, insofar as this was contrary to the usual communist antagonism toward prior colonial policy. When we were introduced, the librarian displayed a brand new copy of my book on metabolic care with my picture, and handed me a pen to autograph the book. A photographer then took a picture of the event, with Laurie standing at my side. For the aging author of a book then 25 years old, this was flattery in the extreme.

Our fellow China travelers were all from our department and included Nathan Couch in vascular surgery, Herbert Hechtman in intensive care, and Nicholas Tilney in transplantation. Just at the last minute our hosts sent us a cable and told us to bring our wives. Our small group certainly got special treatment and had a chance to learn about Chinese medicine and surgery and visit many Chinese patients, in great detail and with a minimum of fanfare or persiflage.

Our visit took place only 5 years after the wind-down of the Cultural Revolution, which had shaken everything to its roots and was now being referred to as the greatest disaster in Chinese history. A notable superlative. Our host, Dr. Tseng, now Professor of Surgery at Beijing, had during the Cultural Revolution been assigned to a province just northeast of Tibet where he dug in manure fields and made irrigation ditches. He and two or three of his colleagues quietly started a small hospital there. At the time of our visit they were still helping to run that hospital 2,000 miles away in a rural land of peasants and few modern conveniences. It no longer had to be kept a secret from the government.

The Chinese smoke cigarettes excessively. Maybe this is the cause of their vascular disease. Every morning, when starting hospital rounds, we attended a little sit-down ceremony with the director of the hospital and possibly the mayor. In front of each of us was a cup of steamy hot water with green tea leaves floating on top. When the leaves got soaked and sank to the bottom, the brew was ready to drink. Four cigarettes had been placed on the saucer and you were supposed to smoke them. The Chinese admired the fact that most Americans did not smoke any more and acknowledged that smoking was a health problem in which the Chinese had made no progress whatsoever, whereas the United States somehow had.

Our host, Professor Tseng, died of carcinoma of the lung only a year after our visit. He was a far-sighted leader of surgery, and his death was a tragic loss to Chinese surgery. His son studied at Johns Hopkins and later became a member of the faculty of Harvard Medical School. Tseng's wife, Qin-sheng Ge, is a distinguished endocrinologist who visits us here on occasion. One of their grandchildren is named Francis Moore Tseng. Zhu-ming Jiang, one of Dr. Tseng's staff, has been a research fellow in our lab and that of Doug Wilmore on several occasions.

While we were in China, official enthusiasm for acupuncture was already on the wane. According to our host, publicity about acupuncture had been advanced during the Cultural Revolution because it appeared to be anti-Western, was contrary to conventional teaching, and was considered peculiarly Chinese. For my own part, I was always impressed with the nature of acupuncture's effects. Operations around the face and chest could apparently be carried out under acupuncture anesthesia alone. This success sent a message about the nervous system that we did not understand. To explain this, people liked to mutter something about gate theory (how sensations from one irritant could block out sensations from another, even pain). There was little hard evidence to back up such ideas. Within 2 years of our visit I was disappointed to find that the Chinese were no longer doing research on acupuncture. The special unit in Shanghai had been closed. In the United States, research on acupuncture had largely been abandoned. Although there were always plenty of people to defend it, there was precious little insight into its use. Acupuncture is something we should learn more about but seem now to have stopped the effort.

Despite my defense of acupuncture as requiring more study, I was disillusioned to see it being used in China for everything from headache to asthma. A patient with old poliomyelitis and a withered, useless limb would be treated by acupuncture, hoping it would make her better and bring back the kilograms of missing muscle. The patient usually felt better, we were told, but all the doctors recognized that there had been no change. Even the Chinese had a limit on the wanton use of acupuncture; it did cost something after all; even in a communist state, economic reality must sometimes rule. There was a rule that no patient could come in for acupuncture more than five times.

A famous American journalist, James Reston, had undergone an abdominal operation in China a few years previously for acute appendicitis. Our friend and host, Dr. Tseng, had been the surgeon. The American press got the idea that the operation was conducted under acupuncture anesthesia. I had been doubtful about this, since even at that time the Chinese pointed out that the muscle relaxation so necessary to abdominal surgery was rarely attained with acupuncture. Now we got the straight story. Dr. Tseng told us that regular Western-style anesthesia had been used, and that the acupuncturist had been called in only to help ease postoperative gas pains. Dr. Tseng was one of the many Chinese surgeons we met who spoke realistically (and disparagingly) about acupuncture. He made it clear that even in the case of Mr. Reston he was not sure the acupuncture helped much and noted wryly, "Gas pains always go away anyway."

Although the events of Tienanmen Square in 1989 were unforeseen during our visit in 1982, roots of discontent were already strong. There was a clear desire on the part of the university community—not only the students—to shake off a restrictive and vengeful government. And yet, when that uprising came, many university people we knew rather surprisingly opposed it. Some of our friends were among that conservative group, along with the majority of Chinese. While they might have agreed that there was some justification for the democratic movement, to them, stability of the Chinese government, culture, and economics was far more important than democratic reforms at this difficult time. Now a few years later (1995) there may be traces of some slight liberalization even among the Chinese intelligentsia. But precious few.

Back Home

While it is typical for travelers to recall their trips abroad with sentimentality and nostalgia, our visits to many of the universities in this country have given us equal pleasure, and the experiences have been just as instructive.

One of the pleasures of academic life is that you meet people from all over the United States and the world. Wholly aside from teaching, research, or sharing new knowledge, this eclectic brotherhood makes the academic life enjoyable. It makes for notable memories to operate with a strange surgeon in a strange country and despite difficulties to find that you both share the same basic language of anatomy and surgery.

Of memorable visits in this country, I will select one to tell here because of its special nostalgia. In Chapter 3 I told about how one of the surgeons who influenced me as a child was Frederick Christopher, a leading surgeon of Evanston and Winnetka. He had taken care of me because of that injured knee. He was the author of one of the first textbooks of minor surgery and later of a standard large surgical text, now edited by David Sabiston of Duke University. It was therefore a thrill for me to be asked to give the first Frederick Christopher Memorial Lecture at the Evanston Hospital about 40 years later. Quite a few friends of mine from high school had gone into medicine and came to hear the talk. Others came because they also had been cared for by Dr. Christopher. I told of the pleasure of growing up there and of having Christopher as my surgeon. I ended by showing a slide of that picture from his book showing my injured left knee at the age of 14.

This brought down hoots and hollers from the audience. After the meeting, I was inundated by friends who had grown up in Winnetka. They showed me pictures from the same textbook, pictures that Christopher had taken of their left ear, their fractured finger, or their facial burns. Of such is the fellowship of patients.

Our visits on this continent have ranged from Bangor to San Diego, Seattle to Tampa, Halifax to Vancouver. Always congenial, always hospitable, always something to learn and surely to tell about on your return. Of such is the fellowship of surgeons.

BOOK NINE

Big News

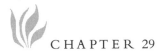

CHAPTER 29

1963 and a Cover Story

The year 1963 was the kickoff for the second half. I was halfway through my responsibility for the Department of Surgery of Harvard Medical School at the Brigham Hospital. Although it was the year of my 50th birthday, neither Laurie nor I thought of it as any kind of a milestone, because I had not yet given any thought as to when I would seek relief from all those committee meetings. I knew that my Harvard tenure as university full-time professor would end after my 67th birthday. This specified retirement date (soon to be revised and then revoked) went back in university tradition many years. Since I had received my first Harvard appointment in July 1941, I was part of the old guard and the old system and thus subject to this old rule. That academic retirement was 18 years off: June 30, 1981. Like all dates that lay far in the future, it bore little resemblance to reality. The year 1963 was one of national tragedy: at the end of that year we lost our young and charismatic president to a senseless assassin. But it was also a year of triumph: we did our first human liver transplant. And it was the year *Time* magazine gave our department front-cover treatment.

Family Still Growing

In 1963, Nancy, our eldest, was 27 years old and had presented us with two Hill grandchildren (Lucius Tuttle III and Elizabeth Thayer Hill),

305

two more yet to come (Peter Isham and Susannah Wyatt Hill). While a sophomore at Bryn Mawr, she had married a young gentleman, Lucius Hill, the son of a near neighbor in Brookline. Luke had graduated from Yale and was then a second-year medical student at McGill. Nancy therefore transferred from Bryn Mawr to McGill. In 1958 they both graduated on the same day: he from medical school, she from college. He became a Brigham surgical resident. In 1963 they lived near us in Brookline with their new family, and he was soon to start up surgical practice in Exeter, New Hampshire, which then became their home. In 1993 their oldest son Lucius and his wife Wendy became the parents of my first great-grandchild, Harry Bartlett Hill.

Peter, our eldest son, had graduated in 1957 from Milton Academy, long considered a prep school for Harvard College. During Peter's senior year, the Harvard recruiter had made a strongly negative impression on the Milton graduating class, whereas the man from Yale had charmed them all. So, possibly for the first time in history (and maybe the last), many of the graduates of Milton Academy decided to apply to Yale. After finishing up at Yale (1961), Peter decided to return to Harvard to earn his Ph.D. in biophysics with James Watson. He was studying in the Harvard Biology Department at the time Watson won the Nobel Prize for the description, with Crick and Wilkins, of the double-helical structure and chemical bonding of DNA. We always enjoyed Peter's story of coming into the classroom that day in early October and seeing written on the blackboard in the mock lettering of a 10-year-old child, "TEACHER WON THE NOBEL PRIZE."

After this sojourn at Harvard, Peter did his postdoctoral work in Geneva and then at Cambridge (on the Cam, not the Charles) before returning to a faculty position in biochemistry and biophysics at Yale (1969). Within a few years he was given tenure (1976) and took his 3-year term as department head from 1987 to 1990. Peter Moore married Margaret Murphy in 1966. They have two children, Catherine Huston and Philip Wyatt Moore.

In 1963, our next oldest daughter, Sally, was about to complete her studies at Swarthmore College, following which she did graduate work at the University of Chicago (1964). She then married Richard Agassiz Warren (1965), son of Richard Warren, a close friend and mem-

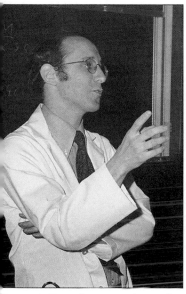

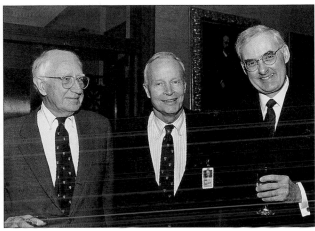

Steven A. Rosenberg, a graduate of Johns Hopkins Medical School and the Brigham Surgical Residency program, now Chief of Surgery at the National Cancer Institute.

John Mannick (*center*), FDM's successor as Professor and Head of the Department, first at Peter Bent Brigham Hospital (PBBH) and then at the newly merged Brigham and Women's Hospital. On his right is FDM, on his left is Nicholas Tilney, the first Francis D. Moore Professor of Surgery.

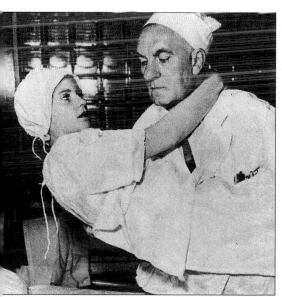

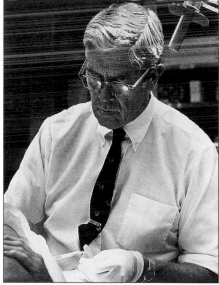

Adolph Watzka, operating room orderly through the regimes of Cushing and Cutler and into the early years of FDM. Strong, gentle, and skilled in managing very sick patients, Watzka never wore a facemask in the operating room. If questioned about this, he stated that he "never breathed there."

John R. Brooks, early arrival at PBBH with FDM and for many years assistant to FDM in administration of the Department of Surgery. Brooks later became the Frank L. Sawyer Professor and Head of Surgery for the Harvard Health Services in Holyoke House, Cambridge.

Plate 17

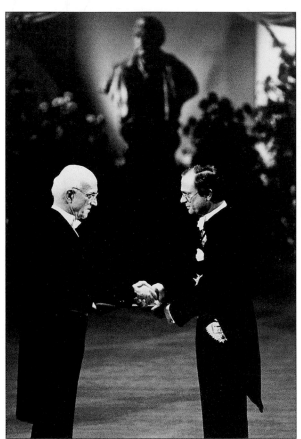

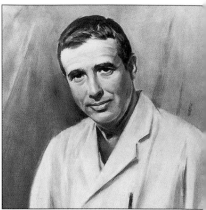

David Hume, who performed the first set of human kidney transplants between unrelated persons.

Joseph Murray receiving the Nobel Prize from the King of Sweden in December 1990, in recognition of his early successful transplant operations.

The first successful kidney transplantation in man, performed on an identical twin with his brother as donor, on December 23, 1954, at PBBH. The patient's head (hidden by the anesthesia screen) is at the lower right. Joseph Murray, the surgeon, stands on the patient's right. Opposite Murray is the assistant, John Rowbotham; to his left is Edward Gray, and to the surgeon's left is Dan Pugh. Roy Vandam (back turned) is the anesthetist. To the upper right is the circulating nurse, Edith Comisky. The scrub nurse (*above left*) is Miss Rhodes.

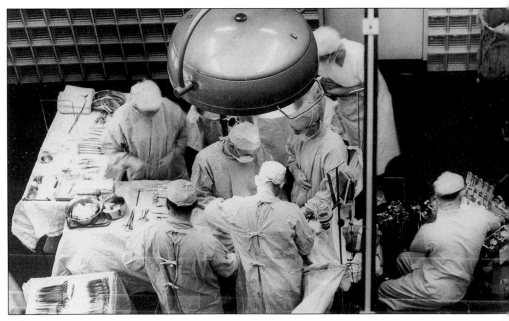

Plate 18

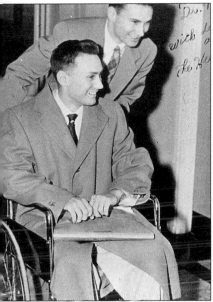

The Herrick twin donor (Ronald) pushes his recipient brother (Richard) in a wheelchair on their way home, January 1955. Both look healthy after their historic operation.

Sir Roy Calne of Cambridge (*left*) and Tom Starzl of Pittsburgh celebrating Sir Roy's 25 years at Cambridge. The two leaders of transplant science are drinking tea from laboratory jugs because the teacups ran out.

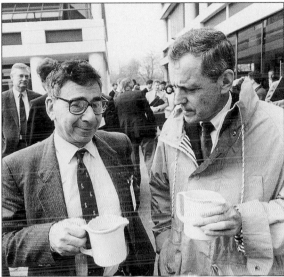

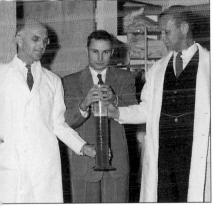

Transplantation humor: "Who owns this urine?" Holding the cylinder containing the precious fluid is the donor (the patient's twin brother) who claims it was his kidney that made the urine. On the left, Joseph Murray (the operating surgeon) claims his patient's urine. To the right, also claiming the urine, is J. Hartwell Harrison, who removed the kidney to make its urine available to the patient. The patient (not shown), whose urine it might now appear to be, seems to have no claim at all.

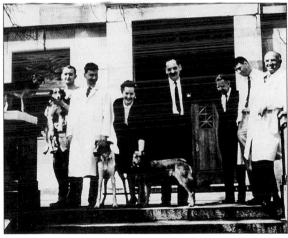

Canine recipients of transplanted kidneys, enjoying company on the veranda outside the surgical laboratories of Harvard Medical School (HMS), 1960. Under azathioprine immunosuppression, these animals are healthy and well. Dr. George Hitchings (*center*) and Dr. Gertrude Elion (*to his right*), the researchers who synthesized this drug, along with Dr. Donald Searle (*to his left*), Medical Director of Burroughs Wellcome, are visiting the lab. Dr. Joseph Murray (*far right*) and several members of the team, including Ted Hager (*second from right*), Larry Ayres (*far left*), and Roy Calne (*second from left*), are also enjoying the scene.

Plate 19

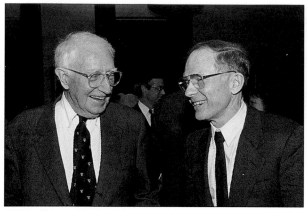

FDM talking with Daniel C. Tosteson, the present Dean of HMS, about 1990.

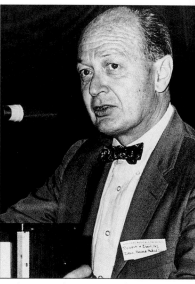

George Packer Berry, who succeeded C. Sidney Burwell as Dean of HMS in 1950.

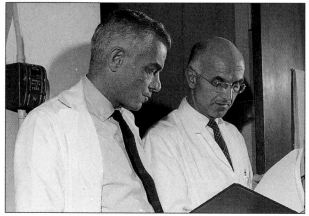

John Merrill (*left*) and Joseph Murray (*right*), collaborators with Hume on transplant research, about 1963. Merrill, a member of George Thorn's medical service at PBBH, was responsible for all patients with chronic renal failure and was in charge of dialysis on the artificial kidney.

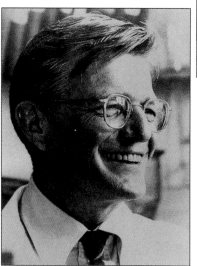

Robert H. Ebert, Dean of HMS (following George Packer Berry) and architect of the Harvard Community Health Plan.

Paul Snowdon Russell, long-time director of surgical transplantation and research at the Massachusetts General Hospital.

Plate 20

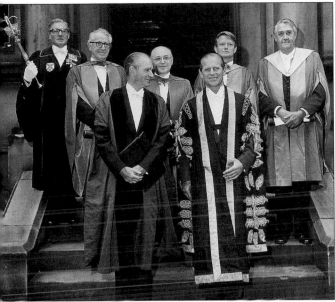

FDM receives an honorary degree at the University of Edinburgh, June 25, 1976. This event marked the 250th anniversary of the founding of the faculty of medicine at Edinburgh. The two robed gentlemen standing in front are Sir Hugh Robson (*left*), Principal and Vice Chancellor of the University, and Prince Philip (*right*). Behind them are the four honorands (*from left to right*). FDM, Professor William Goslings of the Netherlands, Robin Irving of the University of Otago (New Zealand), and Professor Henry Harris of Oxford.

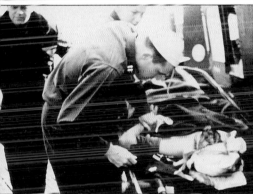

rly morning in Korea, 1952. Scene at a Mobile rmy Surgical Hospital (MASH #8209), site of the rgical research unit under Colonel John M. Howard. helicopter has brought in a wounded man.

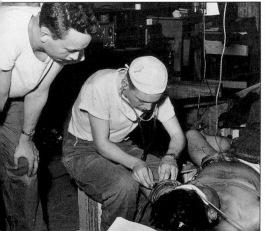

Cover of *Time*, May 6, 1963. The story was written by Gilbert Cant and Ruth Mehrtens.

Care begins for another casualty. The detailed study by Col. Howard of a few such wounded men made it possible to give better care to many without research.

Plate 21

The Moores and the Robs about 1950. Charles Rob was Professor of Surgery at St. Mary's Hospital in London. The Moores were visiting his department as part of the Brigham–St. Mary's exchange. Mary Rob is standing in front of FDM, on the left, and Laurie Moore is on the right.

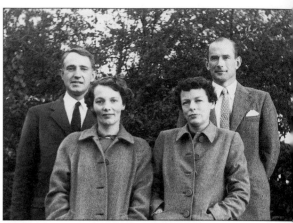

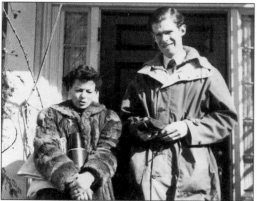

Laurie with Bent Friis-Hansen, a visitor and laboratory collaborator for several years, early scholar of body composition in children, and later Director of Pediatrics at Copenhagen.

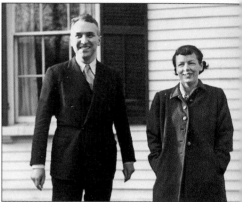

André Monsaingeon with Laurie. André, a collaborator and visitor on several occasions, headed the surgical unit at l'Hôpital Paul Brousse, south of Paris, and was later Dean of the University of Paris School of Medicine at Orly.

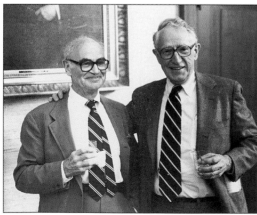

Reminiscing about the "good old days" are Roy Vandam, Professor and Head of Anaesthesia at the Brigham, and FDM at the time of his retirement.

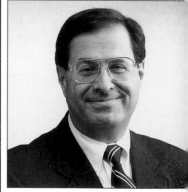

Michael Zinner, the new Moseley Professor, took up his work in July 1994, succeeding John Mannick. Zinner is the seventh Moseley Professor, and the tenth in the "old line" stretching back to the early Warrens and the Revolutionary War.

Plate 22

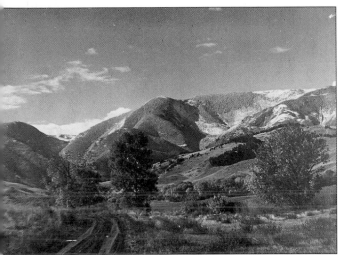

Wyoming, 1934. Coming along the ranch road in early September, with snow on the mountains ahead.

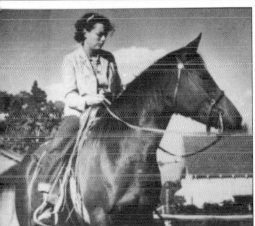

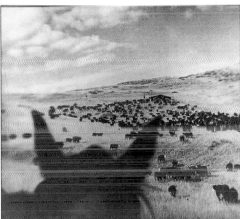

...urie on her favorite horse, "Babe" — the product an unusual Shetland/Arab cross.

Cattle roundup as seen by (and from) a horse.

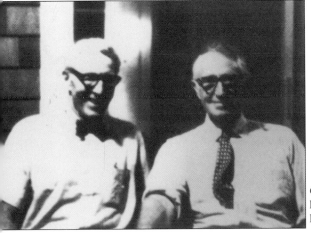

Codgers. Fisher Howe III (*left*), life-long friend and confidant, is having a laugh with FDM, about 1985.

Plate 23

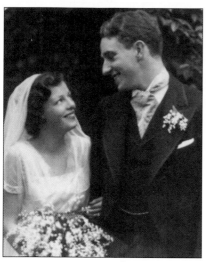

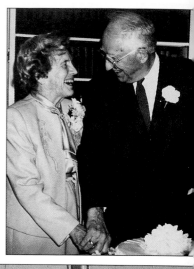

Two weddings. On the left, Laura Bartlett and Francis Moore, June 24, 1935. On the right, Katharyn Saltonstall and FDM, May 13, 1990.

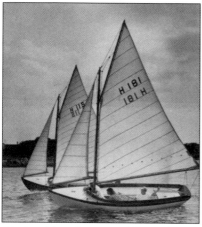

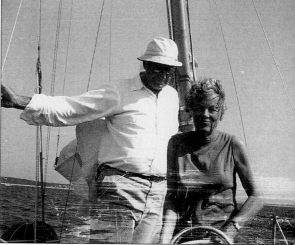

Marion, Massachusetts, and Buzzards Bay, about 1960. Two small boats (Herreshof 12-footers) racing in the harbor. *Sea Worm*, the Moore boat (H-181), is "covered" by Pratt's *Wee Capa* (H-115). How to get out of this fix? Son Peter at the tiller, FDM puts some heavy weight forward by the mast, daughter Sally to leeward.

Laurie at the wheel of *Angelique* while FDM offers some free advice.

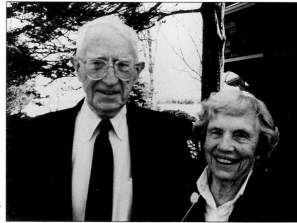

FDM and Katharyn in 1994, about the time of their fourth wedding anniversary.

Plate 24

ber of our faculty and staff. Dick was a teacher of high school students. Sally is a musician and an artist. She has started a new program called the Vermont Institute for Teaching the Arts (in 1989) to provide home-room teachers in small community schools with more tools and background to instruct their young charges in art and music. She creates her own art from home-made paper and has taken her turns as president of the local school board. Dick and Sally Warren have three children: Peter Agassiz, Rebecca Pepper, and Samuel Bartlett Warren.

In 1963, Caroline (Ceci), our youngest girl, was at Sarah Lawrence College, where her mother had received more learning in 2 years than I had in 4 on the banks of the Charles River. Ceci also had a fine college experience, graduating in 1966 from Sarah Lawrence before entering graduate school at Columbia (1967 to 1969) and becoming a city planner in New York City under Mayor Lindsay (from 1971 to 1977). Now she is Assistant Head for Communications and Enrollment at the Day School in New York, where she has been on the faculty since 1981. In 1965 she married James Tripp, a lawyer with the Environmental Defense Fund. They have two boys, Benjamin Baldwin and Zachary Daniels Tripp.

Meanwhile, our youngest, FDM, Jr. (Chip), 6 years younger than Caroline, was in 1963 struggling with the travails of secondary education at Browne and Nichols School in Cambridge before moving to Choate School in Wallingford, Connecticut. After Choate, Chip attended Harvard College (1972) and then Harvard Medical School (1976). He is now Associate Professor of Surgery at Harvard and the Brigham, pursuing the same schizoid combination of research and clinical surgery that his father did. His research in molecular immunology, elucidating the chemical details of the immune process, is a matter of great importance in surgery, not only in transplantation but also in immunity to infection. He and Carla now have six children ranging from 6 to 16 years old: Kyle Crescenzi, Lynsey Jean, Hadley Huston, Colby Daniels, Alessandra Laura, and Francis Colcord Daniels Moore.

Department Still Growing

In our surgical department many exciting changes were taking place in 1963. Staff and faculty were continuing to grow in numbers and international distinction. Private practice, while small and consistent with an academic's time limitations, continued to be challenging and rewarding. Although our department at the Brigham had succeeded in acquiring more hospital beds by new construction, we still needed an entirely new hospital (which would be many years in coming, as described in Chapter 30). On the side of research progress, we had completed the three signal transplantation operations carried out by Joseph Murray and others of our staff (1954, 1959, and 1962), making ours the leading transplant center in the world. I had started my work on liver transplantation. In 1963, we published our global summary of body composition, *The Body Cell Mass and Its Supporting Environment*. The King of Arabia and his entourage had been our patients. Possibly most important was the fact that the practical summary of our metabolic studies on surgical patients (*Metabolic Care of the Surgical Patient*), published in 1959, had now been translated into several languages and had attracted a large sale. It was read by medical students and surgical residents in many countries and was frequently quoted in the surgical and medical literature.

Attention from the Press

Whatever the significance of all this, the local press had started to pay a good deal of attention to our department, particularly with transplant operations, the opening up of new additions to the hospital, and the visit of Ibn Saud (Chapter 26). The *Boston Globe* and *The New York Times* mentioned our work from time to time.

In January 1963, I received a call from Gilbert Cant, then the medical editor of *Time*. We had become acquainted because the magazine had done a couple of other stories on surgical matters, and he had sought my advice about their interpretation. He was a knowledgeable and agreeable person. Also a sailor. He told me that *Time* was going to run a major story on recent advances in surgery and wanted to get the full story on my department, among others. I had no inkling that this was going to be the lead story, and I told him we would be happy to cooperate. He assigned Ruth Mehrtens (later Mrs. John Galvin), a young science reporter, to cover the story. Ruth came to Boston frequently. She immersed herself in both ancient and modern surgical history and visited various departments of surgery over the country where important advances were taking place.

In a month or so, Cant asked me to go into town to have a portrait painted in color by one of the magazine's artists. The portrait was painted using tempera, sort of a plastic material, and was clearly typical of *Time* cover portraits. I expressed the thought to him that there were other surgeons in the country who might better have their portrait painted for this purpose. He adroitly agreed; this was a good way of making it seem indefinite, thus keeping me in the dark as to specific plans for the cover.

I went over the stories about various aspects of surgery with Ruth. We tried to achieve accuracy, but somehow the story of David Hume's early kidney transplantations got projected into 1954, and he was identified as the surgeon in that first identical twin operation instead of Joe Murray. I am not sure who owed the apology for this error to Joe Murray, but we both felt responsible.

The article had not yet appeared when Laurie and I went off to Mexico, where I attended a surgical congress. We had never been to Mexico before and enjoyed our visit tremendously, especially because of the kindness of many interesting people and the remarkable antiquity of so many things in Mexico City. If somebody finds a seventeenth-century church in New England, they declare it a historic place. In the center of Mexico City you can find a huge cathedral that dates back to the earliest years of the sixteenth century. On a May morning in Mexico I went to a newsstand and picked up a copy of *Time*, that picture on the cover and the entire story within.

Not many people knew where we were when the issue of May 3, 1963, was put on the newsstand. Nonetheless, the telephone began to ring in our hotel room and continued to ring (back home) for several weeks.

When one of their own achieves some sort of special public prominence, people have an ambivalent reaction. On the one hand, they are proud that their profession—in this case, physicians in general and surgeons in particular—is receiving favorable attention. On the other hand, some are apt to feel envy or jealousy. Others may consider themselves or their friends more worthy of such prominent mention, for example the head of their own department or the founder of their hospital.

Among the latter, there are always some who feel that the media attention was sought out by the recipient of that attention and is just another example of his general malfeasance and criminal desire for notoriety. Stated otherwise, reactions ranged from sweet grapes to sour grapes and then to grapes of wrath.

In due course any feeling of resentment passed off. While I can understand and forgive all sorts of negative reactions on the part of my colleagues, I was pleased and surprised that the great majority of them responded with kindness, were thrilled, and gave me the sort of backing you need when you are suddenly thrust into a spotlight position of unwonted and unwanted prominence.

So we went on with our work much as before.

As did Laurie, who was interested in the political process, in current events, and in the League of Women Voters of Brookline. As an active member of the league, Laurie was assigned the role of official observer at the meetings of town government. Meetings of the league were often held at our house, and whenever I could assist her with some audiovisual preparations, to help her presentations, I did so. Then I joined up. It may come as a surprise that quite a few men are members of the League of Women Voters.

The Year Ends in Tragedy

I never knew John Kennedy personally; he was 4 years younger and in a later class at Harvard College. On one occasion in the middle 1940s the Boston Chamber of Commerce had selected several young men whom they regarded as "coming up fast" for special achievement awards and held a dinner in their honor. I met JFK at that dinner because both of us had been selected for one of the awards. He was a Massachusetts senator at the time. His Republican opposite number was Leverett Saltonstall.

Nearly everyone remembers where they were when they heard of Pearl Harbor and, 22 years later, when they heard of the death of President Kennedy. On that November day in 1963, I was idle, waiting for ducks to drop into our decoys on a small promontory (Browne's Point) bordering Merrymeeting Bay in Maine. Richard Warren was there with me. Mrs. Erle Browne, the wife of the farmer who was our guide and owned the point, came rushing out the half mile or so from the house. "The president's been shot!" was her only statement, and she rushed back to her farmhouse. We picked up our gear, ran back to the house, and watched the T.V. for a moment or two. Then we hurriedly threw our heavy clothes in the back of the car and drove home, listening all the way to the nonstop radio account of the tragic events in Dallas. An era of immensely high hope for all of us, led by one of our own generation, now killed in the line of duty, seemed all at once uncertain and tragic. While we would forever grieve over this tragedy, just then the best thing to do was to get back to work.

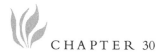

CHAPTER 30

The Urge to Merge;
A New Teaching Hospital
for Harvard

(1958-1980)

Hospitals in small towns and rural communities do not like to merge, no matter the pressure of economic reality or the attraction of shared services. Like magnets of the same polarity, nearby community hospitals repel each other strongly. Each is the pride of its community, the crowning achievement of its board, the hallowed hospice for ills and injuries, scenes of the birth of babies who later grow up to become board chairmen.

When you are a patient in a small community hospital (as I have often been), you can understand their point. These are comfortable places, with kind people looking after you. Everyone knows everyone else. There is a personal flavor. Such hospitals are essential to the operation of the entire American system of medical care. Their function is to give the care at which they excel and then seek further help from others when necessary. In many cases, the smaller hospitals could do their task better if they joined forces, the way high schools in small communities began to do about 75 years ago. Together they could provide a more complete menu of shared services and lose fewer patients to the big hospitals in the nearest city.

By contrast, large urban hospitals (including teaching hospitals) are anxious to merge. While the same local chauvinistic pressures, loyalties, competing physicians' interests, and cheerleader enthusiasm of the ladies' auxiliaries will struggle to avoid merger, cooler heads usually prevail. Economies of scale, shared use of extraordinarily expensive equipment, greater prestige, specialists, and drawing power are now measured in millions of dollars. Balance sheets speak louder than local pride. In many of our large cities over the past five decades, such hospitals have been merging by the dozens to form better balanced units.

Time to Expand

In the 1950s, after several years at the Brigham, it seemed clear that the clinical sciences and arts—as they had developed after World War II—had rendered our hospital, at 250 beds, too small to fulfill its mission as a teaching hospital. Many argued that in voicing this opinion I had been overly impressed by the size of my alma mater, the MGH (then about 850 beds), and its breadth of clinical services—almost impossible to achieve in a smaller hospital. The stand-pat arguments pointed out, as all would agree, that the accomplishments of the Brigham, however small its size, were world-renowned and would doubtless continue to develop, as indeed they did. We all agreed that large size alone did not spell quality of care. Nonetheless, I was sure that the time had come to expand.

Mine was not the only voice to push this need for broader shoulders and major change. Money was scarce. Our hospital was experiencing a hard time financially. Our deficits were impressive and the annual charitable fund drives barely made them up. Our ancient and honorable endowment was about gone. One of our leading trustees actually wanted to close the hospital! Some of the staff wanted to shrink it even further, making it just a small research institute. To me, this would have been a fatal mistake. That way lay disaster. Such a small research institute certainly would have lost my interest entirely and (I am sure) that of many others. My voice, while not the only one, was one of the most persistent. And rightly so, as Surgeon-in-Chief. Surgery fills lots of beds, uses all the labs, the operating room, intensive care, blood bank, rehab. Surgery serves a very broad population of patients with urgent but varying demands and uses the whole hospital organism, not just one corner. The surgical voice carries some special clout. Despite antagonisms and the

313

many enemies I made (most of them temporary), things began to move our way in the late 1950s.

In 1958, in the surgical office, we quietly held the first organizational meeting designed to bring three of these hospitals together. Later this number became four. This was a meeting of George Van Sicklen Smith, William H. Baker Professor of Gynecology and head of clinical and research units in gynecology at the Free Hospital for Women of Brookline; Duncan Reid, William Lambert Richardson Professor of Obstetrics, who was in charge of the busy obstetrical service at the Boston Lying-In Hospital; and myself. The three of us were all surgeons at heart. We knew that our three surgical units could coexist and function peacefully and cooperatively in one building, strengthened by sharing essential services, working in more modern facilities, and with a better balanced nursing and support staff. Soon the Robert Breck Brigham Hospital, a specialized facility for medical and orthopedic care of rheumatic diseases, under its leaders K. Frank Austen in medicine and Clement Sledge in orthopedics, joined our effort toward a new combined hospital.

Twenty-two years later, in July 1980, we admitted our first patient to the new hospital. The Harvard Medical School now had a new 800-bed general hospital across the street from its science quadrangle, complementing the MGH down at the old harborside 4 miles away and helping the school and its biomedical science departments to enter a new century. And our hospital was able, now, greatly to expand its services in clinical surgery, teaching, and research. And expand it did, under the leadership of my successor as professor and head of surgery John Mannick.

Not many readers will be interested in what went on between conception in 1958 and delivery 22 years later, or in the details of how four Boston hospitals—often rivals—actually got together to form what is now known as the Brigham and Women's Hospital. Mergers of teaching hospitals are awkward but commonplace. While the details of each are different, they do go through rather similar steps. I will tell a little bit about the one leading figure who emerged, who could see the economic, legal, clinical, and educational implications. He was Mr. F. Stanton Deland, the lawyer-trustee who later became President of the new hospital, who worked with four separate Trustee boards, three Harvard medical Deans, and the Massachusetts State Legislature to make it all happen.

The Harvard Family of Hospitals

Peter Bent Brigham, Esquire, a successful Boston merchant, was by birth a Vermonter. In 1877, having become affluent through his labors (labors largely of brain rather than hand) and through the acquisition of some valuable Boston real estate, he was able to bequeath a large sum of money to endow a hospital. This hospital was to be called the Peter Bent Brigham Hospital and was to be built immediately adjacent to the Harvard Medical School to care for the sick poor of Suffolk County. During the 25 years that the Brigham endowment was accruing interest, the Harvard Medical School moved from the Back Bay to its present site on Longwood Avenue, and the Brigham Trustees bought a spacious 14-acre field across from the medical school, on Francis Street.

The grand opening of the hospital was in 1913, and within 25 years the Peter Bent Brigham Hospital achieved a worldwide reputation based largely on the work of its staff and its first Surgeon-in-Chief, Harvey Cushing. Despite its initial wealth, the hospital soon became as poor as the proverbial church mouse. This poverty was said to have come about owing to clumsy management of real estate and railroad holdings exacerbated by the onset of the Great Depression in 1931, 18 years after the hospital opened.

The brother of Mr. Peter Bent was Mr. Robert Breck Brigham. Not to be outdone by his older and somewhat wealthier brother, he also endowed a new hospital in Boston, the Robert Breck Brigham. Instead of being across the street from the medical school on what we might call the "plains of Longwood," it was up on nearby Parker Hill, looking out toward Boston harbor in the distance. It opened its doors in 1915, and by 1970, the Robert Breck Brigham Hospital had achieved a remarkable preeminence in medical and orthopedic care as well as basic biological research in rheumatic joint diseases.

Much older than either of the two Brigham hospitals was a nearby hospital that provided the obstetrical care for women and neonatal care for their newborn babies. This was opened in 1865 as the Boston Lying-In Hospital, a quaint name based on the fact that women in labor prefer to lie down on the way to the hospital. By the turn of the century the Boston Lying-In Hospital was the leading obstetrical hospital in New

England, concentrating on the birthing care for thousands of women each year. These patients were largely of the Protestant and Jewish faiths by custom, not by exclusion. Catholic women often chose to be cared for at one of the several Church-affiliated hospitals.

Larger and more ancient than these hospitals beyond the limits of downtown Boston was the Massachusetts General Hospital, founded in 1811 and admitting its first patient in 1817. Right from the start it covered nearly all clinical phases of medical care. The one major exception was obstetrics. By the late 1920s and early 1930s, the MGH had a capacity of around 850 beds and included a small psychiatric wing (the Hall-Mercer Hospital), wedged into the larger general hospital, a gynecologic unit (the Vincent Memorial Hospital), and a pediatric unit (the Burnham), which also had merged into the MGH. Immediately adjacent was the Massachusetts Eye and Ear Infirmary. In the view of most people the whole complex was a single hospital unit famous for both the breadth and the excellence of its care. The MGH was my professional home for 10 years, and I cherish a great affection and respect for its eminence despite my being cast as a leader of its smaller rival. This great hospital, the MGH, with its closely allied Eye and Ear Infirmary, was the dominant force among the privately endowed trustee-operated hospitals of New England. The cluster of seven hospitals around the Longwood area could become a clinical force balancing to the west of Boston the downtown strengths of the MGH and the Boston City Hospital, but it would be somewhat larger in the total number of beds and closer to the Harvard Medical School.

Merger of four of these into one would strengthen the work of the whole area through shared services, cross-fertilization in teaching, and shared support of research.

In gynecology there was yet another hospital to be included. Just beyond the plains of Longwood, on the river formerly called Muddy (now distinguished as The Fenway), was the Free Hospital for Women of Brookline. This hospital was established by local endowment for the specific purpose of providing gynecologic care to the needy women of Brookline (a suburb virtually surrounded by Boston) and nearby Roxbury (a part of Boston). It became a center for gynecologic surgery and for research on reproductive physiology and endocrinology and was one of the smallest and most specialized of the Harvard-affiliated teaching hospitals.

Several hospitals on the plains of Longwood shared facilities and services with the Brigham and were supportive in this new conjunction of their neighbors. These hospitals included (in addition to those already mentioned) the Beth Israel, Children's Hospital, Boston Psychopathic (a state hospital), and New England Deaconess. The Deaconess had been a private hospital of high quality that was largely unassociated with Harvard surgery until 1963, when William V. McDermott, Jr., Cheever Professor of Surgery at Harvard Medical School and Director of the Sears Department at Boston City Hospital, moved that surgical service to the Deaconess. From that time forward, the Deaconess became a major collaborator in research and in undergraduate and graduate surgical teaching at the medical school. Bill McDermott was the only Harvard professor during those 50 years to start up a new Harvard Department of Surgery. Before his retirement in 1985, he brought his department to international eminence.

A Leader Emerges from the Crowd

If a merger is to succeed, it needs a leader. During the preliminary first step, in which the Lying-In merged with the Free Hospital, such a leader emerged and Stan Deland first showed his mettle. He led Trustees and staff of both hospitals through a maze of obstacles to merge these two into a new entity, the Boston Hospital for Women (BHW). It was on the basis of this achievement (in 1965) that his talent was recognized and he rose through the ranks of trusteedom to assume the leadership position that later became so important.

With the new BHW firmly in place, it was clear that the next step—merging the BHW with the two Brigham hospitals—would be welcomed by those who felt (as Smith, Reid, and I had since 1958) that the two Brighams should join forces with the Lying-In and the Free. Their shared orthopedic, medical, and surgical services should round out the whole. This struggle for union embodied several salient features common to all hospital mergers.

There were severe tugs of war among the staff: stand-pat versus change. These differences were soon resolved. Our neighbors were quite understandably concerned at the sudden appearance of a new giant in their midst. The women's auxiliaries, so much the soul of each hospital family, at first were wary of merger but now work together as one. Jealousy between the members of the several boards of trustees was keen. This was a surprise to me and quite a contrast to the rapidly emerging sense of unity among the professional staffs. Real estate is a problem in many hospital mergers, but the old Peter Bent Brigham was land-rich. We had extra property on which new construction could start promptly. Most of all we needed a helmsman to guide these four hospitals through those tortuous 22 years from that first joint meeting to a new hospital ready to admit its first patient.

In this new venture Deland continued his leadership. He was a Boston lawyer, Harvard College class of 1936, Harvard Law 1939, who displayed a unique combination of understanding and good humor mixed with the determination and legal and political know-how needed for such a massive public venture. I had known Stan since college days and was immensely pleased and confident of our success by dint of his appointment as Board Chairman.

Under his guidance the merger agreement was signed in 1971 and from there things moved rapidly forward. It was Stan who asked Thomas Dudley Cabot, a distinguished senior citizen of Boston, long a benefactor of Harvard University and its hospitals, to be in charge of our fund drive. While Stan was supremely effective, he could not have accomplished this four-way merger without the help of Charles B. Barnes, John Lowell, George Kuehn, Lawrence Damon, the Alan Steinerts (père et fils), Joseph Powell, and the other presidents and chairmen of the four constituent boards. They all deserve full credit for their important contributions to the formation of this new member of the Harvard hospital family.

Coasting to a Grand Opening

The rest of the story is less complicated. The requisite millions of philanthropic dollars were gathered. While the sinking fund was established, the bond issues were floated. The new hospital was built as a tower consisting of four round, linked units, resembling a cloverleaf as seen from above. By its detractors it was likened to four large beer cans full of square holes. Now almost 15 years old, it is one of the more successful new hospital buildings in the United States. The architect, Bertrand Goldberg, deserves an architectural laurel wreath for his achievement.

For a long while during its early gestation, the project was referred to as the hospital complex (often disparagingly as the "complex hospital"). Then it became the Affiliated Hospitals Complex. Then the Affiliated Hospitals Center, Inc. After the building was built, a name was still needed. Finally, one was selected by Stan Deland and his trustee executive committee: The Brigham and Women's Hospital (BWH). This name combines the interests of all four of the participants, acknowledging the two Brigham hospitals and the two women's hospitals that made up its whole.

In July 1980 the new hospital was opened, and by a supreme effort over the course of 48 hours, hundreds of patients were moved into their new rooms in the 16-story tower. On the first evening, a patient with acute appendicitis entered the emergency ward and the first operation was carried out. Stan Deland donned a surgical "monkey suit" and was in attendance for that landmark event.

Tragedy at the Moment of Triumph

Thus it came about that Stan Deland, more than any other one person, brought about this merger. He lived to see his new hospital become a reality, increasing satisfaction among those who, years before, had threatened to disrupt the project. Gradually a new Board of Trustees was created from the four original Boards.

A practicing lawyer, Stan was the exceptional hospital trustee who understood enough law to put through new state charters as part of the merger; enough politics to keep the mayor, governor, and legislature on our side; enough human values, humor, and good will to assuage dissension; and enough clinical common sense to realize that the whole project had but one purpose: the care of the sick. This was the main reason for its existence, despite the pressures of its two strong subsidiary missions of teaching and research. To achieve this objective he worked with three successive Deans of the Harvard Medical School: George Packer Berry, Robert H. Ebert, and finally Daniel C. Tosteson.

In July 1987 Stan Deland, only 73 years of age, died rather suddenly of a recurrent lymphoma. He had been Chairman of the Board of Overseers of Harvard University and President of our hospital, had merged four hospitals and built a new one to make a glorious new hospice for patients and students alike. John McArthur, Dean of the Harvard Business School, succeeded Stan as Chairman of the Board. H. Richard Nesson has been the President and Chief Executive Officer.

The year of his death, his wife Susan Deland, with our help, established a fellowship in Stan's name to provide an educational opportunity for young clinicians who might wish to go into hospital administration. But equally important, and as it turned out somewhat more frequently, it offered a clinical opportunity for observation and immersion in medical care for those individuals with a legal, business, or administrative background who wanted to learn the administration of a teaching hospital.

As a result of Stan Deland's efforts, one corner of Boston has been rebuilt. The Harvard Medical School has a major new clinical and research center. Patients from all over the world have access to that remarkable combination of wisdom and mercy, science and humanism that has characterized these four hospitals—now merged into one—since their earliest beginnings over 100 years ago.

As this book nears completion, a new merger is under way between the two Harvard hospital giants, MGH and BWH. Just what the anatomy and physiology of that huge organism will be and how each partner will continue true to its own genes remain for the future. The merger that went before may provide some guidance to a new generation expressing the urge to merge.

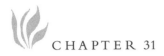

CHAPTER 31

A Nobel Prize for Joseph Murray

(1990)

In October 1990, two years after Laurie's death, Kathie and I went to San Francisco for the annual meeting of the American College of Surgeons. We had been married less than 6 months, and this was an occasion where I was introducing her to the phenomenon of a large surgical meeting in a delightful city where we would surely meet and dine with a great many of our friends in American surgery, as well as many from abroad.

Early Monday morning, October 8, we were awakened by a call from Susan Lang, my secretary in Boston. It was then about 8:30 AM in Boston, and she asked the age-old question, "Have you heard the news?"

"What news?"

"Dr. Murray has been awarded the Nobel Prize," she replied. I got a few more details before announcing this remarkable news to Kathie.

Within the next half hour we received several more telephone calls, either from officials of the American College of Surgeons who wanted to arrange a reception for Joe—the first surgical Nobelist since Huggins, 44 years before—or from friends and reporters. We were able to contact Joe quite early, though as I recall he had checked in only the night before and had heard about the award only a few moments before Susan's call.

There was great excitement among surgeons, not only those at

321

the meeting, but throughout the world. This excitement spread of course to all Harvard Medical alumni and all transplanters. Somehow, the Nobel award casts a glow of pride over all those associated with the recipient through their field of science, their professions, or their institutions.

Joseph Murray's partner in the prize, E. Donnall Thomas of Seattle, had been a resident in medicine with George Thorn at the Brigham at the same time the identical twin transplant had taken place (1954). In fact, Don had written a consultant's note in the record. His Nobel Prize–winning work had been in bone marrow transplantation, recognizing the many ways in which he had made this procedure safer and more reliable.

On a cold, dark December afternoon in 1990, Kathie and I sat in the State Theatre in Stockholm, in our best formal garb, long gown for her, white tie and tails for me. We watched while Joseph Murray was called from his seat on the stage to receive a sheepskin from the King of Sweden along with a medal designating him as the recipient of one of the two 1990 Nobel Prizes in physiology or medicine. His citation was read in Swedish, translated into English, summarizing his pioneer work in kidney transplantation.

We were pardonably proud not only because of Joe's remarkable work, but also because I was possibly the first American professor of surgery to witness that prize being awarded to a staff member, a teacher on his faculty, a man who had done the honored work in his laboratories and in the regular line of study and surgery.

Alfred Nobel

The story of Alfred Nobel, the Nobel Foundation, and the establishment of the Nobel Prizes has been told on many occasions with various emphases. Possibly the most engaging detail is that attested to in the official history. This is the story of Alfred Nobel reading his own mistaken obituary, an item published in a Swedish newspaper on the occasion of his brother's death. Evidently the reporter got the two Nobels mixed up and wrote an elaborate account of how Alfred had stabilized dangerously explosive gunpowder by spacing out the particles with diatomaceous earth so it would maintain its explosive power but would be easier and less dangerous to handle. The new explosive powder was called dynamite. And how, over the years, dynamite had been used for the building of inter-ocean canals and epic structures throughout the world, and it was Nobel's hope that his discovery would benefit mankind. But the paper also emphasized how this discovery revolutionized gunfire, artillery, and bombs and had led to the deaths of hundreds of thousands of young men. Alfred, very much alive, was shocked at what the world would think of him after his death. So he resolved to do some good. He endowed a foundation and made possible what has become the prototype of all honorary awards. The Nobel Prize is large in amount, is overlain with great ceremony, is given in several fields of endeavor, and is unmatched worldwide in prestige.

The Karolinska and the Prize

The Karolinska Institute of Stockholm had known of the work being done in our department for many years. In 1960 I had been invited to participate as a scientist in the celebration of their 150th anniversary, as mentioned previously. Their professor of surgery at the Karolinska, Jack Adams Ray, was a friend of ours, and we have had many Swedish visits and visitors over the years.

Although this background has nothing whatsoever to do with the selection by the Nobel Committee of two transplant scientists (Joseph Murray and E. Donnall Thomas) for the prize in 1990, it does account for the fact that I was one of many university department heads in this country asked annually to submit a Nobel nomination in physiology or medicine. Over the years I had nominated several American, British, and French surgeons with whose work I was well acquainted. When the committee asks a representative of some special field of study for nominations, they of course expect him or her to know of the outstanding people in that field and to discriminate among noteworthy discoveries as to which are of Nobel caliber.

The Nobel Committee has clearly been aware of progress in the field of transplantation and in the underlying study of immunogenetics and pharmacology. Prizes in this area have included those awarded to Alexis Carrel (1912) for his study of kidney transplantation in the cat and the method for suturing blood vessels (Chapter 19), to Peter Medawar and

MacFarlane Burnet (1960) for their studies in immunogenetics, and to George Hitchings and Gertrude Elion (1988) for the chemical engineering of highly specific drugs (Chapter 20). Among the drugs cited by the Nobel Committee was azathioprine, the use of which in transplantation was pioneered in our department. In fact, even before the Nobel recognition of Joseph Murray, we had dedicated a new laboratory in immunogenetics at the Brigham to those two pioneer workers most prominent in this field: Hitchings and Murray. Baruj Benacerraf, Jean Dausset, and George Snell had been awarded the prize in 1980 for their work on the histocompatibility gene that recognizes self versus nonself when new proteins are introduced into the body.

Previous surgical Nobelists given the prize for work by their own hands in their own fields of surgery have been few. In addition to Carrel, there was the Swiss surgeon Theodor Kocher (1909), recognized for his work on the thyroid, and Charles Huggins, a surgeon at the University of Chicago (1966), for his work showing the close association between the male sex hormone (testosterone) and the growth of cancer of the prostate. Several other surgeons have been recognized as being part of Nobel Prize teams, although their work was not a part of their regular clinical studies.

Attending the Ceremony

The Swedish, like the British, enjoy laying it on with public ceremonies of pomp and circumstance. The Nobel ceremony is one of their greatest annual events, and the entire celebration lasts about 10 days.

At this time of year (December), the sun as viewed from Stockholm does not get more than a couple of inches above the horizon. The nights are long, cold, damp, and intrinsically gloomy, while the days are very short. What better time to have this huge, colorful, exciting international celebration with several events attended by leading figures from all over the world? It is a time for fancy clothes, evening gowns, and medals pinned to wide red stripes from shoulder to bellyband for the European gentlemen. But in point of fact, none of that is why the ceremony is held in December. It happens to be the time of Alfred Nobel's birthday, and he designated this as the time for the event.

Our trip to Sweden was largely uneventful save for the fact that I forgot my pants. I discovered this crippling omission on Sunday, the day before the big ceremony. In Sweden, stores are open on Sunday. When I got to the men's dress-clothes department, a cheerful young lady said, in perfect English, but with a charming Swedish smile, "Well, well. Another American who forgot his trousers!" This is what most people would call tact.

Suitably attired, we attended the festivities. Joe's scientific presentation of his work was well done, modest, giving credit to his colleagues and predecessors. George Thorn and many members of the Murray family were present to enjoy the ceremony.

Kathie looked marvelous in her floor-sweeping gown and long, white gloves, an item I thought had disappeared from our society when I ceased to attend Boston debutante cotillions. We danced at the formal ball after the banquet. One of the Murrays' daughters-in-law is a singer (as is Joe's wife, Bobby) and had performed in Sweden before. So as a specialty of the ball, she sang some jazzy American pieces in Swedish and charmed the large gathering.

The banquet itself is held in the huge town hall, said to be the largest single-room banquet hall in the world. The 1,800 guests were precisely arranged by field of study and therefore possibly prior acquaintance. We were seated among friends and not too far from the young and sparkling queen, diamond tiara and all, and the rather stiff and formal young king.

This Nobel ceremony seemed a long way from the smelly dog lab in which the first experimental transplants had been done, the workaday world of developing organ transplantation, the gloom of death and failure, and our excitement in the successes of our long-surviving animals and, later, patients.

BOOK TEN

Things Do Change

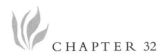

CHAPTER 32

Ethics at Both
Ends of Life

In the last quarter of this century, following the Supreme Court decision in the case of *Roe* v. *Wade* (1973), the social and surgical management of pregnancy termination took on a new face. It became yet another ethical enigma for physicians and surgeons, a major change in the ethical awareness of our era. It has touched all people, especially women, and all surgeons and physicians. From the viewpoint of gynecologists and obstetricians, who so often witnessed the tragic disasters associated with self-induced abortion and abortion parlors, the relocation of this surgical procedure to the realm of hospital care with sterile precautions seems to be such a tremendous improvement that it has outweighed other considerations. Saving lives and ending misery is not a new concern. Gynecology was an integral part of our department. If a department of a hospital is put in the position of providing this service, then it should be done right, both surgically and ethically.

It is important for everyone, including the opposition, to realize that few women ever really want an abortion. A woman may need one and ask for one. But she does not really want it. Certainly not the young girl embarrassed by her life-changing fix. Or the mother of five who feels she just can't carry another pregnancy or afford that sixth child. Neither wants to abort her own offspring. She may even have been through the experience before but still does not want it. In many instances, religious zealots overrate the importance of their ideological bias and seek to force on everyone a policy that fits their own personal needs. They are not the only ones who do not want an abortion.

During our medical school days and in the early years of my surgical work, pregnancy terminations were of the utmost rarity in hospitals, being done only to save lives in critical emergencies such as when the mother had tuberculosis, a heart attack, or epilepsy. And then, often in the second or third trimester. By contrast, we saw many disasters of illegal abortions, especially overwhelming pelvic infection (infection around the uterus) due to septic abortions. Such infection was always destructive, if not lethal, always resulting in infertility.

One Saturday morning, a few years after *Roe* v. *Wade*, Somers Sturgis and I were walking into the operating room and looking at the day's schedule. Pregnancy terminations were carried out on Saturdays. There were six of them that morning. At larger hospitals there might be even more. Of course we knew this was going on, but nonetheless we looked at each other in wonder and amazement. We just couldn't believe how widely accepted surgical abortion had become. Nurses and other hospital staff who did not wish to participate in these procedures were never required to do so, nor were they questioned about their reasons. It is important that most of those patients did not fit the customary image of the college girl in trouble or the high-school girl who drank too much. Instead, they were apt to be mothers who wanted to do some family planning but were about 3 months too late. Now that the liberalizing (yes, liberal) view of enabling abortion has been expressed and endorsed as widely as it has been in this country, crossing all political, regional, ethnic, and religious barriers, no political forces of repression or restriction seems likely to hold it back. Better to keep it legal and make it safe. I have no objection to social safeguards such as parental permission for minors and a waiting period with, under specified circumstances, spousal consent.

Through these troublesome years I have gained respect for the view that we should not take young lives, but let us not make those lives in the first place. Let us pursue birth control and improve education for young people. Let us brave the scorn of a younger generation by talking out loud about these issues. Let us encourage personal devotion, commitment, and love as necessary accompaniments of sex. We favor marriage over informal cohabitation. These are important solutions, each of them only a partial one, to the problem of illegitimate pregnancy, unwanted children, and abortion.

The taking of life is not the only issue in abortion. Rather, it is the avoidance of a life not validated by love and care. Other countries do it differently. Far better legal abortion in the United States than septic abortion here or female infanticide in the Far East. In India, female children are sold out to prostitution or enforced marriage. Better than either are love, caring, and commitment as an integral part of sex.

The Near Miss of a 23-Year-Old Mother

The case of an illegal abortion gives an idea of where such convictions come from for our generation of surgeons. Cases like this help explain my advocacy of legal, clean, safe surgical abortion as a right of choice for American women.

The patient was a 23-year-old woman who had been divorced. During her marriage she had borne four children. Since then she had been pregnant on two additional occasions, both pregnancies being terminated by illegal abortion. The year was 1964, 9 years before *Roe* v. *Wade*. Now, in the fourth or fifth month of her seventh pregnancy, she went to an abortion parlor. At that time a frequent method of inducing abortion in the underworld was the infusion of Lysol or soapsuds into the vagina. Upon her request, a pressurized soapsuds douche was administered. As might be expected, no sterile precautions of any sort were taken.

The next day the patient began to have chills and abdominal pain and was admitted to the Brigham on March 5, 1964. Her blood pressure was low, her pulse rapid, and she had ceased to make urine. On pelvic examination, the uterus was large and extremely tender, with the feeling of crepitus. Crepitus is the sensation you get by running your hand over something filled with a lot of small bubbles. (During World War I, the feeling of crepitus under the skin of a wounded man indicated that bubbles of gas were forming within the tissues in the region of the wound. This was gas gangrene, a common occurrence in that war, less frequent now. Ominous, often lethal.)

As is typical of septic shock, her blood pressure was low (80/40).

Her temperature was low rather than high, a dangerous sign indicating that the patient's resistance to infection was fading. Her white blood cell count should have been very high but was very low (another bad sign), and she was anemic. Waste products were accumulating in her blood because her kidneys were not working. That she already had lung trouble was evidenced by a low oxygen tension in her blood. She was panting and trying to breathe, air hungry. Pelvic examination had confirmed that she did indeed have an infection of the type produced by the Welch bacillus, *Clostridium perfringens*, the gas bacillus. X-ray showed bubbles of gas in the uterus. The blood culture was positive, meaning that these anaerobic organisms grew directly from her blood on culture. Given this overwhelming and deep-seated anaerobic gas bacillus infection with kidney failure, a fatal outcome seemed inevitable.

One of our residents at that time, Robert H. Bartlett, was taking care of her. He consulted with experts in obstetrics and in infectious diseases and sought the use of the new high-pressure oxygen chamber at the Children's Hospital Medical Center next door. She was given penicillin, streptomycin, and antitoxin against tetanus and gas bacillus infection. An emergency operation was performed in which her damaged uterus was removed. As soon as the operation was completed she was taken to the hyperbaric oxygen chamber.

About 20% of the air we breathe is oxygen. High-pressure oxygen chambers employ 100% oxygen at 2 atmospheres pressure. This means that the partial pressure of oxygen within the chamber is almost 10 times higher than it is in the air we breathe. High oxygen tensions are toxic to anaerobic bacteria. The term anaerobic means that the bacteria are able to live without oxygen; oxygen is poisonous to them. After the oxygen treatment, she was prepared for dialysis on the artificial kidney because of her kidney failure. This remarkable combination of aggressive steps in treatment led to her recovery. On the 12th postoperative day her kidneys started to work again, and on the 40th postoperative day, after a long convalescence, she went home, well and healthy.

My only role in the care of this patient was in encouraging Bob Bartlett and the staff to take the necessary steps and for him to follow his own remarkable insights. That the patient recovered so beautifully was entirely due to his vision, imagination, and aggressive care. He is now Professor of Surgery at the University of Michigan.

That this young woman had such a terrible, life-endangering episode was due in part to the fact that legal abortions were not yet available. But this crisis was also traceable to the fact that her emotional life was out of control, with repeated pregnancies and repeated abortions. She was an exploited, confused, struggling orphan of our social controls long before she had this abortion. Although we sought the advice of psychiatrists and social workers while she was with us, they did not hold out much hope of redesigning her life.

It has been said that the quality of a society is measured by the care it gives to its least fortunate members. We gave this unfortunate young woman care that returned her to life. We could only hope that she would lead her life better in the future than she had in the past. While the statistics were against rehabilitation, she surely would never become pregnant again.

A case like this makes us stand in awe of the complex and fateful ramifications of reproduction in our society. And it shows again, as do several of the other cases described in this book, how medicine and science, for all their high-tech complexity, can help humble, low-tech people in distress. And how clean surgery to terminate pregnancy is to be much preferred over the filthy manipulation of illegal abortion.

Helping Life at Its End

At the other end of life there has also been a change during our years of surgery. But this has been a change more in the thinking of the public than in the ethical awareness of physicians and surgeons who have embraced these problems and tried to help solve them for many years.

Doctors of our generation are not newcomers to this question. Going back to my internship days, I can remember many patients in pain, sometimes in coma or delirious, with late, hopeless cancer. For many of them we wrote an order for heavy medication to be given regularly by the nurses. Morphine by the clock. We were assisting with a softer exit from this world. Nurses helped willingly. This was not talked about openly, and little was written about it. It was essential, not controversial.

According to the press, another reason this problem has become so urgent now is that with such measures as assisted respiration, assisted heartbeat, and an artificial kidney, we are able to keep people alive long after they otherwise would have died. These patients, some of whom have long since lost their desire to live, have attracted lawsuits and court actions and have brought headlines on this matter to the public view.

It is my conviction that although such patients on complex life-support systems have focused attention on the matter, they are but a tiny fraction of the total population for whom this matter of preserving unacceptable existence becomes urgent and urgently demands a solution. Many patients who want surcease from life are not being kept alive, either by machines or by the machinations of physicians or family. They have managed to survive too far into the progress of disease by dint of their own efforts, better hygiene, and nutrition. While doctors may not have been guilty of keeping them here, they need guidance on helping them leave.

Another concept that has brought this problem into focus has been the definition of brain death, that is, defining death as having occurred when the brain no longer shows any activity. This definition of death was established by the Commission headed by Harry Beecher in 1953. The group was asked to define death legally, morally, and biologically—not only to clarify the answer to the medical-legal question "When is a person actually dead?" but also to decide at what point the human body could become available for the donation of its precious anatomical resources to give other people a better life. This definition of brain death was primarily based on prolonged, irreversible coma. It stated, in essence, that if the brain was long dead, the person was also dead.

Soon this reality was extended to include people who might have been in coma for only a few minutes but who had suffered irreversible and irreparable physical destruction of the brain by a bullet or blunt injury, as in a shooting or an auto crash. I believe it is a tribute to the level of education of the public both here and in Western Europe that the concept of brain death was widely accepted within a decade.

Going back to Chapter 1, where we saw the human body as a dwelling place for a person's mind and soul, the concept of "brain death" helps move our thinking along. As soon as you understand the meaning of brain death, you begin to appreciate the converse meaning of "brain life." The brain can be alive in a suffering person, while the rest of the dwelling place itself is in such wreckage and is the source of such anguish that the person should be allowed to leave that dwelling place by achieving brain death. No human being should be required to remain very long in the terrible situation of fearing death and at the same time wanting it to come as soon as possible: a living mind seeking brain death.

This matter has now reached the stage where all physicians should declare their credo, at least to themselves. It is my credo that assisting people to leave the dwelling place of their body when it is no longer habitable is becoming an obligation of the medical profession. It is part of the doctor's job. This new job for the physician is being defined against a rapidly moving backdrop of changing images that include doctors doing this publicly and possibly illegally; new laws being proposed in some states and nations making it legal, acceptable, and possible; families who want to pull the plug or remove the tube; and anguish over the suitability of physicians' behavior in helping soul leave body. Inevitably, both society and the law will come to accept a variety of solutions. Broader ranges of acceptability will develop in a decade or two.

It is best to approach a struggle with clear views of the obstacles ahead. As this matter moves closer to practical reality, we can be sure of two things. First, that many will be bitterly opposed to any social and legal acceptance of the physician caring for patients in death, assisting them to leave their bodies by achieving brain death. This will become as emotional an issue as pregnancy termination and rather similar to it in pitting personal choice against unremitting life preservation. It will involve a similar struggle between available choice and stand-pat bias. There will be strong feelings and deep human awareness of potential abuse and misuse. While we can expect headlines about doctors undoing a tradition that goes back to Hippocrates, there will be a strong public awareness that such a step is often essential to the doctor's historic mission of care and caring for human life, its quality as well as its duration. Events have broadened the physician's responsibilities. Now we must often hurt before we can heal. In the future we will be called upon to heal by declaring the dwelling place uninhabitable.

Second, we can be sure from the very outset that when physicians' care in death becomes either commonplace or publicly accepted, this privilege will occasionally be abused.

The best way to bring the problem into focus is to describe two patients whom I cared for in the later years of my clinical work who exemplify the many problems of this genre. The basic human understanding that went into their care and the thinking of those near them have a strong bearing on this problem of the ethics, ways and means of care, in death. Experiences like these have been weathered by many families, physicians, and surgeons of our era. These two epitomize many similar challenges in my surgical years.

A 65-Year-Old Woman with a Fractured Pelvis

The patient, formerly a nurse, had sustained a fractured pelvis in an automobile accident. A few days later her lungs seemed to fill up with a process that at first was called pneumonia, but soon other causes became more likely. She stopped making urine and her heart began to act up with dangerous rhythm disturbances. Her blood pressure began to fall. She was transferred to our hospital, to the Bartlett Unit.

On admission she was only intermittently conscious and became unable to oxygenate her blood adequately. An endotracheal tube was placed for assisted breathing, and with machine assistance she achieved higher oxygen tensions in her blood. With a slow, low-volume transfusion, her blood pressure picked up. She was placed on dialysis for renal failure. She improved but was neither fully conscious nor aware.

The mystery of what was going on in her lungs was hard to solve. In people with fractures of the pelvis, bone marrow fat sometimes leaks out into the circulation and produces a disorder called fat embolism. Because she might also have had some such transport of fat to her lungs, she was placed on an anticoagulant, despite its hazards. This helped her. But as her breathing began to improve, her heart rhythm became more erratic and she lapsed into deeper coma. An electrical pacemaker was placed, running from a vein in her neck down into the heart. With the help of this device, she was able to maintain a strong regular heartbeat.

So there she was: in coma, on dialysis every couple of days for kidney failure, intubated, on machine breathing, heartbeat maintained with an electrical device. Being kept alive with all those high-tech machines. Since she was on the Bartlett Unit where I made rounds every day, I was well aware of her precarious status.

One day after rounds I was in my office talking to one of the residents. There was a knock at the door. My secretary said that two relatives of a patient on the Bartlett Unit wanted to see me. I asked her to show them in. Because I had glimpsed them over the last few days, and many of the staff had talked with them at length, I recognized one of them as the husband of our patient, the other as one of her sons.

They sat down with me, looking sad and gloomy. As well they might. They told me that their wife and mother was obviously going to die, that she did not want to die this kind of a death while being maintained by machines. She was a nurse and had told her family that she never wanted this kind of terrible death in the remoteness of a hospital intensive care ward away from her family. Death with dignity, at home if possible, had been her wish.

I told them that while I respected their view, we should all be aware of the fact that she did not have cancer or some other malignant condition. There was nothing intrinsically lethal about her situation. It was precarious. It was dangerous. It was unpleasant. But not necessarily fatal. She did not have severe vascular disease, by which I meant anything resembling a stroke or a heart attack. The disturbed heart rhythm for which she had received a pacemaker was one that often returned to normal, leaving no trace. The sort of kidney failure she had was just the kind for which the artificial kidney was most effective. Many such patients recover their kidney function and a year later have perfectly normal kidneys. Such lungs as hers could also recover completely.

I did not want her family to think I was going to force things on them or could guarantee recovery. They wanted to have her care discontinued, the plug pulled, although they did not use those exact words. They wanted to have all those artificial devices disconnected and let her die in peace and without pain.

I listened attentively, shook their hands, and told them that we did not feel death was imminent and, in fact, she might well recover completely. For the moment at least, we should hang in there. I asked them if they would stick with us for a few more days and invited them to call me or come see me again as often as they wished.

While possibly a bit reassured, they were disappointed. Here was the head surgeon seemingly determined to keep everybody alive, no matter what, just as they had read in popular magazine articles about those misguided doctors. I tried to tell them such was not my philosophy. But you cannot review all of ethical philosophy in a few tense moments. I just said, "Let's give her some more time." Somewhat more content, but still unhappy, they thanked me and left.

About 3 days later her kidneys began to open up. Over the next week, slowly but surely, the patient dug herself out of her troubles. Our diagnosis of fat embolism to the lung was never substantiated by a lung biopsy or by any of the meddlesome methods one might use. In any event, the lungs cleared up just the way fat embolism does. Anticoagulants were stopped. She no longer needed the machine to breathe, and the endotracheal tube was taken out.

When patients start to get very sick, they often seem to fall apart all at once. Everything stops working: a syndrome known as multisystem organ failure. The reverse is also true. When dreadfully sick patients start to get well, suddenly everything starts to pull together at once like an eight-oared crew that has suddenly got it all together with a good coxswain: multisystem organ recovery.

Within a few days the patient's pacemaker could be removed, and she awoke from her coma, albeit a bit fuzzy. She could not remember anything that had happened over the previous weeks. She left the hospital and went home with her family.

I did not happen to see the husband and son again up on the Bartlett Unit, and I didn't even give it much thought, because I knew of course that they were pleased. The younger staff kept in close daily touch with the family. About 6 months later I was again in my office, on a day when I was seeing patients. So it was not unusual when a woman and her husband and son walked in. My secretary asked them if they wanted an appointment. They said yes, they did, but they weren't really patients anymore. They just wanted to see me. To talk.

Doris Lewis, my secretary, was intuitive. She sensed that this was something very meaningful to these people. She vaguely recalled their first visit. So when a gap opened up in the office schedule she told me over the intercom that a woman, husband, and son wished to see me for a few minutes. Somehow I had a flash association and thought of that patient.

The door opened and in walked a gloriously fit woman with her snappy new dress and a large picture hat. She was prancing, almost waltzing. Showing off. The husband was feeling good and smiling. The son trailed in, proud to be with his parents.

They introduced themselves and after some cheery words of appreciation, the father and son asked to speak to me alone. They had planned this. The wife and mother—the patient—went out and sat in the waiting room.

As soon as the door closed, both men became tearful. They didn't quite know what they wanted to say and couldn't really say it. All that came out was, "We want you to know how wrong we were..." and "We're so glad that you did what you thought was right." I knew what they were thinking. No explanations were needed.

I thanked them for their thought and told them again how much confidence I had had in the recovery of their wife and mother. I gave them a few minutes to collect themselves. They left the office quietly, joined her, and departed.

There is a lesson here for everybody. The lesson is so obvious and has such a timely message for all of us that I won't even repeat it. *Res ipsa loquitur.* The facts speak for themselves. Assisting people to leave this life requires strong judgment and long experience to avoid its misuse. It is always a clinical decision, not an ethical, legal, or religious decision, despite the importance of those aspects in getting there.

An 85-Year-Old Woman with Severe Burns

The second patient whose case is relevant here was an elderly lady whose hair caught fire while she was smoking. Elderly women are especially prone to bad burns when they live alone, if they smoke, and especially if they drink and try to operate an electrical appliance. Although we never got the story straight, she had put some sort of liquid or hair tonic on her hair and while smoking had also tried to dry it or blow it with an electric hair dryer. It was not clear just what the source of ignition had been. Maybe a spark. She arrived at the hospital with a deep burn involving her face and the upper part of her chest, the very area that might be exposed in a woman wearing a nightie. Only 15% of her body surface was burned, but a very critical area it was. She was 85.

She had been a sprightly woman, well educated. She was not an alcoholic. She was admitted directly to the Bartlett Unit, and we gave her the usual resuscitation.

From career-long experience I knew that a burn even of this small size including the face and the upper airway (nose and throat) in a woman of this age would surely be fatal. But if my own personal experience was not enough to go on, several statistical and probabilistic analyses had recently been done in which percentage of burn and patient age along with other variables were taken into consideration. Young infants are highly vulnerable to burning. Tiny babies with a burn of only 15 or 20% of their body surface are apt to die. It is for them that heroic removal of the burned skin and replacement with skin grafts from parents may sometimes be life-saving. And at the other extreme of age, as in this patient, small burns are lethal. Even though the patient's heart, lungs, and kidneys seemed to be working pretty well day to day, because of her age they lacked the reserve required to deal with the added burden of such a severe injury.

We had not yet formulated a specific plan for this patient, but we had talked about the options. And we had talked with the nurses. Nurses are of immense importance to any consideration of what should be done for patients with a life-threatening illness. The nurses have a deep sense of what is right and wrong with patients. They know the families. I have had nurses warn me not to pay attention to a family because they were interested in their inheritance rather than their mother's welfare. While that was not the case here, it is an example of why it is important to consult with nurses in such critical situations.

As a remarkable coincidence there was a seminar going on at that time on medical ethics, given by the wife of an official of our university. She was interested in ethics in general as well as the ethics of medical care. The seminar course was given at Harvard College, but upon my invitation she brought some of the participants over to the hospital from time to time to have discussions with physicians. A day or two after our patient was admitted, she asked me if I had any sort of an ethical problem that I could bring up for discussion. I said yes. So, when the patient had been in the hospital about 3 or 4 days, the time was right for me to bring this case up for discussion by these bright-eyed young students.

I described the case of this 85-year-old woman who had a small burn, but one that would surely kill her, a very painful death. Part of the skin of her face and neck would slough off, and she would require skin grafts if she lived long enough. I told them she would probably die in a week or two of kidney failure. At the time I was presenting this case (in the previous 12 hours) her urine output had begun to decline—the first sign of kidney failure.

After I told the students about this agonizing situation, I asked their opinion. Some thought morphine by the clock was the way out. Others were violently opposed to this course and said it would be murder if we didn't do everything conceivably possible to keep the old lady alive as long as possible. Every minute we could. Even in pain. At 85.

No vote was taken. If somebody had suggested a vote, I would have been opposed to polarizing their opinions. After the discussion I made a remark that was, in retrospect, a serious mistake.

I said, "I'll take the word back to the nurses about her and we will talk about it some more before we decide." I did not think twice about making this simple, matter-of-fact statement.

The response was immediate and totally unforeseen, at least by me. The instructor, the ethics expert, and the students were shocked.

"You mean this is a real patient?"

"You mean this is a patient there in the hospital right now?"

I said, "Yes... I thought it would be most important for us to deal with some ethical problems the way they arise in real life."

The ethics class was shocked. I will not record the rest of the conversation except to say that the teacher of ethics was not accustomed to having her prejudices challenged by reality. She wanted make-believe, fantasy, on which to drape her gossamer of theory. I will admit to pique and a flush of anger at her seemingly self-serving desire for simplistic ethical fantasy rather than real-life cases. Why weave fantasies when reality is so fascinating and challenging? Truth is both stranger and more important than fiction. So we did not exactly part happily. Later, we had a chance to talk it over and we remain friends.

In any event, I went back to the ward and met with the nurses. We didn't say or discuss anything new. I made no mention of the ethics class. I did reassure the nurses that it was a good policy always to start out by treating the patient vigorously, as we had done. In this way the patient's family would not worry that we just wanted to let go. In time, the family themselves would come to recognize futility. The nurses were often among the first to sense this.

Curiously, it was some of the younger nurses who were the most aggressive. They were the ones who wanted to continue treatment and start skin grafting right away (she would not have survived a general anesthetic). It was the older, calmer nurses who thought that we should somehow let her go if we could do it mercifully and with the blessing of the family.

Should we ask the patient herself? Febrile, in and out of coma, under drugs, often in pain, hallucinating and disoriented, it would be a cruel mockery of informed consent to ask her if she wanted to stay alive.

Here, as occurs all too often in the elderly, family members were few and far between. Her husband had died some years before. A daughter living in California, age 65, had been unable to afford travel to see her mother for the past several years. Only a grandson in New York could be reached by telephone. He had come up to visit once when she was first admitted, but he fled when he saw her and washed his hands of the whole affair. Since he was the nearest relative, I called him up and told him I thought his grandmother probably wasn't going to make it and would he suggest any other members of the family to talk with. He just said, "No. Do whatever you feel is right."

So, about a day or two later, when she was making little or no urine, her lungs were filling up with fluid because of heart failure and she was suffering terribly, we began to back off on her treatment. When she complained of pain, we gave her plenty of morphine. A great plenty. By the clock.

Soon, she died quietly and not in pain.

A New Task for the Doctor

Neither in this instance nor in the cases of many other terribly sick patients we have helped along to an easy end have I been the least bit disturbed about the ethical problem now termed euthanasia. Maybe I have been too slow and too conservative. Too unfeeling? Don't think so. I hope not.

For patients dying of cancer, I do not believe there is any insurmountable problem if they are in severe pain or in coma, near the end. As the responsible physician, you had better move ahead and do what you would want done for you. And don't discuss it with the world—or any ethics classes—first. Maybe just one member of the family. The doctor should do his duty, which is to give the patient the best possible chance for good minutes, hours, days, but avoid prolonging agony.

The problem becomes far more difficult when the patient does not have cancer, a bad burn, or any other clearly terminal condition. Or when helping a patient leave this world would involve doing something drastic even though the patient is fully conscious and seeking death, with weeks or months ahead, as for some patients with acquired immune deficiency syndrome (AIDS). When patients are in pain or anguished by the necessity of invasive treatment (such as breathing or feeding tubes), they often seek a way out even though they have a good chance of recovery. In such cases, morphine by the clock is definitely not the answer.

The solution to this problem is just as much a part of the physician's charge as is the care of the newborn or the elderly. It is becoming part of our responsibility to help patients safely and painlessly out of this life. I do not know just what form our social understanding of this problem will take. What ways we will find acceptable are still unclear. It will probably not be as simple as assisted suicide. Nor morphine by the clock. Nor pulling the plug, because for most such patients (as pointed out earlier) there is no plug to pull. It must involve legal safeguards. It will involve the family, so long as they can be trusted.

The clergy would like to be involved. I believe that many ministers of the gospel have an insight into such matters, but their importance is limited entirely to those patients who, before they were sick, were personally close to a rector, a priest, or a rabbi and for whom religion was an

343

integral part of their lives. While I welcome the clergy into the sanctum of those who must make these ethical decisions, I am not convinced that any class of people gains a special depth of human insight just because they deliver a sermon every Sunday. It is the patient's relationship to them, rather than any pipeline to revealed truth, that gives the clergy their authority. The clergy should demonstrate through the patient's affection and confidence that they have earned a place in this decision.

Now is the time for guidelines to be drawn and the public to accept some way for desperate patients—those in pain, anguished, or hopeless—who have good enough reason to want to leave their bodily dwelling place to do so. They need social approbation and the assistance of merciful science via their physician to acquire the ways and means of care in death.

Do not forget that most critically ill patients are emotionally upset, often mixed up, sometimes hallucinating, often heavily medicated, rarely getting things straight. If you follow the advice of such a disoriented patient just to console yourself about consent, you may be doing the patient a disservice.

Responsible physicians should join forces with the public to write a new chapter in medical education that places care in death in its proper context. It is tricky. It is dangerous. We need it and people are ready for it. It will relieve more suffering than did the discovery of anesthesia 150 years ago. Physicians today should help lead the public to understanding the nature of this problem and the need for a new solution.

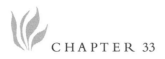

CHAPTER 33

Trying to Retire;
Letting Go Gradually

It was the spring of 1972. I was meeting with Bob Ebert, the Dean, about several matters. So I thought I would spring it on him. After all, he would need several months for his committee to come up with a nominee.

"Bob, in July 1973 I will have been head of my department for 25 years," I said.

"Quite a while," he sparred, wondering what I was driving at.

"I have always said that no major department of a university should be under the thumb of the same person for more than a quarter of a century." I was trying to get on with the matter.

"But you're still doing a great job!" he said, wondering if I was just fishing for some words of praise.

"Thanks," I said. "But I think it's time we got a younger man to run the department." This caught him a little bit off guard. So, he sparred some more, for time.

"When is your Harvard retirement age?"

"June 30, 1981," I shot back. Obviously I had looked up the matter and checked with University Hall. Harvard retirement ages come in different sorts and sizes, and I was one of the older appointees, since my first faculty appointment had been in 1943. So retirement came on the June 30th after my 67th birthday.

345

"That's great! Another 9 years as professor," he said.

"Yes." Now I wanted to drive home the point. "I would like to retire as head of the department next July."

There it was. On the table. He became visibly upset. He seemed surprisingly concerned about it. Somehow I didn't think that I, merely one of his 20 or 30 department heads, would loom very large on his list of worries. He tapped out his pipe. Filled it with new tobacco and tamped it down, slowly. Lit it up. Puffed. Swung around in his chair. This was a ballet Bob Ebert went through whenever he was stalling for time. It was such familiar body language that the students had lampooned it several times in the annual student burlesque. It said, "Give me a moment to think this one over."

"You can't retire now," he said.

"Why not?" I shot back.

"Because I'm going to retire."

I was stunned. In the one-upmanship of conversational poker, he had a royal straight flush! This was totally unexpected. I had thought I was surprising him, but he won.

Bob Ebert had been appointed dean by President Pusey in 1965. He had done a great job, particularly in shepherding the medical school through those difficult years of the late 1960s and early 1970s, years of student uprisings about the Vietnam War and public opposition to the new hospital. He had started up a large health maintenance organization (HMO), or prepaid care plan, known as the Harvard Community Health Plan (in 1969). This was one of the first and most successful of the university-based HMOs. He had had some differences with President Pusey, particularly when students occupied the main offices in University Hall in 1969. Bob Ebert, along with the deans of two or three other graduate schools, had counseled strongly against calling in the police or making any sort of a public nuisance out of this student action, which certainly bordered on violent trespass. Nate Pusey had apparently rejected his deans' advice and called the police anyway. What happened thereafter is one of the darker chapters in Harvard's history: the police threw out the students with considerable violence. There were some cracked heads. Our son Chip was a freshman at Harvard at that time. He and most of the uninvolved students thought that it was not a student riot at all, but a police riot, that the police simply ran amok and took it out on all those rich boys.

I had enjoyed working with Bob Ebert and saw no need to cross him on this point. My plan had been to resign as department head in 1973. Now that was postponed to 1976, still 5 years before my Harvard retirement in 1981.

So it all worked out, and about 4 years after that talk with Bob Ebert I was able to struggle out of some of the responsibility I had accepted so excitedly on July 1, 1948. Laurie and I were much freer to do things together. I welcomed John Mannick, my successor as Moseley Professor, on that same day. He moved into the old Cushing-Cutler-Moore office. I yielded also my precious laboratories next door, which would be as convenient for him as they had been for me.

In 1977 Derek Bok appointed Daniel Tosteson as the new Dean of the Harvard Medical School and in 1978 he took over from Bob Ebert.

Fending Off the Retirement Neurosis

The retirement neurosis is basically a fear of not having anything to do. It affects busy people who are suddenly unoccupied. It also contains a germ of deflated ego. Having a lot of responsibility for many years makes a person feel important. Part of the retirement neurosis comes from a loss of that sense of being a cog in some important piece of machinery.

I was lucky on both scores. I would stay busy by helping raise funds to build the new hospital for which I had been busily working for so many years, taking on new national responsibilities with NASA, becoming the book review editor of *The New England Journal of Medicine*, and chairing the Massachusetts Health Data Consortium (MHDC). President Ford was kind to give me an assist when he asked me to become a member of the Board of Regents of the new federal medical school in Washington, the Uniformed Services University of the Health Sciences (Chapter 27). The MHDC is a free-standing organization based on collaboration of the Massachusetts hospitals to pool their clinical data using a standard method and terminology. This work fitted in with my long-standing interest in national health policy. So I had plenty to do!

The university-hospital committee again went on the prowl for a new Moseley Professor and Surgeon-in-Chief. In 1976 John Mannick was appointed my successor as the sixth Moseley Professor of Surgery at Harvard and the fourth chief surgeon at the Brigham. He was a graduate of the Harvard Medical School, likewise interned at the Massachusetts General Hospital, had been a staff member under one of our Brigham stars, David Hume, then Professor of Surgery in Richmond, Virginia. Mannick was brought to Harvard from Boston University. He was Moseley Professor at Harvard as well as Surgeon-in-Chief at the Brigham until he retired on June 30, 1994. Identification of the next surgeon to fill the Moseley chair did not have to wait too long, as we now welcome Michael Zinner as John's successor. Considering the Brigham tradition, it is fitting that Zinner is a Hopkins trainee but in addition brings us fresh ideas from UCLA, where he pursued his surgical work before coming to the Moseley chair and the Brigham department.

Thus, the tradition of the Moseley Professorship of Surgery at Harvard carries on with flying colors and will soon celebrate the 100th year of its endowment. An important 200th anniversary was celebrated in 1982, because it was in 1782 that John Warren was appointed Professor of Anatomy and Surgery at Harvard. It was also in 1982 that the Harvard Medical School celebrated its bicentennial, and I was thrilled to be the recipient of an honorary doctorate. In 1990 a new surgical chair was endowed at Harvard University, named in my honor. This endowment came from the generosity of hundreds of friends, colleagues, and patients. This professor is to work with the Moseley Professor. In 1992 Nicholas Tilney was appointed the first Francis D. Moore Professor.

To have been one link in this chain of Harvard surgical leadership and to live to celebrate its 200th birthday was a unique privilege for me, as it would have been for any surgeon.

In 1976 the Dean gave me an office on the fourth floor of the Countway Library. It is perfect. Not much bigger than the cabin of a boat, but with a secretary's office next door. I am grateful for this privilege. Imagine in retirement having an office right in the midst of the library and right next to the hospital where you could visit patients and old friends, and then, into the bargain, to have it just one story below the

Journal where you were going to work as Book Review Editor for 12 years.

The New England Journal of Medicine

On several occasions over the course of 50 years, I have been for a time a member of the editorial board of *The New England Journal of Medicine*. The term was usually 3 or 4 years. I served under a succession of distinguished editors including Robert Nye, Joseph Garland, Franz Ingelfinger, Arnold Relman, and now (appointed in 1992) Jerome Kassirer. The *Journal* enjoys a large circulation, something close to 300,000 a larger paid circulation than any other medical journal in the United States. Although the *Journal of the American Medical Association* (JAMA) has a larger circulation, *The New England Journal of Medicine* has entirely a paid circulation.

I went up to see Bud Relman one day in 1981, feeling underemployed, only to have him offer me the job of editing the book review section. I happened to hit the day he was ready to make such a change. A perfect job for a job-vacant retiree. Lucky again.

I accepted this task, worked at it for about 12 years, and enjoyed it immensely. The *Journal* receives 3,000 to 4,000 books annually. My job was to pick the approximately 500 to 550 books to be reviewed each year. And then find other people to review them.

Over the years I had reviewed a good many books and continue to review a few each year. As Book Review Editor it was my job to assign most of the reviews to other desks, and we rarely had a turn-down. We often asked distinguished senior scientists, physicians, pediatricians, and surgeons to review important new monographs in their field. For some of the other books we sought reviews from young people just starting out who were already making a mark in science or teaching.

The conduct of this book review section brought me a small income, always welcome when you are suffering from acute and chronic retirement. It also put me in touch with doctors of all stripes and many scientists over the country and over the world. After 12 years of this enjoyable job, I began to think that maybe they needed a younger man. I am very proud of the fact that Robert Schwartz succeeded me as Book Review Editor of the *Journal*—the same Dr. Schwartz referred to in Chapter 20 who coauthored with Dr. Dameshek that key paper describing for the first time the immunosuppressive potency of 6-mercaptopurine.

As Book Review Editor I was impressed with the large number of medical books published every year. It became my conviction that most of them should be interred in some library soon after birth and spend the rest of their natural lifetimes or, rather, deathtimes there. I became disillusioned with the torrent of books in medicine. So here I am adding a ripple to that torrent.

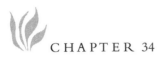

CHAPTER 34

Laura's Death;
A New Life with Katharyn

W hen our youngest son FDM, Jr. (Chip), had finished college and medical school and was married (in 1976), our life, like that of all married couples, underwent a radical change. With the fledglings flown from the nest, our house was quiet. Empty. We rattled around. We moved to a much smaller house. But even there the house seemed vacant.

Despite this (and after 41 years of marriage), the pleasures we enjoyed together never abated. We went together on medical trips. Many visits to England, France, Italy, Scandinavia, Australia, New Zealand, and finally around the world via Australia, Bangkok, and New Delhi. Some years later we had a wonderfully interesting trip to China. Nice to have a wife who knew a bit of Chinese history.

On July 25, 1988, in a sudden, black, summer thunderstorm and thundersquall like the one we had driven through at the start of our honeymoon 53 years before, Laurie's life was ended in a moment of terrible encounter. I was working in my office at the time; the great black cloud from which came the fatal thundersquall could be seen in Boston, coming in from the northwest. I looked at it and still remember a sense of foreboding. She was driving home from Carlisle, northwest of Boston, near Concord. Because of the darkness and the torrential downpour she could not see the fully loaded gravel truck bearing down on her tiny car.

The service in her memory was a simple one, held at the First Parish Church across the street from our home in Brookline. I had asked several young women, close friends of Laurie, if they would help as ushers at the service. Diana Phillips, niece of Rebecca Lewis, one of our closest friends, had become an ordained Episcopal minister. She had also been the chaplain at our hospital and had presided at the wedding of our youngest son, Chip, to Carla Dateo 3 years before. Diana's remarks, the service filled with music, the church filled to overflowing, marked a milestone in our family's life but not an ending for Laurie. A believer in the soul of mankind, I have no trouble with the thought that her memory and her living legacy to her children and grandchildren constitute an eternal life for her as it does for any mother taken away in her prime.

A couple of weeks after Laurie's service, our youngest grandchild was born. One of Laurie's Bartlett family names going back to colonial days of New Hampshire was Colcord. He was named Francis Colcord Daniels Moore. His father is Chip. This young man, who never saw his grandmother, is known as Cord.

A month or so later, Laurie's ashes were put into the earth on the hill above Grafton, Vermont, the village that was the home of my great-grandfather Francis Daniels and his son (my grandfather) Francis Barrett Daniels, and where my daughter Sally Moore Warren and her family now live. My father and mother, who died in 1966 and 1972, are buried in that same small Grafton cemetery. Laurie's father had been buried in Peoria, Illinois, and her mother in Granville, Ohio. Laurie had told us that if anything happened, she wanted to be buried up on the Daniels hill, there, in the old Vermont cemetery. We had then been married for 53 years; she had been part of my life for at least 58 years.

After Laurie's death came a new form of loneliness. Some men simply cannot get along alone. This might be especially true of men who married young, men who have had a happy marriage for many years.

Kathie Saltonstall and her husband William, formerly principal of Phillips Exeter Academy in New Hampshire, had been friends of ours for many years. In 1944, through my friendship with his brother Henry Saltonstall, a classmate, a surgeon of Exeter, New Hampshire, I had been asked to operate on their older son Bill, Jr., for appendicitis. Then, over the years, the acquaintance of the two families had become closer, and in the last 15 years before Laurie's death, Katharyn and Laura were intimate friends. Over the last 10 years, with her husband's progressive sickness, our lives involved many parallel activities in Marion, Massachusetts, especially trying to help with Bill and taking him sailing, despite his illness. On other days Laurie was the crew for Katharyn in races that Katharyn often won, and Laurie could bask in reflected glory.

Katharyn's husband was quite ill and bedridden at the time of Laurie's death. We both had tried to help as best we could with Bill's care. Laurie and I had been worried about Katharyn's stress and fatigue during those hard years of his illness. Katharyn's husband died December 18, 1989, about 18 months after Laurie. Kathie and Bill had been married 58 years.

Katharyn Watson Saltonstall and I were married about 6 months later, on May 13, 1990. We tried to explain to people that although we were newlyweds, we were embarking on our 111th year of happy marriage.

Like Laurie and me, Katharyn and Bill had five children. They had 16 grandchildren, we had 17. Katharyn has two great-grandchildren; a ways ahead of me. Katharyn's younger son, Sam, had worked with us one summer helping to look after our youngest son Chip, who was about 10 at the time. Katharyn is a successful author. *Small Bridges to One World* (1986) is the story of the years she and Bill spent in Nigeria when he was the Peace Corps representative (1963 to 1965), supervising the work and tending to the well-being of almost 750 Peace Corps volunteers there.

The instinctive need for prayer usually arises from fear of the future, of the unknown. But it also arises from gratitude. Prayers of thanksgiving are deeply ingrained in the Christian tradition and have a secure place in American secular culture as epitomized by the celebration of Thanksgiving Day.

Since Laurie's death and my marriage to Katharyn, I seem to have become a more religious person. Katharyn and I attend church fairly regularly, though not quite as steadily as we should. As I enter that Marion church—where we were married in 1990—I have the sensation, and I think Kathie shares it, that we are entering a place where, among other things, we can give thanks to some higher power for our marriage, for finding an end to our loneliness, and for our large and wonderful families.   Our Pastor, Bob Duebber, by his kindness and concern has added immeasurably to these feelings of reverence.   It is said that older people acquire religion because they need it.

One might offer thanks to God (in the conventional sense of the Christian Church), to chance, to the forces of nature, or to the combined coincidence of our two families.   When I hear of men who have lost their wives, or wives who have lost their husbands, I could never wish for them a happier outcome after loneliness and grief than a marriage such as ours.

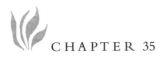

CHAPTER 35

Leisure

Early to the hospital, late home. Sunday morning rounds. In times of despair our children referred to their parents as workaholics. In their more thoughtful moments they could hardly hold to such a view, and Laurie stoutly held up for our side. After all, we had sailed together in Buzzards Bay, ridden horseback in Wyoming, skied, fished, hunted, traveled, and sang with the best of them. We tried to broaden the experience of our children to realms beyond Boston, away from home, following the tradition initiated by our parents years before. Now, all five of our offspring are workaholics in their own way. Each of them attacks the particular problem at hand with fierce determination. While all have found satisfaction in their careers, each family has developed its own pattern of release.

Our hobbies boiled down to sailing and music.

Sailing

While many summers of my youth were spent wielding a lasso or riding a horse on roundups up and down mountains, I had done some sailing as a youth. About 1947 we began to spend some summers at the seashore on Buzzards Bay and became addicted to sailing. Laura, likewise a middlewestern landlubber, also took to the salt water and enjoyed sailing, being crew for Katharyn in the ladies' races, also being the chief cook and bottle-washer on our cruising boat. She was keen of eye and ear. Navigating at night or through the fog, she was the most reliable in getting us where we should go, spotting the lights, hearing the groaners. In addition, she could take the helm and steer a compass course along with the best of them despite winds or tide. Our children took up racing and won their share of trophies.

Many of the hobbies of Americans are complex and demanding, something you have to work hard at. Sailing is an example. Sometimes sailing is beatific in brisk wind on bright water (as in the beer ads), but it can also be grungy work. On one occasion there was a clogged valve (probably valvular stenosis) in the carburetor of our engine. You could only get at it by taking apart the whole afterpart of the boat, exposing the bilge, which could be at times a bit oily, even smelly, and not as clean as we would have liked. It was a very hot day. I was stripped to the waist. Dripping sweat. Leaning down and reaching around in this filthy bilge water trying to locate the valve. Swearing softly to myself. Somebody peered down the hatch and said, "Hi Franny, whatta'ya doin'?"

In a moment of inspiration I replied:

"Yachting."

The Moores and the Delands were the co-owners of a 40-foot Bermuda yawl, *Angelique*. Over the course of 12 or 15 years we did a good deal of ocean racing. As skipper, I conducted *Angelique* to Bermuda, on the Whaler's Race at Block Island, and several times to Halifax. The Halifax Race became our specialty. Most of the time you can't see anything because of the fog. One time we had a major northeast gale. But it was on the Halifax Race that we came closest to some sort of glory. In our class of 40-footers, we were second. Halifax is 365 miles from the start at Marblehead. We were only 38 seconds behind Ted Hood, a yacht designer and genuine pro. We are proud of our silver bowl. It is used to serve potato chips.

There is something especially serene about sailing at night, as you do on long ocean races. It is dark. Maybe a few stars. You are in your bunk up forward. As skipper you are apt to have a small compass there and a flashlight so you can secretly check on the helmsman. But more likely, you are drifting off to sleep on the off watch. There is only an inch of mahogany between your ear and the entire ocean, which gurgles soporifically along the hull. Looking aft you can see up the companion-way where there is the dim red glow of the binnacle light on the compass. And around it faces of family or friends, having a good discussion or argument, laughing, and enjoying themselves immensely as they guide the boat through the night sea. Sailing in the Gulf Stream on the way to Bermuda, flying fish are attracted into the cockpit by the binnacle light, flopping around in that strange place until they are assisted back to their element.

Then there are the storms, the crashes (we were hit full-on by another boat in one race), or the encounters with geology (once we hit a rock during a gale in outer Marion Harbor within sight of our house). If you do a lot of sailing, such things are bound to happen.

While there are many delightful moments in the world of cruising, few surpass the "happy hour." It has been a long day in the wind and sun. Now you are in a secure anchorage. The hook is down. She is swinging kindly. It is the time for some snacks and a few drinks, on deck. The gulls are shrieking around, hoping for a handout, or geese are honking and hoping for their bit of a Triscuit with cheese. And maybe you can see an osprey gliding off to its evening hunt. As the sun sets, small lights go on in the cabins of other yachts around you. If you have been clever, you have fixed the main halyards so they won't slap against the mast. And unless there is somebody on board who snores too loudly for kind words, you are in for a good night's sleep.

Surprisingly, there are actually people who dislike yachting. I remember one horseman who said, "Why should I sleep in a narrow hallway with a toilet at one end and a smelly gasoline engine at the other?" I thought for a little while and said, "Well, you have different functions at the two ends of a horse."

Music

Music provides some of the same kinesthetic sensations and aes-thetic joys as sailing. There is a sheer physical, muscular, pleasure in playing the piano, in the exercise of arms and hands, in hearing nice sounds come out. It does require a fair amount of work. We were pleased that all our children at one time or another played two-piano or instrumental music with me. Some of them clung to their music more than others, but music did become a part of their lives: Peter playing the guitar, Sally as a choral singer in Vermont, Caroline with her two-piano music.

Music began for me at a young age when somebody thought I might be good at playing the piano. I never had any sense of practicing very much. While I was never disciplined or forced to practice, I played at the piano a good deal. During high school and college I was involved in various public performances: musical shows, concerts. Probably only a few of the musical sounds that an amateur makes are very pleasurable to others.

It was in college that I became involved with writing the music for two musical comedies at the Hasty Pudding (Chapter 6). And then later on, both in medical school and afterward, I continued to write some musical comedies. Those various musical comedies were often more comical than humorous. At medical school, John Rock was one of the pioneers in birth control. He was one of our teachers. So one of the jazzy songs of the medical school show in 1938 was *Rock, Rhythm, and Romance*. Here the word "rhythm" had an unusual double entendre: hot jazz and the female fertility cycle. And "Rock" meant Professor John, not a form of swing. In fact, the term "rock" for any sort of music had not yet been coined.

In composing later musical shows I enjoyed the coauthorship and collaboration of several talented people, including David McCord, who wrote the book and lyrics for one of our shows. It was based on the fanciful concept of a hospital that was losing too much money and a bank that was making too much money. Since the hospital needed money and the bank needed a built-in deduction, they merged. The name of the show was *Futures and Sutures, or the Urge to Merge*.

While the tunes for these ventures could hardly be referred to as serious music, they sometimes took the form of more conscientious pieces in the nature of trios or quartets. My musical philosophy defends the concept that all music is joyous, written to provide joy to the listener. True, there are exceptions, such as the requiems. And some of the passionate parts of the oratorios and masses, for example, the tragic *Crucifixus* from Bach's B Minor Mass. Possibly it would be an injustice to Bach, Mozart, Fauré, and Brahms to say that these requiems are intended to give joy to the listener. Maybe it would be better to say that all music provides the listener with an aesthetic experience, usually a pleasurable one. There is no fundamental difference between the music of Bach, Handel, Haydn, Mozart, and Beethoven and that of Gershwin, Porter, Berlin, Copland, or Bernstein. Some are greater composers than others, but all music has the same message of joy in performance and, if well performed, for the listener.

As I grew older, my sailing did not improve any. In fact, it deteriorated. I became very good at losing races. But my music seemed to improve.

About 1975, several of us got together (faculty and students) and formed the Harvard Medical School Music Society, or HMSMS. It was our intention to make the most of the musical talent in the medical school, students and faculty. One of our surgical residents had taught piano in Cleveland for some years and had performed all the Beethoven piano concertos with the Cleveland Orchestra. Another student had been first clarinetist in a symphony orchestra. Still another medical student, a violinist, was the sister of Yo-Yo Ma and, like her talented brother, a delightful performer. At HMSMS we could hear unusual duets and arrangements that the students themselves found and performed. We gave two concerts a year. I used to play piano in some of these concerts, usually playing one of two pianos, or else accompanying students. The performers came entirely from within the Harvard medical family. Now HMSMS is guided by a faculty wife, Annette Benacerraf. I have not played in the concerts so much recently.

"Hey Doc, whatta'ya do in your spare time?" is a question that every doctor (or his wife) is frequently asked. About a month or two before Christmas. Be careful what answer you give. I have a great many recordings piled up from past Christmases, and I have received quite a few life preservers. The former are most enjoyable. I am not sure the latter are much of a tribute to my nautical abilities.

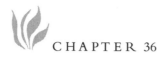

CHAPTER 36

Cool Streams, High Mountains, White Faces: Looking Back

Thissbook should end with sparkling memories of youth. I especially enjoyed the brightness of those Wyoming years, living for a time each year in a part of the world quintessentially American. A part of the West claimed by the white man only since the Battle of the Little Bighorn, 50 years before we first arrived in 1927 and 50 miles away in southern Montana.

From high school years until entering medical school I enjoyed a drastic change of scene every summer. This Wyoming cattle ranch, by name the Horseshoe, had been put together from homesteads around 1890, as were many ranches in that part of Wyoming. In its early years it was a horse ranch providing remounts for the United States Cavalry. Range mares were bred to the remount stallions placed in that country by the army to improve the breed. Buyers sent out by the cavalry then came to pick up the product.

A Ranch Beside the Mountains (with a River Running Through It)

The circumstances of our summers there arose from the rental of the ranch house by my parents for a summer vacation of family and friends in 1927 and again in 1928, followed by their purchase of the place in 1929. They operated it for the next 17 years, and our summers were spent there. Our honeymoon was spent there. It was a bright and shining aspect of our lives until the time when war, medical school, graduate studies, jobs, and a growing family of young children prevented our going there. We last went there for a vacation just before the war in 1941.

The Horseshoe Ranche (the terminal *e* a holdover, it was said, from the Spanish spelling) comprised 5,000 acres on the eastern edge of the Bighorn National Forest near Dayton, Wyoming. The western border of the ranch was the eastern border of the forest. It was also a distinct geologic borderline. To the west the heavily timbered mountains rose abruptly. From this border eastward lay the flat open plains of eastern Wyoming, stretching across the Powder River Divide, the land of the great cattle ranches of the 1880s (a small town there, Ucross, is named after one of those cattle brands), finally bounded by the forests of the Black Hills 150 miles away. This open land is marked by colorful buttes and mesas, pine-bordered rimrock, deep red cliffs, and shale. Rivers come down out of the mountains from melting snow, through limestone canyons, and change to a slower flow. They are lined with huge cottonwoods, making places of coolness and damp shade, of quiet pools for trout. A welcome contrast to the broiling summer heat on the plains. The grateful shade.

The hay and grain raised on these dry plains must be on meadows under ditch. The irrigation system consists of ditches leading from the streams as they emerge from the mountain canyons. Alfalfa is grown on the hay meadows, the standard hay crop of the area, stacked in huge haystacks (10 to 20 tons each), never kept in barns or silos as in New England.

Just west of the ranch, the land abruptly rose almost 5,000 feet in just a mile or so. The altitude at the ranch house was about 3,800 feet. The tops of foothills immediately to the west were at about 8,600 feet. Then, a limestone plateau extended westward for several miles, in the center of which was the granite uplift of the snow-covered Bighorn chain, culminating in a few peaks at 12,000 to 13,000 feet.

Animals, Wild and Tame

Riding on the lower ranch to the east you were on open plains. Immediately to the west we started up trails in the steep mountain canyons. As teenagers, we worked in the hayfields, driving teams, mowers, stackers, and buck-rakes. Hard work in the hot sun, a volunteer effort for the family project. All the heavy machinery was pulled by four-legged horsepower. We raised Belgian draft horses to do this work. Driving these marvelous beasts was a powerful experience.

The wild animals we encountered (always called "game") were intriguing. The bighorn sheep were there no more, although we found their sunbaked white skulls, curled horns intact, in the deep canyons. Buffalo were long gone; we found many of those skulls also. The sheep and buffalo must have been driven into the canyons to escape the predations of the Indians, who in turn were escaping the predations of the white man. Elk, deer, black bear, and coyotes were there in abundance. In the early morning when we left the corrals to enter the pastures along the mountain front to wrangle the horses, we would often surprise these wild animals as we tried to find where the horses had wandered, grazing during the night.

Although there were roads up the mountains, the landscape that we saw still looked much as it must have in the time of Lewis and Clark. Certainly there were fences every few miles. There might be an occasional ranch building. But the general lay of the land—the mountains, forests, buttes, mesas—and the crystal-clear limestone-alkaline mountain water with plenty of trout gave a special charm to this part of the West.

The cattle business at that time was heading into a severe depression. The great drought of the early 1930s, as evidenced by the Okie dustbowl and Steinbeck's *The Grapes of Wrath*, dry farmers gone broke and leaving Oklahoma for California, was reflected in Wyoming by severe drought and an almost biblical plague of huge grasshoppers that lasted for several years. Beef prices were low. Hay prices were high. A bad combination. The 1930s were not good years for cattle ranchers. The economic success of a ranch depended on water rights, irrigation, and a mountain-grazing permit obtained from the U.S. government (which involved a fair amount of politicking) that enabled the rancher to graze his cattle in the national forest during the summer and feed them home-grown hay in the winter. After the roundup in the fall, the steers, dry cows, and old bulls ("baloney bulls") were shipped by railroad to Chicago where they were resold, the prime steers going to the corn-feeding farms of the middle west, the old bulls to the sausage factory.

The cattle in those days were uniformly the white-faced Hereford. On the mountain grazing-ranges, cattle of many owners and from different ranches roamed over large areas of the mountains with no fences. For this reason all ranchers in an association had to agree to purchase bulls of about the same quality.

Much of this has now changed. Huge trucks are used to take the cattle from the ranches directly to the Iowa feedlots without passing through Chicago at all. The Chicago stockyards have disappeared. Overgrazing on both plain and mountain pasture produced loss of ground cover, erosion, and degradation of grass in the mountain meadows. The number of cattle grazing on national forest land (on government mountain permits) has been sharply reduced. Angus, black or red, have partly replaced the white-faced Hereford.

For trips into the mountains we did everything ourselves: tossing the diamond hitch to pack the horses, picketing them at night, hunting for the lost ones the next morning, catching trout for breakfast, cooking, making the paniers of equal weight for balance on the two sides of the packsaddles. Or, in haying time, mowing the hay, sulky-rake, buck-rake, and horse-drawn stacker. The men with whom we worked were never hurried or harried. They got the job done, rested the horses at noon, fed them, ate their box of sandwiches in a cool cottonwood grove by the stream, and taught us how to pace ourselves.

Fine Art

As to the particular crafts of the western ranch hand, his ability to rope horses or cattle at a high gallop is certainly legendary. But of all the things the cowboy could do, there was nothing quite like rolling your own at a full gallop in a high wind. This was an operation carried out under difficulty, with impressive skill, an elegant technique in a learned handicraft. Surgical.

The prevailing form of tobacco for ranchers at that time was a dry, brown, powdery substance called Bull Durham, a reference to Durham, North Carolina, although the residents of that beautiful college town may possibly wish to deny it. The tobacco itself was disparagingly referred to by the locals as the "sweepings from the Lucky Strike factory."

That little cotton sack of tobacco (old print of a Red Bull on the label) was kept in the left upper front pocket of the cowboy's vest (if he was right-handed). A small, yellow cardboard tag was hitched to the drawstring of the tobacco bag, hanging out. Then, at a high gallop in a high wind (left hand for the horse at all times), the procedure was as follows: the bag of Bull Durham was removed and one tiny, fluttering piece of flimsy cigarette paper was withdrawn from the attached paper-packet, shaped like a little trough or gutter in the left hand (also holding the reins) by curling it delicately with the thumb and third finger around the extended index finger. Then, with the horse still at a gallop, still in the wind, tobacco was poured into the cigarette paper by gently agitating the open bag. By seizing the tag-end of the tobacco pack-string in the teeth, it was possible with one hand to close the bag by pulling on the other end and to put it back in the upper left-hand vest pocket. Then the cigarette was rolled dry between the fingers using two hands but guiding the horse around boulders or over streams the while. Finally, when a small, cylindrical object that vaguely resembled a store-bought cigarette had been produced, it was passed across the tongue. Such was the nature of this paper that when moistened it would stick to itself. One end was then squinched together between the fingers, the whole rolled again, and the other end placed between the lips for smoking.

Now came the hard part. A match was taken from the right-hand side pants pocket and struck by scraping it across the slot in a little screwhead that is always found in the central part of the horn, or pommel, of a western saddle. This requires some skill, even when one is standing quietly in the barn. The paper is still wet. Hard to ignite. Once the match is struck and lit, held in one hand, it must be shielded by curling the fingers around it with only minor burns, protecting the flame from the wind. The burning match is brought up to the cigarette, the cigarette lit, and a contented puff taken. This whole operation requires only a short time, possibly 2 or 3 minutes. There are at most six puffs and only a few more minutes left in the smoke. This western horseback ballet, while a routine matter-of-course to the rider (the smoker), could not help but arouse astonishment and admiration on the part of an observant young companion galloping alongside.

Many young men from back East have tried to repeat this themselves, after only a few rehearsals on a horse galloping around in the corral, only to find that this is an art to be neither taken lightly nor mastered quickly. Even standing still on the ground with no wind, there is frustration. You have to keep spitting out the little bits of tobacco that get into your mouth.

Years later we learned that those heavy-smoking ranchers had a high incidence of lung cancer. It took a lot of work to get even a few short puffs out of Bull Durham. Think of the lives it saved.

Good Times Together

Everyone is entitled to enshrine one setting as the place that holds the most cherished memories of youth, of the years when everything seemed possible and the present looked good.

Laurie's family were very liberal in letting her visit my family each summer in the early 1930s. She was a good rider. Mother gave her a spunky little mare called Babe, a cross between an Arab and a Shetland. Small, peppery, lots of energy, very intelligent, never panicked. She was perfect for a small lady. We rode every day either to do ranch work or just for pleasure after supper on long summer evenings. Usually we went with friends. But sometimes alone, getting off and sitting on a pine-needle carpet on some hilltop looking out for miles over a limestone rimrock. It was there we made our plan to get married.

Then we came out a few more summers before medical work occupied 12 months a year. In 1937 we brought Nancy out there as a baby. One or two more brief visits. Then, during the war, mother and father aging, the family moved away, the ranch was sold. Better the book to be closed.

We visit Wyoming only occasionally, these days. Usually for fishing or, like Conrad, in quest of our youth. As you look over the pool and the brush, taking your eye off the fly at precisely the wrong moment, the country ahead is unchanged from our first visit almost 70 years ago. Or when Custer (only a few miles to the north) made that fatal decision in 1876 to send Major Benteen off toward the Bighorn Mountains with his Gatling guns. There were 15,000 Sioux waiting for Custer. They knew he was coming. Then, as you dream of these things, the fish strikes and you miss him. Just to be there, even casting a fly, is a renaissance of body and soul.

Sit down on the bank and drink it all in. But watch out where you sit. Rattlers, too, are just like they used to be all those years ago.

Notes and References

CHAPTER 1—*Medical Student (1935-1939)*

Our medical school courses were arranged so logically that it was difficult, 15 years later, to become enthusiastic about the massive changes in the teaching of medical students introduced after World War II. We had started out with anatomy, both gross (i.e., dissection, anatomy as viewed by the unaided eye) and microscopic (histology). Then came biological chemistry, physiology, pharmacology, pathology. What could be more logical? Or simpler? Each of these was a major course arranged by a professor and department head who gave most of the lectures and whose personality was strongly impressed upon us. It is said that no two people can agree on how to mix a martini. Certainly it is true that no two decades of faculty opinion can agree on how to mix a medical curriculum. Even in our day, medical education in the United States seemed a radical departure compared with that in the British Commonwealth.

We spent 4 months in anatomy. Seemed long at the time. In Great Britain, that would have been regarded as too short—a mere dab—since medical students there spent the entire first year in anatomy and, in New Zealand, most of the first 2 years. In United States medical schools, the emphasis on chemistry and physiology was much stronger than in the Old World. Maybe it was not surprising when, after World War II and the great revolution of applying physiology and biochemistry to patient care, it was America that led the way.

When the next change came, about 1960, our generation (speaking for myself, at least) was a bit shocked at the complete restructuring of the medical curriculum—the so-called "omelettization" of medical education. We were probably being typical and stuffy older conservatives. Pathology was now chopped up into small pieces and mixed in with physiology and biochemistry. Pharmacology disappeared in the Curriculart mixer. The basic preclinical sciences were not presented as disciplines but rather in conjunction with some organ or system of the body (e.g., kidney, brain, liver) or one set of diseases (e.g., injury, infections, tumors). Twenty years later, the takeover by molecular genetics made further changes essential. Do the students emerge better prepared than we were for their hospital work and careers in practice? I would answer "No." But they know about a lot of things we never heard of.

Possibly all students look back on the way they were taught as being the best and most logical foundation on which all education should rest. Any change seems unnecessary, radical, meddlesome, and undesirable. Moral: Never let the alumni run an educational institution.

Professor Bobby Green's version of the quotation from Terence—*Nihil humanum mihi alienum est... nihil anatomicum*—may not have been perfect, but the idea he wished to convey was crystal clear. I am indebted to James Learmonth, a teacher in the British school system, for correcting this back to the original line by Terence (*Heauton Timorumenos*, Act I), with amendment: *Homo sum: humani nil a me alienum puto... [nec anatomici]* ("I am a man, and nothing human is foreign to me ... [nor anything anatomical]").

Reference is made in the text to the "Fabrica" of Andreas Vesalius and the concept of anatomy as being the fabric of the human body. The complete reference:

Vesalius, A. 1543. *De Humani Corporis Fabrica, Libri Septem.* Basel.

CHAPTER 2—*Harvard Medical School in the 1930s*

What is now known as the Harvard Medical School was started up in 1782 as the Medical Faculty of Harvard College. The lectures were open to the public and were given in Holden Chapel. Articles and books on the history of Harvard Medical School include the following:

Harrington, T.H. 1905. *The Harvard Medical School. A History, Narrative, and Documentary, 1782-1905.* Mumford J.G. (ed), New York: Lewis.

Harvard Medical School Faculty of Medicine. 1906. *The Harvard Medical School, 1782-1906.* Boston, private printing.

Beecher, H.K., and M.D. Altschule. 1977. *Medicine at Harvard: The First 300 Years.* Hanover, NH: University Press of New England.

Benison, S., A.C. Barger, and E. Wolfe. 1987. *Walter B. Cannon: The Life and Times of a Young Scientist.* Cambridge, MA: Belknap Press (of Harvard University Press).

The Nobel lecture of John Enders is important in Harvard history not only because of its significance in the global conquest of a costly and lethal disease, but also because of the participation of medical students in the discovery.

Enders, J. F., F. D. Robbins, and T. H. Weller. 1954. *The Cultivation of the Poliomyelitis Viruses in Tissue Culture*. Les Prix Nobel en 1954. Stockholm, The Nobel Foundation.

Two of our teachers wrote autobiographies:

Irving, F. 1942. *Safe Deliverance*. Boston: Houghton & Mifflin.

Zinsser, H. 1937. *As I Remember Him. The Biography of R.S.* Boston: Little, Brown.

Zinsser, H. 1945. *Rats, Lice and History. A Study in Biography*. Boston: Little, Brown.

President Eliot's reforms began early in his Harvard presidency. Richard Wolfe, Curator of Rare Books and Manuscripts at the Countway Library, supplies this account:

> On 1 November 1869, the medical faculty, on J.C. White's suggestion, voted to invite Harvard's new President—Eliot had been inaugurated on 19 October 1869—to attend its meetings.
>
> Accordingly, Eliot appeared at the next meeting, 21 November 1869, and took over the Chair. This one incident is often cited, with some justice, as symbolic of the changes to come at the Medical School. The sharp academic struggle that began in November 1869, in which the school underwent a transition from the old to the new, lasted until October 1871.
>
> There followed reorganization of the school, its curriculum, an upgrading of standards for admission of students, and for the granting of the M.D. degree.

At the time of the U.S. bicentennial in 1976, I contributed a history of American surgery to the Bicentennial Volume published by the Josiah Macy, Jr., Foundation:

Moore, F.D. 1976. Surgery, pp. 614–684. In *Advances in American Medicine: Essays at the Bicentennial*, J.Z. Bowers and E.F. Purcell (eds). New York: Macy Foundation.

Six years later, in 1982, there was a celebration of the Harvard Medical School bicentennial:

Moore, F.D. 1982. In medicina, veritas. The birth and turbulent youth of the Faculty of Medicine at Harvard College. *N. Engl. J. Med.* 307:917-925.

CHAPTER 3—Family Origins, Childhood in the Trenches

The name Hubbard Woods, assigned to a station on the Chicago and North-western Railroad just north of Winnetka, Illinois, was a reference to Gurdon

Saltonstall Hubbard, a New England pioneer of lower Lake Michigan and its environs. In his book he tells of coming to the Chicago area in 1818 as a 16-year-old hunter and trapper, trading with the Indians for valuable pelts of beaver, otter, and mink. This was only 6 years after the Fort Dearborn massacre (1812). He lived to become a leader of commerce and banking and a patriarch of the region. The Hubbard Trail is named after him. His life epitomizes the short span of time that changed this area on the southwest shore of Lake Michigan from a swampy wilderness to a great metropolis and railroad center. Two books tell of Hubbard's adventurous career:

Hubbard, G.S. 1911. *The Autobiography of Gurdon Saltonstall Hubbard: Pa-Pa-Ma-Ta-Be (The Swift Walker)*. Chicago: Lakeside Press.
Hubbard, M.A.: 1912. *Family Memories*. Chicago: Donnelly Printers, Chicago Historical Society.

Frederick Christopher was the surgeon in Winnetka who had pictured my fractured knee in his *Textbook of Minor Surgery*. This textbook (the leader in its time) later went through many editions and was finally succeeded by the huge *Textbook of Surgery* currently edited by David Sabiston, Professor of Surgery at Duke. Christopher was an engaging person, Head of the Department of Surgery at the Evanston Hospital. My contacts as a patient of his were unquestionably part of my drive toward surgery.

His brief autobiography:

Christopher, F. 1957. *One Surgeon's Practice*. Philadelphia: W.B. Saunders Co.

Christopher's textbook legacy:

Christopher, F. 1937. *Minor Surgery*, 3rd ed. Philadelphia: W.B. Saunders Co.
Sabiston, D.C., Jr. (ed). 1981. *Davis-Christopher Textbook of Surgery. The Biological Basis of Modern Surgical Practice*, 12th ed. Philadelphia: W.B. Saunders Co.
Sabiston, D.C., Jr. (ed). 1991. *Textbook of Surgery. The Biological Basis of Modern Surgical Practice*, 14th ed. Philadelphia: W.B. Saunders Co.

CHAPTER 4—Trains, Family Doings, and Travels

The Pullman Company of the 1920s was a vast corporation. With Grandfather as escort, we visited the city of Pullman. Here, red iron ore—the raw material used to build the railroad cars—was brought, freshly mined from the Mesabi Range, by the ore boats docked alongside the huge blast furnaces. The finished product, standing on the tracks a mile or so away, was the "Pullman Palace Car," with its painted Victorian finery and woven tapestry, complete and

370

ready to roll. Even to catch glimpses of this heroic industrial sequence was unforgettable for a third-grader. In 1969, operations in Pullman ceased. At that time a glory, the Pullman manufacturing process is now becoming a relict in the rust belt. Has Boeing taken its place?

In our childhood we were subject to certain health fads espoused by our parents' generation. All who pursue the diet and exercise fads of today, such as "designer" foods or workout machines, will enjoy perspectives from similar activities of 75 years ago.

As mentioned in the text, children were supposed to sleep outdoors on "sleeping porches," no matter what the weather. Sleeping outdoors was healthy. Suburban dwellings built between 1890 and 1940 shared this structural spinoff of a health fad now long gone, and largely forgotten. Many homes had a sleeping porch, maybe even two or three, on the second floor. Plenty of room for everybody. Good ventilation. Fresh air. Like jogging and cholesterol-free, high-fiber foods, this was a health fad exclusively indulged in by those who could afford it, those whose education included warnings of the hazards of doing otherwise (i.e., sleeping indoors).

This physical culture craze centered on the cult of a muscled hero named Bernarr Macfadden. His largely nude figure, muscles clenched and bulging, was on the cover of his books. As little boys we mocked his poses and showed off our muscle-clenching for anyone who had a Brownie camera handy. I am indebted to Diane Fortl of Dedham, Massachusetts, for drawing my attention to the fact that it was in Macfadden's book that outdoor sleeping was raised to the status of a health mandate in 1904. It is refreshing today to view some of the chapter titles: "Building Vital Power With Long Walks," "Vast Importance of Water," "How a Powerful Stomach May be Acquired," "Developing Great Lung Power," and "Perfect Ventilation," the last being best achieved, of course, by sleeping outdoors. Many architects, builders, lumber companies, and blanket manufacturers owed Macfadden a debt of gratitude:

Macfadden, B. 1904. *Building of Vital Power. Deep Breathing and a Complete System for Strengthening the Heart, Lungs, Stomach and All the Great Vital Organs.* New York and Chesham, England: Physical Culture Publishing Co.

CHAPTER 5—A Great School (1919-1931)

Quite a few couples from among the students at North Shore Country Day School later became husband and wife. Laurie and I were not the first. In 1983, about 50 years after graduation, the two of us were given the Stanton Award as outstanding alumni of the school. Never mind honorary degrees or such like matters of high prestige; this was the honor we most enjoyed. They said we won it together.

CHAPTER 6—Harvard College (1931-1935)

Our first 2 years at Harvard College were under the presidency of Abbott Lawrence Lowell. At the start of our junior year (1933) James B. Conant was appointed President of Harvard. He had four careers: chemist, university president, High Commissioner to Germany, and educational reformer. A recent biography by Hershberg, an extensive (900-page) review of Conant's life and times, paints him as a rather stern, uncompromising person who made little of human or family relationships.

My picture of Conant was based on his visits to the *Lampoon* while I was president and his attendance at some of our club dinners. When I was appointed Moseley Professor, I met with him in his office to discuss new horizons for the medical school; new undertakings in medicine, surgery, and science; the Moseley Professorship; and my forthcoming salary. Conant attended the faculty meetings of the medical school quite regularly, the only President in my experience to do so. This biography, which I would characterize as unjustifiably and unnecessarily negative, deals only with Conant's later years:

Hershberg, J.G. 1993. *James B. Conant; Harvard to Hiroshima and the Making of the Nuclear Age.* New York: Alfred A. Knopf.

Our text in organic chemistry:

Conant, J.B. 1933. *The Chemistry of Organic Compounds. A Year's Course in Organic Chemistry.* New York: Macmillan.

Conant's successor as President in 1953 was Nathan Pusey (class of 1928); Pusey was followed by Derek Bok in 1971, who resigned in 1992, and finally by Neil Rudenstine. My most abundant and always pleasurable contacts were with Conant and Pusey.

The department of my concentration, anthropology, was still a unified one in the 1930s. Physical anthropology, paleontology, human evolution, ethnology, ethnography, and even some of what would now be called social anthropology were all in one department. Alfred Tozzer was chair. His daughter, Joan, later married one of our classmates, William Lincoln, and became a close friend. Ernest A. Hooton was in charge of teaching human evolution and physical anthropology. His textbook was an entertaining departure from the usual sober-sided text:

Hooton, E.A. 1931. *Up From the Ape.* New York: Macmillan.

Another work on anthropological philosophy:

Hooton, E.A. 1937. *Apes, Men, and Morons.* New York: G.P. Putnam's Sons.

Hooton acquired some fame among the students because on the lecture stage

372

he imitated the posture and gait of the anthropoid apes. His imitation of a gibbon loping along, arms upraised, grasping for a branch to leap onto, was memorable.

In 1984 we staged a 50th reunion of our 1934 Hasty Pudding Show *Hades! The Ladies!* as the entr'acte in the annual club show at the clubhouse in Cambridge. Alistair Cooke came up to Boston from New York for the occasion. As the curtain opened, he could be seen sitting in his wing chair, fingers clasped in his characteristic pose, saying, "Good Evening. I'm Alistair Cooke." This was the way in which he began each television program of *Masterpiece Theatre*. This moment alone made the entire re-staging of a few scenes from our 50-year-old show worthwhile. Some of our singers were still quite operatic, especially Frank Johnson, who sang "Don't Wait for Roses in The Spring," a song I had written for him 50 years before as a sentimental spoof. Our show presented parodies of some of the Tin Pan Alley music and lyrics still current but possibly most notable in the 1920s: the June-moon-soon, love-dove-above, gal-pal-Sal school of lyrics. This waltz was one such. While the Hasty Pudding Show of 1984 was somewhat more grandiose than its predecessor of 50 years before, it had few personalities to match that of Cooke and few marvelous lyric tenor voices to match that of Johnson.

CHAPTER 8—Surgical Residency at the Massachusetts General Hospital (1939–1943)

Insider accounts of the surgical residency experience at American teaching hospitals are rare, at least in published form. Out of a desire to remedy this, we asked our former residents at the Brigham Hospital to help us summarize their experiences, criticisms, and career outcomes. These notes and letters were set forth in a privately printed summary in 1980:

Moore, F.D. 1980. *Three Surgical Decades. Brigham Surgery and the Residency Program*. Boston, private printing.

Here, in these Notes and References, I have not listed all the interns, residents, and surgical scientists who worked in our department between 1948 and 1981, often as close collaborators and always contributing immensely to the productivity of those Brigham years. Some appear here as coauthors of publications. Others whose work was largely in daily clinical care made our surgical care of thousands of patients both effective and safe. All of us on the staff owed these young surgeons and scientists a deep debt of gratitude.

CHAPTER 9—Death After the Game: The Cocoanut Grove Fire (1942)

The Cocoanut Grove fire acquires historical importance not because of the number killed (490) but because of the research carried out and lessons learned, especially with respect to the pulmonary (lung) injury incurred with burns.

Experiences with the patients injured in the Cocoanut Grove fire occurred at a curiously critical moment in my own surgical career because I had just returned from a fellowship year in research and was going straight on toward the chief residency. I had already completed some research on burns, and this accident offered the massive challenge of putting what I had learned to work, as well as laying the foundation for a lifelong interest in the care of burned patients. I was only a junior resident, 29 years old at the time of the fire, and working under the tutelage of Oliver Cope. One of the major contributions of his productive career was to focus attention on the pulmonary injuries observed in burned patients and to guide their treatment.

The fire also occurred at a remarkably critical moment in the development of wound surgery, i.e., the surgical care of injured, burned, fractured, or otherwise traumatized patients. It was nearly one year after Pearl Harbor, just before the massive engagements of American troops in North Africa, Europe, and the Pacific. Here was an opportunity for a civilian hospital to demonstrate an aggressive approach to seriously injured patients, combining the ancient traditions of emergency surgery with the finest of academic work in surgery: research applicable to the care of the sick.

It is to the everlasting credit of Edward Churchill that he saw this opportunity and led the effort to minimize the loss and suffering from this disaster on the one hand, while making of it a lesson for military surgery on the other. The fruits of his foresight are set forth in the *Annals of Surgery* issue cited below, which was devoted entirely to these patients. Shortly after the fire, he left Boston to become the commanding officer in charge of surgical care of the wounded in the Mediterranean theater.

Even at the time of the fire, Churchill was emphatic about the importance of defining the pattern of injury in any particular engagement or geographical area. From such an understanding should emerge better treatment for each individual patient as well as for the wounded as a group. I do not know when this concept first became prominent in his mind, but he certainly applied it to the Cocoanut Grove fire by outlining the nature of the combined burn and pulmonary injury with the assistance of the Departments of Pathology and Radiology.

Another of Oliver Cope's contributions lay in advocating a simple, nontoxic bandage (boric acid, petrolatum gauze) instead of the sometimes toxic materials such as tannic acid, picric acid, and dyes that had been used for years. Although we did not take the opportunity to show by tracer work the dynamics of absorption of substances through the wound surface, it was Cope's conviction that this occurred and led to his abandonment of tannic acid in the treatment of burns. Only a few years later we were to encounter the same phenomenon of absorption with a vengeance in the application of antibiotics to burns. Several patients became totally and permanently deaf because they had been treated with a surface ointment containing an antibiotic that was dangerously toxic when absorbed through the burned surface. In those early days it seemed inconceivable that enough antibiotic could be absorbed to damage auditory nerve conduction, but it *was* absorbed, in large quantities, and caused severe damage.

The supplement to the *Annals of Surgery* that presented the total MGH experience of the Cocoanut Grove fire:

Ann. Surg. 117(6):801–965, 1943.

Near the time of its 50th anniversary, there was a flurry of interest in the Cocoanut Grove fire that prompted several articles on the subject:

Coleman, T.H., F.D. Moore, O. Cope, and B. Cannon. 1991/92. The night the Grove burned. *Harvard Med. Alumni Bull.* 65(Winter):10–19.
Grant, C.C. 1991. Last dance at the Cocoanut Grove. *NFPA J* May/June, pp. 74–86. (Official magazine of the National Fire Protection Association.)
Bass, J. 1992. No way out. *Boston Magazine*, October, p. 74.

Our article on the redistribution of body water in the fluid therapy in burns was based not only on the Cocoanut Grove experience, but also on the application of radioactive isotopes to document the expansion of the extracellular fluid volume at the expense of the plasma volume in severe burns. This turned out to be one of the first researches to apply isotopes directly to problems in surgical care:

Cope, O., and F.D. Moore. 1947. The redistribution of body water and the fluid therapy of the burned patient. *Ann. Surg.* 126:1010–1045.

Oliver Cope was also one of the first to recommend early immediate excision of the burn and grafting. This method has been especially useful in children:

Cope, O., J.L. Langohr, F.D. Moore, and R.C. Webster, Jr. 1947. Expeditious care of full-thickness burn wounds by surgical excision and grafting. *Ann. Surg.* 125:1–22.

Recently, at the invitation of Andrew Munster (a former Brigham resident), who is in charge of the Johns Hopkins Burn and Trauma Service at the Baltimore City Hospital, I reviewed the history of our knowledge of respiratory injury in burns, placing in perspective the Cocoanut Grove experience and the remarkable contributions of Oliver Cope:

Moore, F.D. 1990. The respiratory tract injury of burns: Lessons from the past, pp. 1–15. In *Respiratory Injury: Smoke Inhalation and Burns*, E.F. Haponik and A.M. Munster (eds). New York: McGraw-Hill.

Dr. and Mrs. Oliver Cope died as these Notes were being composed, in April 1994.

CHAPTER 11—Finishing the Wartime Residency; White Suit to Civvies (1942-1943)

Claude Welch was one of our teachers at the MGH and later Clinical Professor of Surgery at HMS. Recently, he published his autobiography, which presents a delightful account of the MGH during this period, including the episode of the bogus Victorian staff portrait in which several of us participated. It hung on the wall of the surgeons' room for quite a while before anybody discovered it was a phony. Commentary (with pictures) about many of the people mentioned here are included in Welch's engaging story:

Welch, C.E. 1992. *Twentieth Century Surgeon: My Life in the Massachusetts General Hospital.* Boston: Massachusetts General Hospital.

Edward Churchill received the diaries of John Collins Warren, Harvard's fourth Professor of Surgery and the first Moseley Professor, from Warren's grandson, Richard Warren, for comment and possibly annotation. Churchill responded by writing an important historical book, tracing in detail the course of surgery in the United States in general (and Boston and Harvard in particular) as seen through the eyes of one of the movers and shakers of that period:

Churchill, E.D. 1958. *To Work in the Vineyard of Surgery. The Reminiscences of J. Collins Warren, 1842-1927.* Cambridge: Harvard University Press.

Looking back on his wartime work 25 years previously, Churchill wrote a brief account of the Italian campaign, including his activities in Sicily and Anzio:

Churchill, E.D. 1972. *Surgeon to Soldiers.* Philadelphia: J.B. Lippincott Co.

J. Gordon Scannell, a long-time friend and associate, was one of Churchill's most devoted pupils in thoracic surgery and has maintained a continuing interest in Churchill's surgical and intellectual accomplishments. He has recently published a brief story of Churchill's study year abroad, his *"Wanderjahr."* This is based on Churchill's account of his travels shortly after World War I, when he made personal contact with many eminent European surgeons and physiologists:

Scannell, J.G. 1990. *Wanderjahr. The Education of a Surgeon. Edward D. Churchill.* Boston: The Francis A. Countway Library of Medicine.

Among Churchill's many papers, two seem especially notable. First is his account of removal of a lobe of the lung to treat chronic infection (bronchiectasis).

His safe performance of this hazardous operation brought him an international reputation:

Churchill, E.D., and R. Belsey. 1939. Segmental pneumonectomy in bronchiectasis. *Ann. Surg.* 109:481–499.

The second is a delightful analysis of the history of surgery as a tension between the Graeco-Roman-French-British humanistic tradition of patient care and the rigid, intensive, research-scientific approach of the German universities in the nineteenth century:

Churchill, E.D. 1947. Science and humanism in surgery. *Ann. Surg.* 126:381–396.

CHAPTER 12—Patient Outcomes, Ernest Codman, and Clinical Research

Many philosophical discussions have attempted to define the nature of surgery and its relationship either to medicine as a whole or to what is now termed internal medicine, meaning by that the work of physicians (internists) who do not operate in the care of adult patients, but who serve adults in much the same way pediatricians serve children.

All physicians alike, be they pediatricians, surgeons, internists, psychiatrists, family practitioners, radiologists, or anesthetists, work from a massive reservoir of factual learning in human biology, now termed cognitive knowledge. Surgeons must master an understanding of a large segment of this knowledge of man and of his diseases. In addition, the surgeon must also master his craft, his handicraft. A skill.

It is therefore not surprising that among these several medical callings one has brought to perfection those methods by which some diseases can be treated by manipulation, by removal or anatomical rearrangement through what is now termed a surgical operation. The performance of operative surgical technique is demanding enough to occupy the full attention of one segment (about 20%) of the medical profession.

Despite its basis in all of biomedical science, the separation of surgery as a mode of treatment from the rest of medicine has given rise to many books, analyses, and reveries. Probably few of these are more trenchant than that written just after the turn of the century by Allbutt:

Allbutt, T.C. 1905. *The Historical Relations of Medicine and Surgery to the End of the Sixteenth Century; An Address Delivered at the St. Louis Congress in 1904.* London: Macmillan.

Dr. Churchill first called my attention to this small book that tells about the increasingly clear separation of medicine and surgery. It was written by a physician practicing what we would now call internal medicine, which in 1905 he termed "inner medicine." He expresses regret that he and his colleagues had lost their ability to deal with these diseases directly, personally, by their own hands. He writes

> The chief lesson of the Hippocratic period for us is that, in practice, as in honor, medicine and surgery were then one. The Greek physician had no more scruple in using his hands in the service of his brain, than had Pheidias or Archimedes; and it was by this cooperation that in the fifth century an advance was achieved which in our eyes is marvelous. As we pursue the history of medicine in later times we shall see the error, the blindness, and even the degradation of the physicians who neglected and despised a great handicraft. To the clear eyes of the ancient Greeks, an art was not liberal or illiberal by its manipulation but by its ends. As because of its ends the cleansing and solace of the lepers by St. Basil, St. Francis, and Father Damien was the service of angels, so also Hippocrates saw no baseness even in manipulations....

The clarity of Allbutt's vision has been borne out by the fact that the great leaders of surgery have been those who shared a broad view of all biomedical science but superimposed upon it their surgical skills. By the same token, the greatest of physicians are those who greet and understand surgery as a collaborator in the treatment of illness, calling upon surgery as they might call upon any other arm of therapy when it is needed. In contrast, the less elevated of our surgical profession carry out their technology with little view to the underlying biology, while the less talented of those practicing "inner medicine" regard it as a defeat or disaster if their patient comes to the surgeon. Mutual knowledge and respect form the most effective bond between these two major approaches to the treatment of human illness.

Now, 90 years after Allbutt's book, the *academic* branches of medicine and surgery in our medical schools are being separated by a widening gulf that could become worrisome, because it involves teaching the new generation.

The surgeon, be he senior professor or lowly intern, is brought into close contact with the patient and the patient's family by the hands-on personal intimacy bred of the operation itself. In even the most academic of teaching hospitals, with its laboratories and lecture halls, the surgeon is a clinician, a practitioner.

By contrast, many academic physicians (internists) have become so oriented toward research, especially in molecular genetics, that they (the faculty) see patients but rarely, if ever. One month on the ward or in the clinic does not a clinician make; private practice is often minimal or nonexistent. Inevitably, the teachings by such faculty members in internal medicine transmit more excitement about molecular genetics than about patient diagnosis or care. Are we spawning a generation of hands-off internists? Possibly most disturbing is the growing lack of role models for excellence in patient care in the groves of academic medicine.

A formal approach to the evaluation of errors and complications in surgery (likewise in medicine, pediatrics, psychiatry, and radiology) inevitably attracts comment. Fox and Swazey have been particularly interested in this subject:

Fox, R.C., and J.P. Swazey. 1974. *The Courage to Fail: A Social View of Organ Transplants and Dialysis.* Chicago: University of Chicago Press.

In 1979, Charles Bosk, a medical sociologist at the University of Pennsylvania, published his monograph on medical error, invoking a sociological authority-stratum theory of error confession and classification. Although this interpretation is more theoretical than real-life situations would attest, his book title inspired our expression, "Forgive, but do not forget."

Bosk, C.L. 1979. *Forgive and Remember. Managing Medical Failure.* Chicago: University of Chicago Press.

Early in this century, Ernest Amory Codman drew up the currently used classification of surgical errors and complications:

Codman, E.A. 1914. The product of a hospital. *Surg. Gynecol. Obstet.* 18:491–496.

About 30 years after my contacts with them, I enjoyed looking back on the careers of both Walter B. Cannon and Ernest A. Codman and wrote the following (presented as an address to the Boston Surgical Society on the occasion of the award of the Henry Jacob Bigelow Medal, November 5, 1973):

Moore, F.D. 1975. Surgical biology and applied sociology: Cannon and Codman fifty years later. *Harvard Med. Alumni Bull.* 49(Jan/Feb):12-21.

The terrible price paid for surgical error, mishap, and complications was borne in on us daily by telephone calls seeking admission to our intensive care ward, the Bartlett Unit. Nathan Couch and Nicholas Tilney worked with me in analyzing the common threads so often interwoven in these miscarriages of surgical care, often in very complex cases:

Couch, N.P., N.L. Tilney, and F.D. Moore. 1978. The cost of misadventures in colonic surgery—a model for the analysis of adverse outcomes in standard procedures. *Am. J. Surg.* 135:641-646.

Couch, N.P., N.L. Tilney, A.A. Rayner, and F.D. Moore. 1981. The high cost of low-frequency events. The anatomy and economics of surgical mishaps. *N. Engl. J. Med.* 304:634-637.

My first article in *The New England Journal of Medicine* resulted from an unusual encounter with a rare infectious disease:

Moore, F.D., C.S. Sawyer, and G.S. Blount, Jr. 1944. Tularemia in New England. A review of eighteen cases with the report of two additional cases. *N. Engl. J. Med.* 231:169-173.

My first publication in the *Journal of the American Medical Association* was based on a national study of drug toxicity:

Moore, F.D. 1946. Toxic manifestations of thiouracil therapy (a cooperative study). *JAMA* 130:315-319.

Throughout this century, duodenal (and gastric) ulcer has been a prime concern of both internists and surgeons. Now, after all this time, the disease seems to be declining in frequency, while evidence is increasing that a bacterium, *Helicobacter pylori*, is somehow involved in its causation. For several decades before and after World War II, surgical treatment for ulcer that was both safe and effective was an ideal not always attained.

The principal cause of death after subtotal gastrectomy for duodenal ulcer was peritonitis resulting from rupture of the suture line closing the duodenum (i.e., the intestine just beyond the stomach). Several solutions were proposed for this. One of them, by McKittrick, was to carry out the operation in two stages. Not only did this bring sharply into focus the commonest cause of death after this operation, but it also brought up some other important physiologic questions concerning the secretion of gastric acid. This is the only paper in which Richard Warren and I were coauthors, although we worked together on many topics over the years:

McKittrick, L.S., F.D. Moore, and R. Warren. 1944. Complications and mortality in subtotal gastrectomy for duodenal ulcer. Report of a two-stage procedure. *Ann. Surg.* 120:531-561.

Lester Dragstedt, at the University of Chicago, was the first to carry out vagotomy for duodenal ulcer. As described in the text, I began studies on this topic in 1942 without knowledge of his work but had become fully aware of his pioneering effort, and was grateful for his experience, by the time my first patient was operated upon:

Dragstedt, L.R., and F.M. Owens, Jr. 1943. Supradiaphragmatic section of vagus nerves in treatment of duodenal ulcer. *Proc. Soc. Exp. Biol. Med.* 53:152-154.
Moore, F.D., W.P Chapman, M.D. Schulz, and C.M. Jones. 1946. Transdiaphragmatic resection of the vagus nerve for peptic ulcer. *N. Engl. J. Med.* 234:241-251.

The following year we reported some of the physiologic effects of severing the vagus nerves:

Moore, F.D., W.P. Chapman, M.D. Schulz, and C.M. Jones. 1947. Resection of the vagus nerves in peptic ulcer. Physiologic effects and clinical results, with a report of two years' experience. *JAMA* 133:741-749.

Having worked with both gastrectomy and vagotomy and having seen many patients treated by nonsurgical means alone, I felt it was clearly important to compare the three. Horatio Rogers and I started out rather ambitiously with 1,000 patient records from the Massachusetts General. Only three of these patients were lost to follow-up. We and our collaborators, Brooks, Erskine, Richardson, and Peete, wound up with the 997 cases mentioned in the title of the paper. When subtotal gastrectomy could be carried out with a low mortality, the results more than justified the investment of time, cost, and effort even though digestive changes over the long term were sometimes a severe problem. Even in nonsurgical management (alkali powders and pills) there was still some intrinsic risk of perforation, obstruction, or hemorrhage. The two treatments (surgical and nonsurgical) could be directly compared. Our platitudinous conclusions from this laborious study were (1) each case is different and (2) clinical judgment is important. But there was a third major conclusion. While obvious to the sophisticated reader, this was never stated clearly enough. This was the skill factor. Pick your surgeon carefully! Not everyone could carry out this operation with a low mortality and morbidity:

Moore, F.D., W.P.J. Peete, J.E. Richardson, J.M. Erskine, J.R. Brooks, and H. Rogers. 1950. The effect of definitive surgery on duodenal ulcer disease. A comparative study of surgical and non-surgical management in 997 cases. *Ann. Surg.* 132:652-680.

Under Dr. McKittrick's guidance I managed the postoperative ulcerative colitis clinic at the Massachusetts General Hospital. We saw a large number of patients with this disease and wrote several papers, in one of which we sought to identify some of the judgmental factors in selecting elective surgery for these patients:

McKittrick, L.S., and F.D. Moore. 1949. Ulcerative colitis. Ileostomy: problem or solution? *JAMA* 139:201-207.

CHAPTER 13—The National Research Council and Isotope Research (1941-1942)

The concept of making a radioactive dye led to that wonderful fellowship year with Joseph Aub, my introduction to biophysical research, and then several decades spent in the study of body composition and the biology of convalescence. At least one element in this sequence had its origin in our pathology course, where Valy Menkin told us how certain dyes tended to concentrate in abscesses:

Menkin, V. 1929. Studies on inflammation. I. Fixation of vital dyes in inflamed areas. *J. Exp. Med.* 50:171-180.

After 6 months of hectic and intensive work, our first research was rather surprisingly crowned by at least a modicum of success. Lester Tobin was able to synthesize a radioactive dibrominated derivative of trypan blue. We could induce the abscesses in rabbits. It all worked out well enough so only a few months later we presented our findings at a scientific meeting. Although we were unaware of it at the time, this would have to be listed as one of the first successful efforts to apply radioactive isotopes for external detection of a disease process (now called nuclear medicine). This article was followed by our description in animals of the concentration of this radioactive dye in tumors:

Moore, F.D., and L.H. Tobin. 1942. Studies with radioactive di-azo dyes. 1. Localization of radioactive di-brom trypan blue in inflammatory lesions. *J. Clin. Invest.* 21:471-481.

Tobin, L.H., and F.D. Moore. 1943. Studies with radioactive di-azo dyes. 2. Synthesis and properties of radioactive di-brom trypan blue and radioactive di-brom Evans blue. *J. Clin. Invest.* 22:155-160.

Moore, F.D., L.H. Tobin, and J.C. Aub. 1943. Studies with radioactive di-azo dyes. 3. The distribution of radioactive dyes in tumor-bearing mice. *J. Clin. Invest.* 22:161-168.

About 5 years after we had completed our radioactive dye work, and after the first human studies using isotope dilution for the study of burns and body composition, we published a review article about the use of isotopes in surgical research:

Moore, F.D. 1948. The use of isotopes in surgical research. *Surg. Gynecol. Obstet.* 86:129-147.

Arthur Solomon, an early advocate of isotope research and of applying biophysics to medical research, later became director of the Laboratory for Biophysics in the Department of Biochemistry under A. Baird Hastings. In 1940 he had written an account for the public, which was helpful to us as neophytes in the field:

Solomon, A.K. 1940. *Why Smash Atoms?* Cambridge: Harvard University Press.

In undertaking a year in fundamental research, learning how to use the new methods of nuclear physics for the study of surgical illness, I was crossing a bridge from the bedside to the laboratory, from the operating room to the world of basic science. In any medical field it is important for some clinicians to cross this bridge and bring back to the bedside whatever they can find out there.

The Latin *pontifex* (later shortened to "pontiff") refers to the ancient ecclesiastical concept of bridge-tending for churchmen bringing the word to earth from heaven.

In my address as President of the Society of University Surgeons in 1958, I pointed out that such a bridge-tending surgeon often finds himself caught in the middle of the bridge. He is accused by his associates of not spending enough time in the operating room, while his scientific associates know full well he is not really one of them. So he is an illegitimate hybrid, and he must learn to live with the appropriate sobriquet.

By taking a year or two at the NIH or other laboratories, thousands of young clinicians in many fields have tended that important bridge and have lived quite happily with their bar sinister.

Moore, F.D. 1958. The university in American surgery. *Surgery* 44:1-10.

CHAPTER 14—Body Composition and the Stuff of Which We Are Made; The Body Cell Mass

Our first paper laying the foundation for our work in body composition and paving the way for the application of multiple isotopes to measure several elements of body composition was published in *Science* in 1946:

Moore, F.D. 1946. Determination of total body water and solids with isotopes. *Science* 104:157-160.

The principle of measuring total solids in solution depended upon the dilution of radioactive isotopes, not in a body fluid, but rather among their sister isotopes. In scientific parlance, this required measuring the specific activity of the radioactive isotope. Our first paper on the use of this principle for measuring the total potassium of the body:

Corsa, L., Jr., J.M. Olney, R.W. Steenburg, M.R. Ball, and F.D. Moore. 1950. The measurement of exchangeable potassium in man by isotope dilution. *J. Clin. Invest.* 29:1280-1295.

Details on total body water measurement were published at the same time:

Schloerb, P.R., B.J. Friis-Hansen, I.S. Edelman, A.K. Solomon, and F.D. Moore. 1950. Measurement of total body water in the human subject by deuterium oxide dilution. With a consideration of the dynamics of deuterium distribution. *J. Clin. Invest.* 29:1296-1310.

Soon we had perfected the method for measuring both sodium and potassium using the two appropriate isotopes simultaneously:

James, A.H., L. Brooks, I.S. Edelman, J.M. Olney, and F.D. Moore. 1954. Body sodium and potassium. I. The simultaneous measurement of exchangeable sodium and potassium in man by isotope dilution. *Metabolism* 3:313-323.

Isidore Edelman was a junior member of our group but soon showed himself to be a remarkably gifted scientist. He later became Professor of Biochemistry at Columbia College of Physicians and Surgeons in New York. Six years after our first description of how to analyze body composition in *Science*, we published a follow-up study relating how the methods had improved:

Edelman, I.S., J.M. Olney, A.H. James, L. Brooks, and F.D. Moore. 1952. Body composition. Studies in the human being by the dilution principle. A progress report. *Science* 115:447-454.

Then, to make this method more readily available to other laboratories, we published a "cookbook" paper describing in detail exactly how the procedure was carried out:

McMurrey, J.D., E.A. Boling, J.M. Davis, H.V. Parker, I.C. Magnus, M.R. Ball, and F.D. Moore. 1958. Body composition: simultaneous determination of several aspects by the dilution principle. *Metabolism* 7:651-667.

Standards and measurements for permissible radiation dosage were in their infancy in the period 1946 to 1956, when we established normal compositional values by studying healthy volunteers, including our own families. The idea that life on Earth once existed in a radiation-free environment was exploded by 1960 with increasing knowledge of cosmic radiation and unavoidable background radiation from the Earth, especially that of radium, radon, uranium, and their decay products. In addition, all living cells since the dawn of evolution have been bombarded by their own naturally radioactive potassium—a factor that may have accelerated evolution by favoring mutations:

Moore, F.D., and K.S.R. Sastry. 1982. Intracellular potassium: ^{40}K as a primordial gene irradiator. *Proc. Natl. Acad. Sci. USA* 79:3556-3559.

The greatest unknown in body compositional analysis was the weight of the bones that hold us up, the skeleton. Compared with the other tissues of the body, the skeleton is dry, dense, large, and therefore heavy. It is heavier in men (especially athletic men) than in women. In slight and less athletic women, it is remarkably less prominent than in men both chemically and by weight and becomes even lighter, smaller, and less dense with osteoporosis after the menopause. We worked out a method for estimating the weight of the skeleton by isotope dilution. It was in connection with this work that we analyzed the body of a patient who had offered her earthly remains to our laboratory specifically for this purpose, as described in the text:

Moore, F.D., J. Lister, C.M. Boyden, M.R. Ball, N. Sullivan, and F.J. Dagher. 1968. The skeleton as a feature of body composition: values predicted by the isotope dilution and observed by cadaver dissection in an adult female. *Hum. Biol.* 40:135–188.

Seventeen years after that initial paper in *Science*, we were able to publish in book form both the method and the results of body compositional studies over a wide spectrum of injury and disease:

Moore, F.D., K.H. Olesen, J.D. McMurrey, H.V. Parker, M.R. Ball, and C.M. Boyden. 1963. *The Body Cell Mass and Its Supporting Environment; Body Composition in Health and Disease.* Philadelphia: W.B. Saunders Co.

About 15 years later, a young Spanish surgeon and scientist, Jesus Culebras, came to work with us. Using the most modern isotope technology, which had changed drastically in the 25 years since we began the work, he checked out the body water method using the dilution of tritium (radioactive hydrogen of weight 3.0). Although not terribly exciting scientifically, these analyses and carcass desiccations to reconfirm an old method were truly a labor of love. Many accepted methods or standard dogmas of research need to be checked out or reestablished every few years or discarded if they do not stand the test of time. This important work, supporting the validity of our old method, was published in 1977:

Culebras, J.M., G.F. Fitzpatrick, M.F. Brennan, C.M. Boyden, and F.D. Moore. 1977. Total body water and the exchangeable hydrogen II. A review of comparative data from animals based on isotope dilution and desiccation, with a report of new data from the rat. *Am. J. Physiol.* 232(1):R60–R65.

Our studies of body composition and the metabolism of water and salt led directly to an appreciation of the importance of the patient's response to injury and surgery in determining the most suitable treatment after injury, shock, burns, and fractures. In 1948 I was asked to summarize the use of fluids, salts, and nourishment in surgical patients and published a paper in the *Journal of the American Medical Association* that anticipated our future work in the biology of convalescence:

Moore, F.D. 1949. The adaptation of supportive treatment to the needs of the surgical patient. *JAMA* 141:646–653.

The late Tom Randall of New York and Providence was long a close friend and key contributor to our knowledge of water and salt metabolism in surgical patients:

Randall, H.T. 1952. Water and electrolyte balance in surgery. *Surg. Clin. North Am.* 32:445–469.

CHAPTER 15—Getting Well; The Response to Injury and the Nature of Survival

The concept of an evolved response to injury consisting of a series of physiological changes favoring survival and hastening convalescence can be traced back to three influences. The first was gained from our studies in medical school under Walter Cannon, most especially from the book in which he summarized his view on a similar topic:

Cannon, W.B. 1915. *Bodily Changes in Pain, Hunger, Fear and Rage.* New York: D. Appleton & Co.

The second influence came from the work of David Cuthbertson, a Scottish veterinarian-physiologist who described the changes in body protein after injury using changes in nitrogen excretion as a proxy for body protein and was later knighted for this work. In Cuthbertson's first study (carried out 10 years before World War II), he showed clear changes in protein metabolism after injury:

Cuthbertson, D.P. 1930. The disturbance of metabolism produced by bony and non-bony injury, with notes on certain abnormal conditions of bone. *Biochem. J.* 24:1244-1263.
Cuthbertson, D.P. 1932. Observations on the disturbance of metabolism produced by injury to the limbs. *Q. J. Med. [N.S.]* 1:233-246.

The third influence was the work of Fuller Albright, who in so many ways and for so many people set the standard for metabolic research in our era:

Albright, F. 1942-1943. Cushing's syndrome. Its pathogenic physiology, its relationship to the adrenogenital syndrome, and its connection with the problem of the reaction of the body to injurious agents ("alarm reaction" of Selye). *Harvey Lect.* 28:123-186.

Our first publication dealing with the natural history of convalescence and the chemical changes in the body that set the stage for recovery was a book of case studies of chemical and metabolic change, done with Margaret Ball, my chief laboratory technician. Based on measurements in patients and using a standardized method of charting (inspired by the metabolic charts of Fuller Albright), the reader could for the first time see at a glance the sequence of nitrogen (protein) loss followed by gain, with appropriate changes in water and salt, after severe injury:

Moore, F.D., and M.R. Ball. 1952. *The Metabolic Response to Surgery.* Springfield, IL: Charles C Thomas.

In 1952, shortly after the publication of that first book on metabolism in surgery, I was asked by the Excelsior Society (a group of officers who had served in the Mediterranean theater under Dr. Churchill) to give the first E.D. Churchill Lecture. In that lecture I tried to summarize our growing picture of the normal sequence of metabolic changes after severe injury:

Moore, F.D. 1953. Bodily changes in surgical convalescence. I. The normal sequence—observations and interpretations. *Ann. Surg.* 137:289-315.

About 4 years after the Churchill Lecture, I was asked by the Harvey Society to summarize our studies on the natural history of convalescence with particular reference to endocrine changes, i.e., the hormonal changes that occur after injury. Here was an opportunity to assemble what was known at the time about the interrelationships among an injury or a wound, the function of the endocrine glands, and metabolic changes within the body: an overall picture of the normal biology of convalescence. This was 14 years after Albright's Harvey Lecture (cited above) had clearly anticipated these findings:

Moore, F.D. 1956-1957. Metabolism in trauma: the meaning of definitive surgery—the wound, the endocrine glands, and metabolism. *Harvey Lect.* 52:74-99.

George H.A. Clowes, long-time friend and worker in surgical metabolism both at Harvard and at Brown, described a leading candidate for the wound hormone that I had postulated in my Harvey Lecture:

Clowes, G.H.A., Jr., B.C. George, C.A. Villee, Jr., and C.A. Saravis. 1983. Muscle proteolysis induced by a circulating peptide in patients with sepsis or trauma. *N. Engl. J. Med.* 308:545-552.

While this general view of metabolism after injury has stood the test of time, many additional changes in endocrine function and cellular biology—unheard of in 1956—have been shown to be important in the response of the body to injury and surgery.

A couple of years after the Harvey Lecture, following a long period of labor pains, I finally delivered the "big green book" to the Saunders Company, setting forth many aspects of metabolic change after injury and relating them to the everyday care of surgical patients. This was my only commercially successful book. It was read widely, translated into Spanish, Polish, Japanese, and probably Russian, though we never knew that for sure. Even today, when I visit with surgeons, I am still pleased to see this book on their shelves:

Moore, F.D. 1959. *Metabolic Care of the Surgical Patient.* Philadelphia: W.B. Saunders Co.

John Dusseau of Saunders helped us to produce that large book in an attractive format and with many illustrations. He helped me with several projects over the years and has given me valuable advice about the publication of this story.

About 30 years after our first work on the subject, I was given an opportunity again, this time in 1975, to summarize the present state of our knowledge about the biology of convalescence. With Murray Brennan, soon to assume his responsibilities as Chief of Surgery at Memorial Sloan-Kettering in New York, I wrote an up-to-date summary:

Moore, F.D., and M.F. Brennan. 1975. Surgical injury: body composition, protein metabolism and neuroendocrinology, pp. 169-222. In *Manual of Surgical Nutrition, Committee on Pre- and Postoperative Care, American College of Surgeons*. Philadelphia: W.B. Saunders Co.

An important aspect of the growing knowledge of nutrition, biochemistry, and metabolism in surgical recovery was the development of total intravenous feeding. Although we had used this method and it was described in the big green book cited above, we had not carried out the fundamental research to prove its effectiveness. This had first been done by Fuller Albright, with whom I had worked as a junior member of the staff at the MGH during the war. His description of total intravenous feeding of a surgical patient is as follows:

Albright, F., E.C. Reifenstein, and A.P. Forbes. 1944. Effect of total intravenous feeding with mixtures of protein hydrolysate (Amigen) and glucose on the metabolic data of a patient before and after a bone operation, pp. 168-176. In *Macy Conference on Metabolic Aspects of Convalescence Including Bone and Wound Healing*, E. C. Reifenstein (ed), Eighth Meeting, New York, NY, October 13-14.

Albright's studies showed the brisk increase in nitrogen excretion (despite constant protein intake) after operation and an increase in glucose excretion (despite constant carbohydrate intake).

But even Albright's work lacked some of the detail that can be achieved only through experiments in laboratory animals. These experiments were carried out by Jonathan Rhoads with his collaborators Wilmore, Dudrick, and Vars, who for many years had been trying to improve nutrition in surgical patients. Their work was summarized in 1968. Almost immediately following this publication, the word on total intravenous feeding spread over the world, finding a special usefulness in infants born with disorders of the gastrointestinal tract, in people suffering severe wounds, and in those debilitated because of cancer or chronic infection. Few events in the field of nutrition and metabolism have changed worldwide practice as much as this publication by Rhoads and his group:

Dudrick, S.J., D.W. Wilmore, H.M. Vars, and J.E. Rhoads. 1968. Long-term total parenteral nutrition with growth, development, and positive nitrogen balance. *Surgery* 64:134.

Recently, Jonathan Rhoads has summarized this era of nutrition in surgery:

Rhoads, J.E. 1994. Memoir of a surgical nutritionist. *JAMA* 272:963-966.

CHAPTER 16—Two Harvard Hospitals: The Brigham and the General; A Candidate for Promotion (1947-1948)

Several histories of the MGH have been published. One of the most recent discusses particularly its recent corporate evolution and financial arrangements. The books by Faxon tell a little bit more of the philosophy of the MGH and of the study of human illness as a means toward understanding normal human physiology:

Castleman, B., D.C. Crockett, and S.B. Sutton. 1983. *The Massachusetts General Hospital, 1955-1980.* Boston: Little, Brown.
Faxon, N.W. 1949. *The Hospital in Contemporary Life.* Cambridge, MA: Harvard University Press.
Faxon, N.W. 1959. *The Massachusetts General Hospital, 1935-1955.* Cambridge, MA: Harvard University Press.
Myers, C.W. 1929. *History of the Massachusetts General Hospital, June 1872 to December 1900.* Boston, private printing.

In celebration of the 50th anniversary of the founding of the Brigham, the poet David McCord (long-time friend and a patient of mine) wrote a history, making use of the term Fabrick of Man, first coined in 1543 by Vesalius, to denote the work of a hospital:

McCord, D. 1963. *The Fabrick of Man. Fifty Years of the Peter Bent Brigham. The Corporation of the Peter Bent Brigham Hospital.* Portland, ME: Anthoensen Press.

CHAPTER 17—Surgical Professors, Ancient and Modern

No books have been written that cover adequately the entire span of surgical research and teaching at the Harvard Medical School over the course of two centuries. Although Beecher and Altschule (see Notes for Chapter 2) covered all of Harvard medicine over three centuries (going back to the first colonists), the surgical story is pretty well buried in the text.

The Truax book is a story of the Warren family of surgeons:

Truax, R. 1968. *The Doctors Warren of Boston; First Family of Surgery.* Boston: Houghton-Mifflin.

John C. Warren and Edward Warren also wrote of their work and their family:

Warren, J.C. 1846. Inhalation of ethereal vapor for the prevention of pain in surgical operations. *Boston Med. Surg. J.* 36:375-379.
Warren, E. 1874. *The Life of John Warren, M.D.* Boston: Noyes, Holmes & Co.
Warren, E. 1860. *The Life of John Collins Warren, M.D.* Boston: Ticknor & Fields.

The textbook of surgery by our contemporary, Richard Warren:

Warren, R. 1963. *Surgery.* Philadelphia: W.B. Saunders Co.

Several books and many articles have been written about Cushing and his work. The Fulton biography is the standard:

Fulton, J. 1946. *Harvey Cushing. A Biography.* Springfield, IL: Charles C Thomas.

The forces that shaped Cushing's life and the remarkable variety of advances that came from this most productive of America's surgical researchers make a fascinating story:

Moore, F.D. 1969. Harvey Cushing: General surgeon, biologist, professor. *J. Neurosurg.* 31:262-270.
Moore, F.D. 1993. The universities in Cushing's life. In *Harvey Cushing at the Brigham.* P. Black (ed). Park Ridge, IL: American Association of Neurological Surgeons.

Nicholas Tilney wrote several articles on the history of surgical research and on Harvey Cushing:

Tilney, N.L. 1980. Harvey Cushing and the surgical research laboratory. *Surg. Gynecol. Obstet.* 151:263-270.
Tilney, N.L. 1986. Harvey Cushing and the evolution of a polymath. *Surg. Gynecol. Obstet.* 162:285-290.

In addition to his work on the heart (described in Chapter 23), Elliott Cutler's major contribution was in systematizing the teaching of surgical technique. He and Robert Zollinger developed an atlas of surgical operations to help young people learn how to carry out operations safely. This book was first published just at the time when our class started internship in 1939:

Cutler, E.C., and R.M. Zollinger. 1939. *Atlas of Surgical Operations.* New York: Macmillan. (Subsequent editions 1949, 1961-67.)
Zollinger, R.M., and R.M. Zollinger, Jr. 1993. *Atlas of Surgical Operations*, 7th ed. New York: McGraw-Hill. (Previous editions 1975, 1983, and 1988.)

A practice that started many years ago but is now rapidly gaining momentum is the use of a lighted telescope, or endoscope, to view and manipulate the anatomy involved. This method was originally used to sever adhesions in the pleural cavity as early as 1940. Richard Sweet, a thoracic surgeon on the MGH staff, often used this technique as part of collapse therapy (such as pneumothorax) in tuberculosis. Tubes for viewing the interior of the stomach, esophagus, bladder, and colon have been used for 100 years. In the past decade electronic transfer of such images to a T.V. screen has revolutionized this field. Gallbladder surgery, hernia repair, and even removal of the appendix or of the cancerous colon have fallen within the reach of endoscopic surgery. Two or three small incisions replace the long skin incisions of previous years.

In view of Cutler's atlas of 50 years ago, it is perhaps fitting that a new atlas—this time of endoscopic surgery—has now emerged from the Brigham staff:

Brooks, D.C. (ed). 1994. *Current Techniques in Laparoscopy*. Philadelphia: Current Medicine, 1994.

Cushing's operating room orderly, Adolph Watzka, stayed on to work under Cutler and then in the Moore regime until his death in 1956. Adolph emigrated from Bohemia as a teenager in 1912. In 1917 he came to Boston and arrived at the Brigham in answer to a "help wanted" ad.

In my annual report for 1956, at the time of Adolph's death, I included a brief description of his life and remarkable career:

Signing up as a hospital orderly, Adolph soon showed his skill in mechanical things, his extraordinary devotion to work, and his ability to solve difficult problems in the operative handling of patients. Miss Madden, the Operating Room Supervisor, appreciated his unusual talent and devotion. He also took the eye of Dr. Cushing and was soon employed in the operating room.

For almost forty years, the operating theater of this hospital was his abode. He worked under three Chiefs of Surgery. It is little wonder that Adolph appeared to be a remarkable person to a doctor who worked with him day in and day out for several years. For many patients who saw him only during a few moments of anxiety or apprehension as they were being moved from their bed to the operating table, he was a big, heavy-boned, homely man who, with great strength, achieved complete gentleness, telling the patient exactly what to do to avoid pain or discomfort and with a comforting word.

In this work his skill was truly surgical. No move was wasted, nothing was done that was unnecessary, everything that was needed was accomplished. He often worked with antique equipment and many house officers concluded that Adolph used the oldest operating table in the operating room out of sentimental preference and because he was the only individual who could possibly work its heavy and corroded controls. Others found it difficult to work with him because his standard of perfection was so high that few could attain it.

The Brigham has always been noted for the perfection of surgical technique. For visitors, it was therefore remarkable to see a large orderly come into the operating room, lift a patient and move that patient around, adjust the table or carry out other steps, with no face mask. Adolph felt that a facemask limited the freedom of his breathing and that it was unnecessary if he was careful. He rarely spoke in the operating room and if quizzed on this point, stated that of course he never 'coughed or breathed heavily.' There was a day when surgeons operated without rubber gloves or facemasks; Adolph was our last link with this bit of history.

To an individual who has worked all of his life in a job that he loves, the terror of old age lies in the fear of crippling illness and withdrawal to lonely strangeness. Although the end came much too soon for Adolph Watzka, it found him happily at work in the operating room at 7:45 AM on April 14, 1956. Thus passed from the scene a man who made a humble chore into a fine profession, and in so doing taught an important lesson to hundreds of young doctors who must also find devoted service in what often is a humble role in the care of the sick.

In one of his last years, he was asked by his family what he would like to do if he lived his life over again. He said 'I would like to be a surgeon.'

An illustrated article featuring Adolph's story appeared in *Collier's Magazine*:

Dineen, J.F. 1951. The hospital orderly they call "Doctor." *Collier's*, December 1, p. 27.

CHAPTER 18—*Young Man at a Young Hospital (1948)*

Mr. Arthur Porritt, a New Zealander as well as a London surgeon of great charm and ability, served as sergeant surgeon to the Queen and was knighted because of his distinguished war record and his long service on the British Olympic Committee. He was later appointed Governor General of New Zealand, the first native New Zealander to receive this honor. He was firmly ensconced at Government House in Wellington when Laurie and I were houseguests there. On the basis of this service he was made a Lord; later, as one of the four surgical Lords, he greeted a group of us from the American College of Surgeons for a reception at the House of Lords (1974). His appointment to the Olympic committee came about on the basis of his victorious career as an Olympic runner. As mentioned in the text, it was in those Olympic years that he met J. Murray Forbes of Boston (also an Olympic runner) and later joined with him in supporting our Brigham–St. Mary's resident/registrar exchange program in 1950. Porritt's career as a runner was well known; in fact, in the motion picture *Chariots of Fire* the reference to the speedy New Zealander was a reference to Porritt. Lord Porritt was Pro Tem at the Brigham on two occasions, once with Elliott Cutler as chief and once with me.

The Brigham–St. Mary's exchange of surgical residents between Boston and London began in 1949 and brought new skills and experience to young surgeons from both sides of the Atlantic for almost 20 years. Despite the British and American collaboration, it was actually two Canadians, Keith Eric Rogers and

Felix Eastcott, who were the first to cross. Eastcott, long a leader of the staff at St. Mary's, with an office on Harley Street and eminence in British vascular surgery, has visited the United States often, both as an Honorary Fellow of the American College of Surgeons and as a friend of many American colleagues. For a time he was Acting President of the Royal College of Surgeons of England.

The heal-in at Boston City Hospital was in essence a strike or job action carried out by the interns and residents and was mimicked (if rather faintly) at other Boston hospitals in the late 1960s. The inspiration for this came from Philip Caper, a young left-leaning physician of the "white suit, clenched fist" stripe in those antiestablishment years. It was his idea to stir up the hospital administrators, not by going out on strike (which would have left many helpless patients bereft), but rather to do just the opposite: admit them all! So swamped, with their beds overwhelmed by not-very-sick people seeking hospitalization, the hospital administrators quickly capitulated and gave the white suits a raise, hoping the clenched fists would go away.

Philip Caper later became a Senate staff aide to Senator Kennedy and developed computer software to document geographical differences in the utilization of medical and surgical procedures.

Since about 1975, interns and residents have received pay that, although hardly generous, recognizes their public service while they are in a learning mode and helps them eke out a living with the help of spouse and parents.

CHAPTER 19—*Rejection, The Twins, and Radiation (1950–1961)*

CHAPTER 20—*The Advent of Drug Immunosuppression (1958–1962)*

CHAPTER 21—*The Liver: Transplanting the Body's Largest Organ (1957–1965)*

CHAPTER 22—*Broadening Scope; New Problems;* Nonnumquam, Nocere Est Renovare

The Notes and References for these four chapters on transplantation are presented together. The references include papers and books on the development of transplantation at Harvard, the Brigham, and around the world between 1950 and 1970.

The remarkable case of the "arm kidney" has never been described fully in the literature. As mentioned in the text, after the patient's death from acute hepatitis, the case was written up to document the complete healing of the kidneys:

Burwell, E.L., T.D. Kinney, and C.A. Finch. 1947. Renal damage following intravascular hemolysis. *N. Engl. J. Med.* 237:657-665.

While I was gathering material to write *Give and Take* (cited below), I asked Charles Hufnagel if he would send me his own account of the arm kidney episode. The letter that follows was his response to this request:

When I was the Cabot Fellow (working in the Surgical Research labs at Harvard) I spent considerable time working with transplantation of the kidney and had also developed a technique for rapid freezing of blood vessels. I had a considerable group of animals with transplantations of the kidney, and at the same time we were working with adrenal transplantation. From time to time, we had been on the lookout for a patient in whom a kidney transplant might be needed, as an urgent and desperate measure to save her life.

In this case everyone was quite sure that the patient was not going to open up with urine output, and was almost dead. Dr. Ernest Landsteiner was the Urologic Resident at the time. After a series of consultations it was finally agreed that the patient should have a transplant from a cadaver to see if she could be tided over this problem long enough to get well.

Accordingly we solicited the help of Dr. David Hume, who went hunting for a prospective donor. We were fortunate in being able to obtain a cadaver kidney later the same day. The kidney was removed under aseptic conditions and taken immediately to the patient.

Because the patient's condition appeared extremely critical, there was some administrative objection to bringing the patient to the operating room. In the dark of night—about midnight—when the kidney had been obtained immediately after the death of the donor, our little group (Landsteiner, Hume, and myself) proceeded to one of the end rooms on the second floor, and by the light of two small gooseneck student lamps prepared to do the transplant.

The brachial artery and a large vein in the antecubital fossa were isolated. The anastomosis was accomplished very rapidly in spite of the unusual conditions in which we were working. The kidney itself with a short segment of the remaining ureter was wrapped in sterile sponges and covered with sterile rubber sheeting, leaving only the tip of the ureter exposed. An attempt to bury the kidney beneath the skin was made, but because of the position of the vessels, a considerable part of the kidney was still uncovered. The entire area was kept warm with the use of the same gooseneck lamps. Immediately the kidney began to secrete urine.

Needless to say, we hovered closely about for a considerable number of hours. As usual, however, at the Brigham in those days, as the light of morning dawned, our duties called us to more routine and mundane things. The kidney continued to secrete urine, and by noon of the next day, the patient herself began to show marked improvement. She began to become more alert and by the following day was entirely clear in her mind. The day after the transplant the ureter began to show signs of swelling, and a portion of it was removed to allow for better drainage of the urine. By the following day the kidney was showing evidence of decreasing output, and because of the great improvement in the patient, it was elected to remove it. I am not quite sure as to the exact time sequence, but two or three days after the removal of the kidney, the patient began to enter a diuretic phase and her subsequent recovery was relatively uneventful.

It was only shortly after this that the enthusiasm for plastic materials and the knowledge of the surface properties of plastics made possible the development of a more efficient artificial kidney so that the use of short-term transplants was not pursued with any vigor, even though we continued to try to solve the problems of the long-term homotransplantation. In those days it was very difficult to engender any clinical enthusiasm for transplantation because the opposition to trials in this direction was very great. It certainly is much easier today....

When I first arrived at the Brigham 2 or 3 years later, this episode had already become surrounded by myth; within 2 years we were going ahead with the Hume series of clinical transplants, and I am very grateful to Charles Hufnagel (who died in 1989) for sending me this note in 1962, while his memory of the matter was still so clear.

About 1947, immediately following the arm kidney episode mentioned above, the development of the artificial kidney became basic to the care of renal failure at the Brigham Hospital. The classic paper that first described this work and formed the basis for future work in the field was published in the Netherlands during the war:

Kolff, W.J., and H.Th.J. Berk. 1944. The artificial kidney. A dialyzer with a great area. *Acta Med. Scand.* 117:121–134.

When George Thorn received the plans for the artificial kidney from Kolff, there was one nagging design defect still to be resolved. The elaborate rotating drum machine leaked blood at the rotator coupling. Such a leak would also be a dangerous entry point for bacteria. Thorn sought the help of Carl Walter, an innovative surgeon on the Brigham staff with a remarkable gift for engineering improvements in medical technology. He developed the leak-proof, bacteria-proof coupling that made this machine both safe and effective. Later in his inventive surgical career, Carl developed the plastic blood transfusion apparatus now used worldwide and made many improvements in the machinery of operating rooms and the safety of sterilization equipment.

With its improved design, the Brigham-Kolff artificial kidney was employed widely and, with the clinical record of Thorn and Merrill as a guide, remained the standard dialyzer in the United States for many years. The role of the artificial kidney in the treatment of renal failure was central to the development of kidney transplantation and to the Hume series, our first exploration of that new field.

The Hume unmatched-cadaver-kidney series was described in a special supplement to the *Journal of Clinical Investigation* in 1955. Here will be found the story of all those patients, including that first patient whose kidney was put in the normal position of the kidney, which was never again attempted in the thousands of subsequent cases. Here also is told the story of the last patient of that series, the doctor from South America, whose long survival set the stage for the work of Joseph Murray and John Merrill:

Hume, D., J.P. Merrill, and B.F. Miller. 1952. Homologous transplantations of human kidneys. *J. Clin. Invest.* 31:640-641.
Hume, D.M., J.P. Merrill, B.F. Miller, and G.W. Thorn. 1955. Experiences with renal homotransplantation in the human: report of nine cases. *J. Clin. Invest.* 34:327-382.

Joseph Murray's work in kidney transplantation, starting with the identical twins, was described in a series of articles published over several years. Upon receiving the Nobel Prize, Joe, like all other Nobel laureates, had the opportunity to summarize his work. Here will be found not only that story but the references to much of the earlier work:

Murray, J.E. 1991. *The First Successful Organ Transplants in Man.* Les Prix Nobel, Stockholm: Norstedts Tryckerie AB, The Nobel Foundation.

In 1964 I published a brief history of transplantation, hoping this might be of interest as the story of a scientific discovery more recent than some of the ancient examples so often used in high school and college courses. Then, in 1972, this book was updated (as a sort of second edition) to include several additional developments, most especially transplantation of the liver and heart:

Moore, F.D. 1964. *Give and Take. The Development of Tissue Transplantation.* Philadelphia: W.B. Saunders Co.
Moore, F.D. 1972. *Transplant: The Give and Take of Tissue Transplantation (revised edition).* New York: Simon and Schuster.

Thomas Starzl, working first in Chicago, then at Denver, and later in Pittsburgh, established in the latter two cities major centers for transplantation that became preeminent in the world for the numbers of transplantations carried out, for the development of new drugs for immunosuppression, and for the teaching of the surgical methods of transplantation. He tells his story in a recent autobiography:

Starzl, T.E. 1993. *The Puzzle People. Memoirs of a Transplant Surgeon.* Pittsburgh: University of Pittsburgh Press.

Key references in the early history of transplantation follow. These include the pioneering work of Alexis Carrel, now almost a century ago, the studies of Peter Medawar during the war, and initial reports from our department:

Carrel, A. 1905. The transplantation of organs. A preliminary communication. *JAMA* 45:1945-1946.

Carrel's Nobel lecture 78 years before Murray's, on a closely related topic:

Carrel, A. 1913. *Suture of Blood Vessels and Transplantation of Organs*. In Les Prix Nobel en 1912. Stockholm: Imprimerie Royale, P.A. Norstedt & Soner.

The original reports of surgical research by Gibson and Medawar that laid the foundation for immunogenetics and transplant science:

Gibson, T., and P.B. Medawar. 1942-1943. The fate of skin homografts in man. *J. Anat.* 77:299-310.
Medawar, P.B. 1944. The behavior and fate of skin autografts and skin homografts in rabbits. (A report to the War Wounds Committee of the Medical Research Council.) *J. Anat.* 78:176-199.

The studies from war-torn London that clearly described reversible kidney failure after severe injury, or the "crush syndrome," incurred during the incessant bombings of that city:

Bywaters, E.G.I. 1944. Ischemic muscle necrosis: Crushing injury, traumatic edema, the "crush syndrome," traumatic anuria, compression syndrome; a type of injury seen in air raid casualties following burial beneath debris. *JAMA* 124.1103-1109.

The three classic papers describing the transplants upon which Dr. Murray's Nobel Award was based:

Merrill, J.P., J.E. Murray, J.H. Harrison, and W.R. Guild. 1956. Successful homotransplantation of the human kidney between identical twins. *JAMA* 160.277-282.
Merrill, J.P., J.E. Murray, J.H. Harrison, E.A. Friedman, J.B. Dealy, Jr., and G.J. Dammin. 1960. Successful homotransplantation of the kidney between nonidentical twins. *N. Engl. J. Med.* 262:1251-1260.
Merrill, J.P., J.E. Murray, F.J. Takacs, E.B. Hager, R.E. Wilson, and G.J. Dammin. 1963. Successful transplantation of kidney from a human cadaver. *JAMA* 185:347-353.

Had John Merrill and David Hume been living in 1990, it is a fair guess that they would have shared the Nobel award with Joseph Murray.

The references listed below tell of the advent of drug immunosuppression as well as the early work of Calne, Mannick, and the French workers:

Schwartz, R., J. Stack, and W. Dameshek. 1958. Effect of 6-mercaptopurine on antibody production. *Proc. Soc. Exp. Biol. Med.* 99:164-167.
Schwartz, R., and W. Dameshek. 1959. Drug-induced immunological tolerance. *Nature* 183:1682-1683.
Calne, R.Y. 1960. The rejection of renal homograft: inhibition in dogs by 6-mercaptopurine. *Lancet* 1:417-418.

Calne, R.Y. 1961. Inhibition of the rejection of renal homografts in dogs by purine analogues. *Transplant. Bull.* 28(2):445-461.

Mannick, J.A., H.L.J. Lochte, C.A. Ashley, E.D. Thomas, and J.W.A. Ferrebee. 1959. Functioning kidney homotransplant in the dog. *Surgery* 46:821-828.

Michael Woodruff, a Scots surgeon who was Head of the Department of Surgery in Dunedin, New Zealand, was an early pioneer in immunogenetic research as well as clinical transplantation. Woodruff carried out the latter when he returned as Professor and Head of the Department of Surgery at the University of Edinburgh, succeeding Sir James Learmonth:

Woodruff, M.F.A., and B. Lennox. 1959. Reciprocal skin grafts in a pair of twins showing blood chimerism. *Lancet* 2:476-478.

Early reports from the French work:

Küss, R., M. Legrain, G. Mathé, R. Nedey, and M. Camey. 1962. Homotransplantation rénale chez l'homme hors de tout lien de parente. Survie jusqu'au dix-septième mois. *Rev. Fr. Etud. Clin. Biol.* 7:1048-1066.

Hamburger, J., and J. Dormont. 1968. Functional and morphologic alterations in long-term kidney transplants, pp. 201-214. In *Human Transplantation*, F. T. Rapaport and J. Dausset (eds). New York: Grune and Stratton.

C. Stuart Welch, Professor and Head of the Department of Surgery at Tufts, carried out experimental liver transplantation in the dog in the early 1950s, placing the liver in a new position in the abdomen:

Welch, C.S. 1955. A note on transplantation of the whole liver in dogs. *Transplant. Bull.* 2:54-55.

In Welch's experiments, the animal's own liver was left in place and intact. Because the object of many liver transplantations in man includes the removal of a diseased liver, our initial experiments involved removal of the entire liver and its replacement by a transplant. The purpose here was to place the new liver in the normal position of the old one and evaluate its function chemically and physiologically. Our work on liver transplantation began in the laboratory in 1957:

Moore, F.D., L.L. Smith, T.K. Burnap, F.D. Dallenback, G.J. Dammin, U.F. Gruber, W.C. Schoemaker, R.W. Steenburg, M.R. Ball, and J.S. Belko. 1959. One-stage homotransplantation of the liver following total hepatectomy in dogs. *Transplant. Bull.* 6:103-107.

Moore, F.D., H.B. Wheeler, H.V. Demissianos, L.L. Smith, O. Balankura, K. Abel, J.B. Greenberg, and G.J. Dammin. 1960. Experimental whole organ transplantation of the liver and of the spleen. *Ann. Surg.* 152:374-387.

Tom Starzl began to experiment with liver transplantation in his laboratory in Chicago at the same time we did in Boston. His early work was carried out as a part of his studies at Northwestern University School of Medicine, then continued when he moved to Denver:

Starzl, T.E., T.L. Marchioro, R.T. Huntley, D. Rifkind, D.T. Rowlands, Jr., T.C. Dickinson, and W.R. Waddell. 1964. Experimental and clinical homotransplantation of the liver. *Ann. N.Y. Acad. Sci.* 120:739-765.

Roy Calne did his early liver transplantations while based in Cambridge, England, working collaboratively with the medical hepatologist and staff at King's College Hospital in London. Before going on to human work he studied liver transplantation extensively in the pig and showed that in this species liver transplantation was not followed by an intense rejection process:

Calne, R.Y., H.H.O. White, D.E. Yoffa, R.M. Binns, R.R. Maginn, R.M. Herbertson, P.R. Millard, V.P. Molina, and D.R. Davis. 1967. Prolonged survival of liver transplants in the pig. *Br. Med. J.* 4:645-648.

Calne's early experience in man was covered in his paper in 1968:

Calne, R.Y., and R. Williams. 1968. Liver transplantation in man. I. Observations on technique and organization in five cases. *Br. Med. J.* 4:535-548.

Our first liver transplantation patient (in 1963) was reported in the book *Transplant: The Give and Take of Tissue Transplantation* (referred to above). In 1969 a conference on liver transplantation reviewed the world experience about 6 years after the first two clinical transplants by Starzl and our group, respectively. Over 90% of all the liver transplantations carried out in the world at that time had been done by Starzl and Calne:

Groth, C.G. 1969. *World Statistics of Liver Transplantation*. Presented at the Cambridge Liver Transplantation Conference, April 10, 1969.

Tom Starzl's book tells of the early developmental phase of liver transplantation:

Starzl, T.E., and C.W. Putnam. 1969. *Experience in Hepatic Transplantation*. Philadelphia: W.B. Saunders Co.

Starzl set a high standard for all transplanters by using the immunogenetic cross-hybridization of organ transplantation to cast light on the chemical and in some cases genetic background of certain diseases involving the liver. As Starzl's work has progressed, he has introduced an important new immunosuppressive drug (FK506), has revealed through transplantation some insights into inherited enzymatic disorders, and has demonstrated through cell tracking that cells from donor organs (the dendritic cells of lymphatic origin) migrate to other sites in the new host and may be the key to the acceptance of foreign tissue (chimerism):

Starzl, T.E., A.J. Demetris, M. Trucco, C. Ricordi, S. Ildstad, P.I. Terasaki, N. Murase, R.S. Kendall, M. Kocova, W.A. Rudert, A. Zeevi, and D. Van Thiel. 1993. Chimerism after liver transplantation for type IV glycogen storage disease and type 1 Gaucher's disease. *N. Engl. J. Med.* 328:745-749.

Our only venture in this field was the demonstration by transplantation that one of the important immune proteins (the third component of complement) is produced entirely in the liver:

Alper, C.A., A.M. Johnson, A.G. Birtch, and F.D. Moore. 1969. Human C′3; evidence for the liver as the primary site of synthesis. *Science* 163:286-288.

Alan Birtch demonstrated the importance of blood flow alterations in the rejection response to transplanted liver:

Moore, F.D., A.G. Birtch, F. Dagher, F. Veith, J.A. Krisher, S.E. Order, W.A. Shucart, G.J. Dammin, and N.P. Couch. 1964. Immunosuppression and vascular insufficiency in liver transplantation. *Ann. N.Y. Acad. Sci.* 120:729-738.

Birtch, A.G., and F.D. Moore. 1969. Experience in liver transplantation. *Transplant. Rev.* 2:90-128.

By moving ahead when an ideal situation arose for the availability of a fresh heart, Chris Barnard scooped his former Minnesota colleagues Lower and Shumway, who by then had moved to Stanford, and reported his first cardiac transplant:

Barnard, C.N. 1968. Human heart transplantation: the diagnosis of rejection. *Am. J. Cardiol.* 22:811-819.

Shumway's clinical work had started at the same time as Barnard's first two human heart transplants in South Africa. Within a short time Shumway could report an extensive series of operations that outstripped other surgeons in the world. Shumway performed a large series of heart transplants in man using standard methods with effective support and a very low mortality:

Stinson, E.B., E. Dong, Jr., J.S. Schroeder, and N.E. Shumway. 1969. Cardiac transplantation in man. IV. Early results. *Ann. Surg.* 170:588-592.

Richard Lower was one of the pioneers working in cardiac transplantation early on, starting first at Minnesota and then with Shumway at Stanford before becoming head of the unit for heart transplantation at Richmond under Hume. He reviewed this work:

Lower, R.R. 1969. Prospects of heart transplantation, pp. 238-247. In *Organ Transplantation Today*, N.A. Mitchison, J.M. Greep, and J.C.M.H. Verschure (eds). Amsterdam: Excerpta Medica.

Four years earlier, Lower had been a collaborator with Shumway and Dong in the dog work that made cardiac transplantation possible. Experiments in dogs had made kidney transplantation possible and were to be the touchstone of success for all major research. This early article was one of the first to be published on experimental heart transplantation in the dog:

Lower, R.R., E. Dong, Jr., and N.E. Shumway. 1965. Long-term survival of cardiac homografts. *Surgery* 58:110-119.

The remarkable role of Wangensteen's department at the University of Minnesota has been reviewed by Simmons:

Simmons, R.L. 1992. The Minnesota story. A brief history of the transplantation program at the University of Minnesota. *Chimera* 4:9-14.

Early reports of transplantation of the lung included the work of Hardy in Mississippi, Blumenstock at the Bassett Hospital in New York, and Derom in the Netherlands:

Hardy, J.D., W.R. Webb, M.L. Dalton, Jr., and G.R. Walker, Jr. 1963. Lung homotransplantation in man. Report of the initial case. *JAMA* 186:1065-1074.

Blumenstock, D.A. 1967. The lung and other organs. Transplantation of the lung. *Transplantation* 5:917-928.

Derom, F., F. Barbier, S. Ringoir, G. Rolly, J. Versieck, G. Berzsenyi, R. Raemdonck, and J. Piret. 1969. A case of lung homotransplantation in man (preliminary report). *Tijdschr. Geneeskd.* 25:109-114.

Transplantation of the pancreas was undertaken to provide the endocrine organ that contains the islets of Langerhans. These islets secrete insulin and would be critical for survival in childhood diabetes. The papers by Lillehei and Reemtsma tell of their work in Minneapolis and New York, respectively:

Lillehei, R.C., Y. Idezuki, W.D. Kelly, J.S. Najarian, F.K. Merkel, and F.C. Goetz. 1969. Transplantation of the intestine and pancreas. *Transplant. Proc.* 1:230-238.

Reemtsma, K., J.F. Lucas, Jr., R.E. Rogers, F.E. Schmidt, and F.H. Davis, Jr. 1963. Islet cell function of the transplanted canine pancreas. *Ann. Surg.* 158:645-653.

Paul Russell, innovative transplanter of the early days, now in charge of immunogenetic research at the MGH, has used genetic manipulation to produce insulin from other cell types:

Selden, R.F., M.J. Skoskiewicz, P.S. Russell, and H.M. Goodman. 1987. Regulation of insulin gene expression. *N. Engl. J. Med.* 317:1067-1070.

Selden, R.F., M.J. Skoskiewicz, K.B. Howie, P.S. Russell, H.M. Goodman. 1986. Regulation of human insulin gene expression in transgenic mice. *Nature* 321:525-528.

Russell, P.S. 1991. Some personal reflections on the development of transplantation, pp. 307-335. In *History of Transplantation: 35 Recollections*, Vol. 17. P.I. Terasaki (ed). Los Angeles, CA: UCLA Tissue Typing Laboratory.

Somers Sturgis and John Brooks of our staff experimented extensively with the transplantation of endocrine organs (ovary, thyroid, parathyroid, pancreatic islet cells) within protective chambers made of Millipore filter material:

Sturgis, S.H., and H. Castellanos. 1962. Ovarian homografts in organic filter chambers. *Ann. Surg.* 156:367-374.

Brooks, J.R., S.H. Sturgis, and G. Hill. 1960. An evaluation of endocrine tissue homotransplantation in the Millipore chamber with a note on tissue adaptation to the host. *Ann. N.Y. Acad. Sci.* 87:482-500.

Brooks, J.R., and J. Levy. 1968. Endocrine transplantation, pp. 271-283. In *Human Transplantation*, F.T. Rapaport and J. Dausset (eds): New York: Grune & Stratton.

Brooks, J.R. 1962. *Endocrine Tissue Transplantation*. Springfield, IL: Charles C Thomas.

As early as 1960 Starzl was experimenting in dogs with multiple organ grafts:

Starzl, T.E., H.A. Kaupp, Jr., D.R. Brock, G.W. Butz, and J.W. Linman. 1962. Homotransplantation of multiple visceral organs. *Am. J. Surg.* 103:219-229.

Thirty years later such transplants in patients met with limited success and were criticized for overextending the available technology. My editorial comment, requested by the editor of *JAMA*, was critical of justifying such operations on the basis of desperation, but at the same time held Starzl and his group as models of complete frankness in their published reports:

Moore, F.D. 1989. The desperate case: CARE (costs, applicability, research, ethics). *JAMA* 261:1483-1484.

The occurrence of malignant tumors in transplant patients is described:

Sheil, A.G.R., A.P.S. Disney, T.H. Mathew, N. Amiss, and L. Excell. 1991. Cancer development in cadaveric donor renal allograft recipients treated with azathioprine (AZA) or cyclosporine (CyA) or AZA/CyA. *Transplant. Proc.* 23:1111-1112.

Penn, I. 1991. Occurrence of cancers in immunosuppressed organ transplant recipients, pp. 53-62. In *Clinical Transplants 1990*, P.I. Terasaki (ed). Los Angeles, CA: UCLA Tissue Typing Laboratory.

Annual reports of transplantation operations and results are available from UNOS (United Network for Organ Sharing) and from Terasaki's reviews:

Terasaki, P.I., and J.M. Cecka. 1994. *Clinical Transplants 1993* (ninth in a series). Los Angeles, CA: UCLA Tissue Typing Laboratory.

Terasaki, P.I. (ed). 1991. *History of Transplantation: 35 Recollections.* Los Angeles, CA: UCLA Tissue Typing Laboratory.

UNOS, Division of Organ Transplantation, Bureau of Health Resources Development, Health Resources and Services Administration, and U.S. Department of Health and Human Services. 1993. *Annual Report of the U.S. Scientific Registry of Transplant Recipients and the Organ Procurement and Transplantation Network—Transplant Data: 1988-1991.* Bethesda, MD: U.S. Department of Health and Human Services.

The data on waiting lists for 1994, presented at the end of Chapter 22, are from the periodical "UNOS Update."

The concept that physicians and especially surgeons often must do harm so that healing can occur is hardly new. It has merely been obscured by the ancient platitude *primum non nocere* (first, do no harm).

Breach of this ancient maxim has sometimes been essential to healing because physicians must often do harm and put the patient at risk so healing may occur. Sometimes the harm is lasting and severe. No one who has been through cancer chemotherapy needs to be told this. Disfiguring surgery in malignancy and the giving of a donor organ by a healthy relative are clear examples of breach of that ancient saying. Hurt, risk, and harm are undertaken so the patient can heal, get well, and return to a normal life.

Although the expression *primum non nocere* is usually ascribed to Hippocrates, it is not part of The Physician's Oath. The authentic reference is to Hippocrates' *Epidemics*, Book I, Section xi (translated by Jones): "As to diseases, make a habit of two things—to help, or at least to do no harm."

To harm has sometimes been essential to healing, to recovery, as in the removal of vital parts of the brain to cure a tumor. In the ancient practice of bloodletting or bleeding, the extent of harm to the patient was often severe and not recognized. Bloodletting, the object of which was to take blood from the vein in front of the elbow, and leeching, in which blood was withdrawn by placing a hungry leech over the vein, were carried out in the hope that the patient would be improved thereby. Galen is alleged to have introduced this practice in the early years of the Christian era, and it lasted until the turn of this century. According to his translators, Galen was both realistic and conservative and cautioned against removing more than an ounce or two (30 to 60 milliliters) of blood.

Like so much of medical mythology, this widespread practice had its origin in a small crumb of truth. In some cases of congestive heart failure, the removal of large amounts of blood (up to 500 milliliters or even more) produces a decongestion of the lungs that must have seemed truly "miraculous" to the ancients. Perhaps we should not be surprised or critical that our ancestors generalized from this to overuse of the remedy. We have often committed the same error; for example, the "penicillin for everything" era of the early 1950s.

The overuse of bleeding was commonplace in the eighteenth century. It was even used for infections such as yellow fever. George Washington's final illness was a severe septic sore throat, possibly of the type caused by the streptococcus. According to most interpretations, extreme bloodletting resulted in his death. Galen's views as well as the care of General Washington are described in the following references:

Brain, P. 1980. *Galen on Bloodletting: A Study of the Origins, Development and Validity of His Opinions, With a Translation of Three Works.* New York: Cambridge University Press.

Jackson, J. 1860. *Memoir on the Last Sickness of George Washington.* Boston: Privately printed.

In major surgery, transplantation, chemotherapy, and radiotherapy, doctors must often do harm so the patient may heal. Sometimes the hurt wins out and the healing fails to occur. Despite such tragedy, the public clearly accepts the fact that severe hazards and physical harm are often necessary for later healing. An educated public will also welcome an updated Latin maxim to express the more realistic relationship between harm and healing in medical and surgical care. I am indebted to G. Bruce Cobbold, teacher of Latin at Tabor Academy in Marion, Massachusetts, for suggesting the phrase *Nonnumquam, nocere est renovare* ("Sometimes, to hurt is to heal"). Here the infinitive serves as an imperative.

I hope the reader will agree that this expression comes closer to the truth, not only in high-tech procedures such as whole-body irradiation for marrow transplantation in leukemia, but also in the seemingly minor interventions such as giving a child with pneumonia an antibiotic known to cause severe side effects.

CHAPTER 23—Opening Its Valves and Then the Heart Itself

In 1924, Elliott Cutler, a junior member of Cushing's staff at the Brigham, attempted to open a narrowed mitral valve surgically. The idea was clear, the method was flawed. Nonetheless, his first patient did quite well for over a year. It was appropriate that 24 years after Cutler's work, Dwight Harken carried out the first large series of successful operations on the mitral valve. These are the two historic articles:

Cutler, E., S.A. Levine, and C.S. Beck. 1924. The surgical treatment of mitral stenosis: experimental and clinical studies. *Arch. Surg.* 9:689-692.

Harken, D.E., L.B. Ellis, P.F. Ware, and L.R. Norman. 1948. The surgical treatment of mitral stenosis. I. Valvuloplasty. *N. Engl. J. Med.* 239:801-809.

The work of Bailey was contemporaneous with that of Harken:

Bailey, C.P. 1949. Surgical treatment of mitral stenosis (mitral commissurotomy). *Dis. Chest* 15:377-397.

John Gibbon's early work under Churchill at the MGH was reported in his first two papers:

Gibbon, J.H., Jr. 1937. Artificial maintenance of circulation during experimental occlusion of the pulmonary artery. *Arch. Surg.* 34:1105-1131.

Gibbon, J.H., Jr. 1939. The maintenance of life during experimental occlusion of the pulmonary artery followed by survival. *Surg. Gynecol. Obstet.* 69:602-614.

John Gibbon, in his account of his early work on the heart-lung apparatus, tells the story of that crucial vigil:

> The idea of attempting to create an extracorporeal blood circuit that could temporarily perform a part of the cardiorespiratory functions occurred to me in 1931. At that time I was a Surgical Fellow at Harvard, working in the newly created surgical research laboratories at the Massachusetts General Hospital, under the supervision of the late Dr. Edward D. Churchill.
>
> In February 1931, a female patient whose gallbladder had been removed fifteen days previously developed a severe pain in the chest in the substernal region. This was accompanied by marked elevation of pulse and respiratory rates and a decrease in blood pressure. A correct diagnosis of massive pulmonary embolus was made and Dr. Churchill had the patient moved to the operating room where she could be continuously observed and operated on immediately should her condition become critical.
>
> At that time no successful pulmonary embolectomy had been performed in the United States and only a very few in Europe. Because the procedure was so hazardous, Dr. Churchill decided not to operate unless it was apparent that death was imminent without operative intervention.
>
> My job in the operating room was to take and record the patient's pulse and respiratory rates and blood pressure every 15 minutes. From 3:00 PM one day to 8:00 AM the next day the operating team and I were by the side of the patient. Finally at 8:00 AM respirations ceased and the blood pressure could not be obtained. Within 6 minutes 30 seconds Dr. Churchill had opened the chest, incised the pulmonary artery, extracted a large pulmonary embolus, and closed the incised wound in the pulmonary artery with a lateral clamp. Despite the rapidity of the procedure, the patient could not be revived.
>
> During that long night, watching the patient struggle for life, the thought

naturally occurred to me that the patient's life might be saved if some of the blue blood in her veins could be continuously withdrawn into an extracorporeal blood circuit, exposed to an atmosphere of oxygen, and then returned to the patient by way of a systemic artery in a central direction. Thus, some of the patient's cardiorespiratory functions might be temporarily performed by the blood circuit while the massive embolus was surgically removed.

Gibbon, J.H., Jr. 1978. Great ideas in surgery: the development of the heart–lung apparatus. *Am. J. Surg.* 135:608–619.

About 20 years after Gibbon began his work on the heart–lung apparatus, designed to remove the entire volume of blood from the veins, oxygenate the red cells, remove the carbon dioxide, and return all that blood under pressure to the arteries, he published a status report:

Gibbon, J.H., Jr., B.J. Miller, and C. Fineberg. 1953. An improved mechanical heart–lung apparatus. *Med. Clin. North Am.* 37:1603–1624.
Gibbon, J.H., Jr. 1954. Application of a mechanical heart and lung apparatus to cardiac surgery. *Minnesota Med.* 37:171–180.

Within a year Gibbon was able to report the first successful application of his pump–oxygenator to surgery in man, after which John Kirklin and Walt Lillehei applied this device to many patients with heart disease, particularly infants and children. The modern era of open–heart surgery had truly begun:

Kirklin, J.W., J.W. DuShane, R.T. Patrick, D.E. Donald, P.S. Hetzel, H.G. Harshbarger, and E.H. Wood. 1955. Intrathoracic surgery with the aid of a mechanical pump–oxygenator system (Gibbon type): report of eight cases. *Proc. Staff Meetings Mayo Clin.* 30:201–206.
Warden, H.E., M. Cohen, R.A. DeWall, E.A. Schultz, J.J. Buckley, R.C. Read, and C.W. Lillehei. 1954. Experimental closure of interventricular septal defects and further physiologic studies on controlled cross circulation. *Surg. Forum* 24 5:22–28.

The concept of using a pump–oxygenator for purposes other than cardiac surgery was especially prominent in our department in the 1970s with the work of Philip A. Drinker and Robert Bartlett. They planned to develop a device of this type for use wholly as an artificial lung, the object being to substitute a machine to oxygenate blood in patients with life-threatening but reversible lung disease. This application of the pump–oxygenator has found its greatest usefulness in newborn infants with respiratory distress syndrome. Philip Drinker's interest in the artificial support of lung function came naturally to him because it was his father, Philip Drinker, who in 1927-29 developed the automatic respirator, later known as the Drinker Respirator, for use in cases of polio. Bartlett carried the work forward in California and then at Ann Arbor as the foremost exponent of this method for treating severely handicapped infants. His record is a remarkable one, with many long-term survivors among infants who would otherwise have died:

Bartlett, R.H. 1990. Extracorporeal life-support in cardiopulmonary failure. *Curr. Probl. Surg.* 27:627–705.

In their most recent article, the Michigan group reports on 20 years' experience in using the extracorporeal life support in 444 critically ill newborn infants. Survival rates in severe respiratory distress (formerly fatal in almost all cases) have risen from 72 to 94%. Here is the successful application of a device invented for the surgical treatment of heart disease being used to help with severe crises in newborn babies. I am sure that Jack Gibbon, were he still alive, would be proud of this totally unforeseen application of the pump-oxygenator he worked so long to perfect:

Shanley, C.H., R.B. Hirschl, R.E. Schumacher, T. Delosh, R.A. Chapman, R.H. Bartlett, and M.C. Overbeck. 1994. Extracorporeal life support for neonatal respiratory failure: 20 year experience. *Ann. Surg.* 220:269–282.

As a research fellow at the Brigham, Charles Hufnagel was a pioneer in many aspects of cardiovascular surgery. The ball valves that he explored so thoroughly in dogs became the prototype later developed by Harken for use in the aortic valve position. Hufnagel later became Professor and Department Head at Georgetown University in Washington, D.C.:

Hufnagel, C.A. 1950. Aortic plastic valvular prosthesis. *Bull. Georgetown Med. Center* 4:128–130.

Ancient history of cardiac surgery includes work by Harvey Cushing. Cushing was an innovator in many fields of surgery and physiology. He carried out some early cardiac surgery in the laboratories at Johns Hopkins:

Cushing, H., and J.R.B. Branch. 1907–1908. Chronic valvular lesions in the dog and their possible relation to future surgery of the cardiac valves. *J. Med. Res.* 17:471–486.

In England, Souttar had carried out work of this type at the same time as Elliott Cutler's efforts but never proceeded with his studies:

Souttar, H.S. 1925. Surgical treatment of mitral stenosis. *Br. Med. J.* 2:603–608.

Harken's wartime work on removal of bullets and shell fragments from the heart was an early report of successful surgery within the heart:

Harken, D.E., and A.C. Williams. 1946. Foreign bodies in and in relation to the thoracic blood vessels and heart. Migratory foreign bodies within the blood vascular system. *Am. J. Surg.* 72:80-90.

The operations carried out by Robert Gross for patent ductus and coarctation of the aorta before and during World War II were milestones in the surgical correction of defects of the heart and great vessels in infants and children:

Gross, R.E., and J.P. Hubbard. 1939. Surgical ligation of patent ductus arteriosus: a report of the first successful case. *JAMA* 112:729-731.
Gross, R.E. 1945. Surgical correction for coarctation of the aorta. *Surgery* 18:673-678.

I am indebted to M. Judah Folkman for details of Robert Gross' early work, as related in the text.
The early work by Churchill on pericardiectomy and the work of Alfred Blalock in rerouting the blood in congenital heart disease also provided essential background for the development of surgery in the interior of the heart. Helen Taussig was a leading scholar of congenital heart disease in children. Her long collaboration with Blalock is an example of the sort of collaboration between a surgeon and physicians, scientists, or scholars in other fields that has produced major advances in surgery:

Churchill, E.D. 1936. Pericardial resection in chronic constrictive pericarditis. *Ann. Surg.* 104:516-529.
Blalock, A., and H.B. Taussig. 1945. Surgical treatment of malformations of the heart in which there is pulmonary stenosis or pulmonary atresia. *JAMA* 128:189-202.

The Department of Surgery at the University of Minnesota under Owen Wangensteen was a center of innovative research in cardiac surgery for several decades after World War II, despite the fact that Wangensteen's own interests lay mostly in the surgical management of duodenal ulcer. Early reports from Minnesota describe the cross-circulation method of supporting the open, quiet heart as well as early adaptations and improvements of the pump-oxygenator:

Warden, H.E., M. Cohen, R.C. Read, and C.W. Lillehei. 1954. Controlled cross circulation for open intracardiac surgery. Physiologic studies and results of creation and closure of ventricular septal defects. *J. Thorac. Surg.* 28:331-343.
DeWall, R.A., H.E. Warden, V.L. Gott, R.C. Read, R.L. Varco, and C.W. Lillehei. 1956. Total body perfusion for open cardiotomy utilizing the bubble oxygenator. *J. Thorac. Surg.* 32:591-603.

Dudley Johnson was one of the first to report an impressive series in which blood was shunted (bypassed) from the aorta to the coronary arteries. This was the coronary artery bypass graft, which, with many variations and improvements, is now used throughout the world to assist people with coronary heart disease:

Johnson, W.D., and D. Lepley, Jr. 1970. An aggressive surgical approach to coronary disease. *J. Thorac. Cardiovasc. Surg.* 59:128-138.

The story of Dwight Harken's life work as surgeon to the human heart would be incomplete without acknowledging the expert work of Anna Mae Fosberg, R.N., Associate in Surgery. Ms. Fosberg was the cardiac technician who operated the pump-oxygenator for him and for his successor, John Collins, from the earliest use of that device at the Brigham (about 1956) until her retirement in 1993. Essential to the success of open-heart programs in all the hospitals that undertake such work is a person, often known as the pump technician, who keeps this complex apparatus clean, safe, and functioning properly. Anna Mae Fosberg, affectionately known as "Scottie," fulfilled this role for almost 40 years and so ably that she became the teacher of many nurses and bioengineers who then filled this role at hospitals elsewhere in this country and abroad.

CHAPTER 24—Adoptive Immunotherapy of Cancer

Our early studies of pituitary removal in the treatment of advanced breast cancer were done in collaboration with Andrew Jessiman and Donald Matson, who performed the operations. While some excellent results were obtained for individual patients, the treatment itself was too taxing, and long-term survival was infrequent:

Jessiman, A.G., D.D. Matson, and F.D. Moore. 1959. Hypophysectomy in the treatment of breast cancer. *N. Engl. J. Med.* 261:1199-1207.

McWhirter, a Scottish radiologist, was one of the early vocal antisurgical advocates. He always carried out radiation therapy without ever questioning whether or not even that was necessary after conservative surgical removal of the breast in very early cases:

McWhirter, R. 1955. Simple mastectomy and radiotherapy in treatment of breast cancer. *Br. J. Radiol.* 28:128-139.

We reviewed the mixing of all these cross currents on several occasions:

Jessiman, A.G., and F.D. Moore. 1956. *Carcinoma of the Breast: The Study and Treatment of the Patient.* Boston: Little, Brown.
Moore, F.D., S.I. Woodrow, M.A. Aliapoulios, and R.E. Wilson. 1967. *Carcino-

ma of the Breast: A Decade of New Results and Old Concepts. Boston: Little, Brown.

Jerome Urban of New York was one of the voices calling for more radical surgical removal of the breast:

Urban, J.A., and H. Farrow. 1963. Long term results of internal mammary lymph node excision for breast cancer. *Acta Union Int. Contre Cancer* 19:1551-1554.

The most successful of our innovations in advanced breast cancer was the combination of surgical adrenalectomy immediately followed by chemotherapy. Some of the few long-term survivals that we obtained resulted from this combination, with these patients living a pain-free existence for 5 to 15 years despite the initial presence of advanced disease:

Moore, F.D., S.B. Van Devanter, C.M. Boyden, J. Lokich, and R.E. Wilson. 1974. Adrenalectomy with chemotherapy in the treatment of advanced breast cancer: objective and subjective response rates; duration and quality of life. *Surgery* 76:376-390.

Early efforts to modify the growth of cancer by means of toxins or immune stimulants go back many years. Although we would now lump all those early efforts under the general rubric of immune modulation in cancer treatment, some of the early workers and authors in this field would hardly agree with such terminology, since they considered these agents poisons or toxins that affected the cancer directly rather than as stimulants of the patient's immune defenses. The work of Bradley Coley, using what were known at that time as Coley's toxins, stands out:

Coley, W.B. 1894. Treatment of inoperable malignant tumors with the toxines of erysipelas and the bacillus prodigiosus. *Trans. Am. Surg. Assoc.* 12:183-203.

Steven Rosenberg's work on adoptive immunotherapy can be traced through his reports:

Grimm, E.A., A. Mazumder, H.Z. Shang, and S.A. Rosenberg. 1982. The lymphokine activated killer cell phenomenon: lysis of NK resistant fresh solid tumor cells by IL-2 activated autologous human peripheral blood lymphocytes. *J. Exp. Med.* 155:1823-1841.

Rosenberg, S.A., J.J. Mule, P.J. Spiess, C.M. Reichert, and S. Schwarz. 1985. Regression of established pulmonary metastases and subcutaneous tumor mediated by the systemic administration of high dose recombinant IL-2. *J. Exp. Med.* 161:1169-1188.

Rosenberg, S.A. 1992. The immunotherapy and gene therapy of cancer. *J. Clin. Oncol.* 10:180-199.

In 1993 Rosenberg published an autobiography describing his work on genetic manipulation and adoptive immunotherapy in cancer. His book presents a fascinating view of both the promise and the limitations of the method. He tells the story of Lieutenant Commander L.G., whose course and recovery (with many additional details supplied to me by Steven Rosenberg) are related in Chapter 24:

Rosenberg, S.A., and J.M. Barry. 1992. *The Transformed Cell*. New York: Putnam.

CHAPTER 25—Korea (1951)

John Howard's book describes his elegant studies at MASH #8209 where the Surgical Research Unit was established:

Howard, J. M., ed. 1955. *Battle Casualties in Korea. Studies of the Surgical Research Team* (Vols. 1-4). Washington, D.C.: U.S. Government Printing Office.

In 1955, nine articles on this subject were published in the March issue of *Annals of Surgery* (Volume 141, Number 3).

CHAPTER 26—Ibn Saud: Caring for the Royal Family of Arabia (1961)

Early in this century, about 1906, Paul W. Harrison was one of the first medical missionaries to visit Arabia and one of the early explorers and ethnographers of the region. His book describes the scene at Dhahran. He remembered that he could not see anything but desert scrub and the burning hot sun. He commented that it was bone-chilling cold at night and broiling hot during the day and that there was no sign of anything to support the activities of human beings in the air, on the ground, or beneath it. He wrote his classic description of the Arabian desert while he was standing on top of the largest oil dome in the world.

The site of the first productive oil well, known as Dhahran No. 1, is now enclosed by a silver fence that celebrates the date when the oil began to flow (1936). Within a few years the Saudi dynasty made the move from camels to Cadillacs and fell prey to the relentless pressure of western economics. The many flaws of western civilization became engrafted on the life of courageous desert nomads.

Harrison's early account was reprinted in 1927:

Harrison, P.W. 1927. *The Arab at Home*. New York: Thomas Y. Crowell.

The son of this exploring Harrison, Timothy Harrison, is a surgeon on the staff of the medical school in Hershey, Pennsylvania. He has followed in his father's footsteps, doing medical missionary work in the Middle East, particularly Lebanon, the Emirates, and Arabia. He married Eliza Cope, the daughter of Oliver Cope, who was so important as a teacher and leader in my early years in surgery at the Massachusetts General.

C.M. Doughty was also a scholar of early Arabic civilization. At the time of my studies in the Department of Anthropology at Harvard College, his books were the source books on the Arabian Peninsula:

Doughty, C.M. 1921. *Travels in Arabia Deserta*. Boston: P.L. Warner.
Doughty, C.M. 1927. *Wanderings in Arabia*. New York: Boni.

The discovery of oil was not the first thing to bring the impact of Western civilization to the Arabian desert. The northwest frontier between Arabia and what are now Syria and Jordan was the scene of the efforts of the British to oust the Ottoman Empire from the Fertile Crescent and Mesopotamia. This heroic story of the desert war in World War I has never been told better than by T.E. Lawrence:

Lawrence, T.E. 1937. *Seven Pillars of Wisdom: A Triumph*. Garden City, NY: Doubleday, Doran & Co.

Many recent American and British visitors have described their reactions to Arabia. One of the recent medical visitors was Seymour Gray, a medical associate of ours at the Brigham for many years. Upon returning from an extensive visit to Arabia, he wrote a revealing analysis of the atmosphere that surrounded the royal family:

Gray, S.J. 1983. *Beyond the Veil: The Adventures of an American Doctor in Saudi Arabia*. New York: Harper & Row.

The Arabian-American Oil Company (ARAMCO) was clearly in charge of United States–Saudi relationships at the time of my visit. This company issued (in 1960) a remarkable handbook for all their employees about to be stationed in Saudi Arabia. It is one of the best reference books obtainable on this subject.

Arabian-American Oil Company (ARAMCO). 1960. *Arabian Handbook*.

CHAPTER 27—The Midnight to Washington: National Responsibilities

Many years of work with the National Institutes of Health included my term as Chairman of the Surgery Study Section. During these years (1958 to 1961) we funneled generous amounts of research support into the development of the pump-oxygenator for cardiac surgery and the earliest immunological studies to make transplantation safer. A retrospective summary of those years:

Moore, F.D. 1961. The Surgery Study Section of the National Institutes of Health. *Ann. Surg.* 153:1-12.

My association with the National Aeronautics and Space Administration (NASA) as a consultant began in 1968 when I was asked to be a member of the NASA committee under Bentley Glass (Dean of the Medical School at the State University of New York at Stony Brook). We were looking into the matter of deconditioning and other physiologic problems that arise during prolonged space flight. While deconditioning consists of changes in the astronauts' body composition that are a major nuisance and at times a hazard, it now seems clear that deconditioning can usually be prevented by engaging in rigorous exercises against spring-loaded resistance. Such conditioning exercise requires special equipment because gravitational force is absent. In the reports written by the Glass committee and its successor, the Robbins committee, we reviewed many of the current issues of space flight:

Glass, H.B., ed. 1970. *Life Sciences in Space. Study to Review NASA Life Sciences Programs.* Washington, D.C.: National Academy of Sciences.
Robbins, F. 1988. *Exploring the Living Universe: A Strategy for the Space Life Sciences. A Report of the NASA Life Sciences Strategic Planning Study Committee.* Washington, D.C.: NASA.

All manned space flights of the Soviets and the Americans, with the single exception of the Apollo (Moon) flights, have been in low Earth orbit, beneath the protective magnetosphere. It is in deep space, beyond this protection, that radiation presents a severe hazard. For several years I devoted my full attention to reviewing this problem. Because no single reference had presented evidence on the severity of the hazards traceable to exomagnetospheric radiation, I prepared a brief review:

Moore, F.D. 1992. Radiation burdens for humans on prolonged exomagnetospheric voyages. *FASEB J.* 6:2338-2343.

CHAPTER 28—Autres Chirurgiens, Autres Moeurs

Visits to other universities were sometimes the occasion of my receiving honorary degrees or honorary fellowships in the surgical colleges and societies of other countries.

One of the first honorary degrees I received was from the National University of Ireland. At that time the aging Eamon De Valera—father figure of the Wars of Irish Independence—was the honorary chancellor of the National University. He handed me my diploma, and it is signed in his shaky hand. This was in 1961. De Valera was an instigator and survivor of the revolution that led to the independence of the Irish Free State, an uprising referred to in England as "the troubles." For everyone in Ireland (with the possible exception of the Anglo-Irish), this was the beginning of modern times in their national life.

Becoming an Honorary Fellow of the Royal College of Surgeons of England has been a source of continuing pleasure, and I always visit there when I am in London. I had the pleasure also of being inducted into the Royal Colleges of Surgeons of Edinburgh, Glasgow, and Canada and of becoming an honorary member of the Polish and Italian Surgical Societies as well as a Fellow of the International Surgical Society. My cherished fellowship in the American College of Surgeons, one of the largest professional associations in the world, goes back to 1946.

Citations for the honorary degrees usually mentioned our work in the biochemistry and metabolism of body composition and of convalescence, improving the care of surgical patients after burns and other injuries, the development of transplantation by my department, and my own work in liver transplantation.

Honorary degrees:

1961	M.Ch. (hon), National University of Ireland
1965	L.L.D. (hon), University of Glasgow
1966	S.D. (hon), Suffolk University, Boston
1975	M.D. (hon causa), University of Göteborg, Sweden
1976	D.Sc. (hon causa), University of Edinburgh
1976	M.D. (hon causa), University of Paris
1979	M.D. (hon causa), University of Copenhagen
1982	D.Sc. (hon causa), Harvard University

For its historical interest, the citation for the Edinburgh degree is reprinted below. The reader will appreciate the unfailing humor of the Scots orator:

Honorary Degree of Doctor of Science
Lauration Address—25th June, 1976
FRANCIS DANIELS MOORE

Lest it be thought that our evangelistic efforts were entirely Antipodean, we recall with pleasure the parts played by graduates from this School in the foundation of several Medical Schools in North America and in the year 1976 it is indeed appropriate that we should honour a distinguished American Surgeon. In Francis Daniels Moore we have one whose name and work are known and respected internationally. He was born at Evanston, Illinois, and graduated M.D. at Harvard in 1939. He rapidly rose to be Moseley Professor of Surgery at the University of Harvard and Surgeon-in-Chief at the Peter Bent Brigham Hospital in Boston. He does not like to be called Professor.

As early as 1941 he was granted a Fellowship by the National Research

Council and towards the end of World War II he and Dr. Oliver Cope published important observations on changes in body fluids in patients suffering from severe burns. He has had a continuing interest in the metabolic processes of those recovering from injury, and he was one of the first to use radio-active and stable isotopes to measure body composition in surgical patients. His monograph on 'The Metabolic Response to Surgery,' written with M.R. Ball as co-author, and his later one on 'The Metabolic Care of the Surgical Patient' are classics.

He did not, however, write Old Moore's Almanac. That was another Francis Moore, also a doctor, but he wrote his classic in 1700. I may perhaps digress further to say that the first record I can trace of an Honorary degree being given in Scotland to a Harvard graduate was as early as 1654 when John Glover, who graduated B.A. there in 1650, was given an honorary M.D. degree by the University of Aberdeen. Harvard College was founded in 1636. We received our charter in 1582. Apart from his work in relation to metabolism, Dr. Moore and his colleagues have made notable contributions in many other fields of surgery—gastro-intestinal disease, cardiac abnormalities, breast cancer and renal transplantation. He has welcomed numerous British graduates to his laboratories and has been a visiting Professor in Edinburgh and in Glasgow. He is an Honorary Fellow of the Royal College of Surgeons in Edinburgh.

Let it not be thought that the interests of Franny Moore (as he is usually known) are limited to surgical practice and research. He is one of the founders of the Harvard Medical School Musical Society and is an accomplished musician, being proficient on the piano and the accordion. At Christmas he leads a carol-singing tour of his hospital, playing on the piano accordion. He is a keen sailor. Riding and mountain climbing are also amongst his habits.

I will not attempt to catalogue the Societies in which he has held office. Francis Moore is a well known figure with many accomplishments and I have the greatest pleasure, Mr. Chancellor, in inviting you to confer on him the degree of Doctor of Science *honoris causa*.

The Glasgow citation (1965):

In his two fields of interest—the metabolic effects of wounding and the problem of the bodily response to homotransplantation—his genius lies in bringing the precise measuring techniques of science to bear on medical problems.

The citation for the honorary degree from Harvard University in 1982 at the time of the HMS Bicentennial Convocation was as follows:

Skillful surgeon, admired teacher, profoundly caring physician. For four decades a leader of Harvard medicine, he has helped thousands to safe passage through complex illness and brilliantly enhanced the successful practice of surgery.

Of other honors and awards, those of particular importance seem to me to include the Blakeslee Award of the American Heart Association. This was awarded upon the publication of my first history of transplantation, *Give and Take*.

The Alvarenga Prize of the Philadelphia Academy recognized the contribution of our first books on metabolism. The Purkinje Medal of Czechoslovakia was presented to me at the embassy in Washington; Hartwell Harrison received the medal at the same time. The Silver Medal of the International Society of Surgery and the Lister Medal of the Royal College of Surgeons of England in London were also examples of recognition abroad of the work of our group.

I was awarded the Gross Medal of the American Surgical Association in 1978. Originally named in honor of Samuel Gross of Philadelphia, one of the founders of the association, this award is now designated the Medallion for Scientific Achievement.

The Nathan Smith Award of the New England Surgical Society was awarded to me in 1989. Nathan Smith was an apostle of medical education in the early years of this nation. He contributed to the founding and growth of several medical schools in New England.

The Beaumont Medal of the Wisconsin Surgical Society commemorates the work of that army surgeon at a frontier fort in Prairie du Chien, who in tending a stomach wound in a trapper (Alexis St. Martin) became one of America's first physiologists. He was a contemporary of Gurdon Saltonstall Hubbard, who, 250 miles south of Beaumont, knew of his work only a few months later (see Notes to Chapter 3).

I was awarded the Bigelow Medal of the Boston Surgical Society in 1974. While I have not spent as much time as I would like in the councils of these societies and academies, I have always found the meetings a good antidote for any self-satisfaction that might creep in. The stream of talent in American society defies description. Such associations enable their members to drink deep of this refreshing spring.

In 1981 I was elected a member of the National Academy of Sciences.

Our trip to China in 1981 brought us close to the matter of acupuncture and into closer friendship with Professor Tseng (of the Chinese National Academy of Sciences), who had operated on the famous American reporter James ("Scottie") Reston for appendicitis in 1971. Was Mr. Reston one of the first eminent American visitors to the People's Republic of China to have a major operation (appendectomy) under acupuncture anesthesia? In his autobiography, reference is made to an appendectomy "under acupuncture," but then a considerable passage is devoted to the consultation with Li Chang-Yuan, doctor of acupuncture at the hospital, seeking treatment for Mr. Reston's postoperative gas pains. Long needles were inserted, incense was burned, and the gas pains went away. Because of our acquaintance with Mr. Reston through the Bill Saltonstalls, I was interested in this detail. On our visit with Professor Tseng I asked about this, and he stated (as he had several times before) that he did not like to use acupuncture anesthesia for abdominal surgery because of its failure to relax the abdominal muscles. He clearly recalled using the procedure in Mr. Reston's case for gas pains but shrugged that off with "... but they usually go away anyway," as mentioned in the text. Whatever actually happened, Mr. Reston recovered and, as a widely read journalist, was able to increase the interest in acupuncture throughout the United States. That he was possibly more enthusiastic about it than his surgeon was 10 years later, epitomizes the changing view of acupuncture among the Chinese themselves after the end of the Cultural Revolution (about 1975). Reston's autobiography:

Reston, J.R. 1992. *Deadline: An Autobiography.* New York: Norton.

Professor Tseng died in 1982. His wife, Dr. Qin-sheng Ge remains a friend and frequent visitor. She is Director of Gynecologic and Reproductive Endocrinology at the Chinese National Academy of Medical Sciences. Their son, Hung Tseng, is a thoroughly American molecular biologist at the University of Pennsylvania, and, as mentioned in the text, the father of Francis Moore Tseng.

CHAPTER 30—The Urge to Merge; A New Teaching Hospital for Harvard (1958-1980)

In 1986, about 6 months before the death of Stan Deland, I was appointed an honorary member of the Board of Trustees of the newly formed (i.e., merged) Brigham and Women's Hospital. As this book goes to press, we are forging a new affiliation with the Massachusetts General Hospital. It appears that this will take the form of a corporate merger, with the two hospitals operating as partners in a chain with one joint Board to govern the merged entity. This is an increasingly familiar hospital organizational pattern in the United States. This MGH-Brigham chain (Partners HealthCare Systems, Inc.) is to include, in addition to the two principal general hospitals, the McLean Hospital and the Spaulding Rehabilitation Hospital, and nursing homes or rehabilitation units that might later be established. Initially, it is planned that the clinical operations of the individual hospitals, and more notably of the two large partner hospitals, will be unchanged.

In a time of stress due to reduced insurance reimbursements, of competition among the urban teaching hospitals themselves, and with community hospitals in bitter price wars, it may turn out to have been wise for these two major hospitals of the Harvard community to join forces. While competing for service contracts (with HMOs or insurance carriers), neighboring hospitals can literally destroy themselves in an effort to ensure occupancy by reducing their day rates and consequently their income. When the era of increased commercialization of American medicine began (about 1975), this self-destructive outcome could scarcely have been predicted. Now, mergers between competitors are an obvious survival strategy being followed in several cities, eliciting a countervailing merger of HMOs, indemnity carriers, and other health-care brokers.

The Brigham-MGH affiliation of 1994 would never have occurred without the prior merger of four hospitals to form the present Brigham and Women's Hospital (BWH), as related in this chapter. The former Peter Bent Brigham

Hospital, with only 250 beds and a shaky financial structure, would not have been a very attractive corporate partner for the huge MGH. If this new merger turns out to be a successful venture in American hospital history, those of us who worked over so many years to bring about the earlier merger creating the BWH will be gratified at this new flowering of our efforts. The continuing growth of the BWH and the success of its mission after its long and laborious birth are due in no small part to the leadership of John McArthur, dean of the Harvard Business School and Chairman of our Board, and of H. Richard Nesson, a native Brighamite who is currently the President and C.E.O.

Looking back on the merger of 1958 to 1980 that brought the four hospitals together to form the BWH, the role of Stan Deland and his fellow hospital presidents is mentioned in the text, as well as the Deans of the medical school in that period (Berry, Ebert, and Tosteson). The account would be incomplete without telling of the remarkably important role of all the department heads in addition to George Smith (gynecology), Duncan Reid (obstetrics), and George Thorn (medicine). Herbert Abrams had been a catalyst for new departures in radiology, Leroy Vandam in anesthesia, Gustave Dammin in pathology, K. Frank Austen in rheumatology, and, as their successors came on the scene with enthusiasm for the new undertaking, Eugene Braunwald in medicine, Kenneth Ryan in obstetrics, Ramzi Cotran in pathology, and Harry Mellins in radiology. Marion Metcalf in nursing, Mary Ellen Collins in nutrition, and Maureen Mac Burney in intravenous feeding services, all of the Brigham staff, took overall responsibility in the new undertaking. Most of these stalwarts who implemented a successful merger of four of Harvard's teaching hospitals to form the BWH are now at or after retirement. A few have died. To all of them the BWH, and now the new BWH-MGH Partners, owes an immense debt of gratitude.

While our decades-long effort to achieve the four-hospital merger was not undertaken with any national objective in mind, it became a part of the national trend to join smaller hospitals together (particularly specialty hospitals) in order to provide a better balance of services more economically to the public. This was and still remains an important objective in national health policy.

As the commercial interests of hospitals have become more dominant, and insurance support of their patient care costs more essential to survival, mergers of smaller community hospitals and private clinics have become increasingly frequent. By regional merger these institutions can maintain a higher level of bed occupancy than they could as single units forced into destructive price competition. Protection of census (i.e., the fraction of beds in use) is overcoming the time-honored avoidance of merger noted among community hospitals at the start of this chapter.

This is an appropriate place to note, however briefly, several other undertakings in health policy that occupied my attention at various periods over the past 25 years: the Study on Surgical Services for the United States, the Harvard Community Health Plan, the Brigham Surgical Group, the Kennedy School of Government, and the Massachusetts Health Data Consortium.

The *Study on Surgical Services for the United States* (SOSSUS) had its origin in several meetings of the Committee on Issues of the American Surgical Association in 1970 and 1971. These led to an uneasy alliance with the much larger American College of Surgeons, based in Chicago and operated by a full-time staff. The two organizations (one small, senior, and voluntary; the other large, all ages, and run professionally) together sponsored and financed this study. George Zuidema, Professor and Head of the Department of Surgery at Johns Hopkins, directed the study. He asked me to join him as co-director of the project and to be in charge of the largest subsidiary section of the study, United States Health Manpower in Surgery.

We enlisted an active group at the Harvard School of Public Health under Professor Osler Peterson and Rita Nickerson, principal research associate (biostatistician), who joined to look at many aspects of surgical training and daily practice. Several years later the massive report was published, as well as its widely available summary:

American College of Surgeons and the American Surgical Association. 1975. *Surgery in the United States: A Summary Report of the Study on Surgical Services for the United States. The Short Form Report.* Baltimore: ACS/ASA.

Several other publications emerged from this study, which was a broad survey of surgeons' activities:

Nickerson, R.J., T. Colton, O.L. Peterson, B.S. Bloom, and W.W. Hauck, Jr. 1976. Doctors who perform operations. A study on in-hospital surgery in four diverse geographic areas. *N. Engl. J. Med.* 295:921–926 and 982–989.

Hauck, W.W., Jr., B.S. Bloom, C.K. McPherson, R.J. Nickerson, T. Colton, and O.L. Peterson. 1976. Surgeons in the United States. *JAMA* 236:1864–1871.

At that time many surgeons were underemployed and their services underutilized. A large number of surgeons were being trained in the residency pipeline, and it was recommended that there be some downregulation of surgical trainee numbers, achieved principally by raising the standards set by the credentialing agencies (the American Boards). This recommendation was not popular. Amidst bitterness that had an adverse impact on me and on the members of our study unit, an attempt was made to discredit the entire study. This attempt was unfortunate and misinformed. Government agencies and later the American College of Surgeons itself became aware of the undesirable effect of an oversupply of surgeons on patient care and costs. Despite this adversity, the importance of assessing the size and training of qualified surgeons in the United States seemed clear. We therefore continued, over the next two decades, to issue periodic status reports on accredited surgical manpower (and now womanpower) in the United States:

Moore, F.D., C.M. Boyden, D. Sabiston, R. Warren, O.L. Peterson, R. Zeppa, D. Heer, and N. Murthy. 1972. The production, attrition, and biologic lifetime of surgeons in relation to the population of the United States: a look into the future through the clouded computer crystal. *Ann. Surg.* 176:457-468.

Moore, F.D., and S.M. Lang. 1981. Board-certified physicians in the United States. Specialty distribution and policy implications of trends during the past decade. *N. Engl. J. Med.* 304:1078-1084.

Moore, F.D. 1982. A community-size model for physician distribution in the United States (Parts I and II). *J. Clin. Surg.* 1:162-173 and 242-255.

Moore, F.D., and C. Priebe. 1991. Board-certified physicians in the United States, 1971-1986. *N. Engl. J. Med.* 324:536-543.

These 20 years have seen some striking changes. After the steep upsweep in the 1970s in numbers of total physicians and percentage of those in surgery, there has been a plateau and most recently a decline in the growth rate of surgery. This has been due to the decline in the number of foreign medical graduates licensed in the United States, an increase in specialty surgery (with a sharp decline in the number of general surgeons), and the growth of two entirely new fields of surgical endeavor that mandate extra training: cardiac surgery and transplantation.

The number of surgeons required by a population is determined by (and sharply limited by) the epidemiology (i.e., the prevalence) of those diseases treatable by surgery. This is a finite need that changes but slowly over decades. A continued sharp eye on the numbers, distribution, and activity of qualified surgeons is essential for any new initiatives in health-care reform in the United States. As I look back on this difficult and, for me, traumatic effort to hold to that standard, I regret only my inability to sell the importance of this work to a few of my colleagues. I was buoyed by the support of thousands of surgeons who by letters or words of support upheld its importance and validity. I was elected President of the American Surgical Association in 1973.

The *Harvard Community Health Plan* (HCHP) grew out of the efforts of Dean Ebert and Jerome Pollack (an experienced labor organizer) to establish in the mid 1960s an academic-based, staff-model, nonprofit, prepaid health delivery plan, later termed a health maintenance organization, or HMO. Our hospital was asked to make available all our residents and emergency staffing provisions (without extra pay) for the subscribers to HCHP.

George Thorn and I complied, but on one major condition: that the benefits of HCHP be made available to all segments of our society. Our nearest neighbors to the south were the minority residents of Mission Hill and Roxbury. They must be included somehow and by some reimbursal mechanism. We did not wish to sponsor another large private clinic serving the middle class on the Mayo or Lahey model, worthy though they were for their time and purpose.

This breadth of coverage became possible because the Office of Economic Opportunity was active at that time as a federal agency sponsoring some healthcare financing for the poor. Our residents, students, and staff would clearly benefit from the added experience and teaching value of this new kind of health mandate in our community.

Gordon Vineyard of our staff has become the Director of Surgery for HCHP. Many staff in all fields, as well as in all the nearby hospitals, now participate in what has become a giant HMO. The care made available to subscribers is excellent thanks to Vineyard and his colleagues, and the plan has prospered. While I have some reservations about what seem to be increasingly restrictive insurance constraints on membership status for patients in the plan, and while many HMOs have drifted downstream, away from the all-inclusive ideals and nonprofit status of their inception, I believe HCHP is a credit to Dean Bob Ebert, Jerry Pollack, George Thorn, and myself, as well as the hundreds of others who joined in its establishment so many years ago. In those ancient times our Dean was a man of vision.

Another matter of medical economics and practice policy, even closer to home, was the organization of the *Brigham Surgical Group* (BSG). After several years of planning, the BSG began its work as a partnership of all the members of our department in 1969. This was the first department-wide faculty group practice in the Harvard Medical School. By pooling the business functions in a central office under a full-time director, we could handle the blizzard of paperwork much more efficiently than in multiple solo practices. At the same time, we could make funds available to younger staff for start-up research as well as provide "perks" and new retirement benefits for the senior staff. Mr. David Heider was our first chief financial officer, followed in 1972 by Douglas MacGregor, who has brought this office to a state of perfection in fiscal management. I am especially grateful to John Brooks, Richard Wilson, and Hartwell Harrison, who helped me draw up the constitution for this group practice, and to the entire staff for their unanimous espousal and support of this project, now about 25 years of age.

One of my most interesting opportunities in the field of health policy was that of working with some of the faculty at the *Kennedy School of Government*, which in the mid 1970s listed health-care analysis and reform as one of several prongs in their multipronged thrust into the areas of sociological and governmental teaching and research.

During that period, Christopher Zook, a doctoral candidate, came to work with me. I had been impressed by the category of illnesses that became extremely expensive to manage because those afflicted must be repeatedly admitted to the hospital for further treatment of an ongoing disease process. These "repeaters" were not patients with cancer or stroke, most of whom sadly died too soon to require extraordinarily expensive care; rather, they were often found to be suffering from more benign but longstanding diseases such as chronic cardiovascular disease, congenital anomalies, diabetes, or chronic neurological or mental impairment. Zook set about a systematic study of this phenomenon and turned it into his thesis, entitled "The High-Cost Users of Medical Care"—an expression that was soon taken up by other workers and became the subject of several subsequent papers:

Zook, C.J. 1979. The high-cost users of medical care. A thesis presented to the Kennedy School of Government for the degree of Doctor of Philosophy in the subject of Public Policy. Cambridge: Harvard University.

Zook, C.J., and F.D. Moore. 1980. High-cost users of medical care. *N. Engl. J. Med.* 302:996-1002.

Zook, C.J., S.F. Savickas, and F.D. Moore. 1980. Repeated hospitalization for the same disease: a multiplier of national health costs. *Milbank Memorial Fund Quarterly/Health and Society* 58:454-471.

Zook, C.J., F.D. Moore, and R.J. Zeckhauser. 1981. "Catastrophic" health insurance: a misguided prescription? *Public Interest* 62(Winter):66-81.

At the same time Chris was working on this aspect of health-care policy, I was beginning my search for hidden causes of expense in U.S. medical care. This led to an examination of the prevalence of profit-making enterprises within American medicine, initially described in an article in the *Harvard Magazine*:

Moore, F.D. 1985. Who should profit from the care of your illness? *Harvard Magazine* Nov-Dec:45-54.

This has been a continuing quest and has led to a conviction that corporate profits in our health-care budget are a cost-multiplying factor virtually unique to the United States. Control of such profits, largely those of insurance companies, would lower the fraction of our Gross National Product devoted to medical care to a level comparable to costs in Europe, Canada, Australia, and New Zealand. As this book is being prepared, we are working with a group at the Harvard School of Public Health seeking to nail down some of the data on profiteering from American medicine—a pursuit that might lead to important national economies. In any such analysis, charitable teaching hospitals and physicians themselves (two groups that have usually been held as largely blameless in the profit matrix) emerge from their cloak of righteousness. Such hospitals accumulated huge surpluses in the 1980s and early 1990s, and some physicians' incomes have soared to a level that many regard as excessive.

Roe, B.B. 1981. The UCR boondoggle: a death knell for private practice? (Sounding Board). *N. Engl. J. Med.* 305:41-45.

The *Massachusetts Health Data Consortium* was established in 1978 by the major public and private health care organizations of the Commonwealth of Massachusetts to provide a standard data set to monitor their occupancy, case mix, and adequacy of service to the public. Elliot M. Stone, a gifted worker in this highly specialized field, has been the executive director since its founding.

Paul M. Densen, professor of community health and medical care, emeritus, was the first president and I, the second (1981 to 1987). This important neutral turf in the "number wars" of health-care providers is needed in every state. It is often done by government. A nongovernmental neutrality seems preferable. I congratulate Elliot Stone and my two successors, Frederick W. Ackroyd (1987 to 1993) and Alvin R. Tarlov, beginning his term in 1994, on their continued refinement of our knowledge of how the hospitals of our state behave.

CHAPTER 31—A Nobel Prize for Joseph Murray (1990)

Accounts of the life of Alfred Nobel and some lore about the Prize and its history are to be found in the following:

Crawford, E.T. 1984. *The Beginnings of the Nobel Institution; The Science Prizes, 1901-1915.* New York: Cambridge University Press.
Crawford, E.T. 1987. *The Nobel Population 1901-1937.* Berkeley: University of California Press.
Sourkes, T.L. 1967. *Nobel Prize Winners in Medicine & Physiology, 1901-1965.* London: Abelard-Schuman.

Recently, a new biography of Nobel has appeared that emphasizes the breadth of his scientific interest:

Fant, K. 1993. *Alfred Nobel: A Biography.* New York: Arcade (distributed by Little, Brown).

Joseph Murray's address on receiving the Nobel award is cited on page 396. At the time of this Award to Dr. Murray, I was asked to describe some of the background at a meeting of the New England Surgical Society:

Moore, F.D. 1992. A Nobel Award to Joseph E. Murray, M.D.: some historical perspectives. *Arch. Surg.* 127:627-632.

CHAPTER 32—Ethics at Both Ends of Life

In the history of science, each new age regards itself as making new and sweeping advances that will revolutionize the world. Each also sees itself as operating with an improved and enlightened ethical view on the relationships between human beings. Accordingly, we regard the second half of this century as absolutely preeminent in both regards: scientific and ethical progress. Within 100 years we will surely be shown to have been operating under some sort of a delusion.

Any ascending logarithmic curve describes a hyperbola, the most recent portion of which appears as a steeply upsweeping slope. Then with longer time coordinates leading to a later date, that steep upswing disappears into the background slope and a more recent upswing appears. That is in the nature of the graphic representation on linear coordinates of any exponential progression or logarithmic hyperbola.

Thus, each age regards itself as the paragon of science. To paraphrase a popular statement, "In the last 50 years more new scientific facts have been discovered than in all previous world history." This same statement could have been made any time in the past 300 years. The same secular conceit is found in ethics. At the founding of this country, the most important new ethical concepts were "all men are created equal" and a government should be directed toward "life, liberty and the pursuit of happiness" of its citizens, remarkable rhetoric from a nation beset with slavery and a subjugated population devoid of opportunity, education, wealth, or equal protection under the law. One of the byproducts of Lincoln's presidency, the Civil War, and the freeing of the slaves was a new ethical view toward citizens with black skin. Who knows what future ethical insights or retrospective judgments will lead to revised opinions about our views of right and wrong today?

Some landmark papers on ethics include the following. In 1966 Henry K. Beecher pointed to the ethical lapses clearly displayed in the published literature on medical research:

Beecher, H.K. 1966. Ethics and clinical research. *N. Engl. J. Med.* 274:1354-1360.

Shortly thereafter, Beecher chaired the Commission that defined death as being the irreversible cessation of cerebral function:

Beecher, H.K., chair. 1968. Report of the Ad Hoc Committee of the Harvard Medical School to Examine the Definition of Brain Death: a definition of irreversible coma. *JAMA* 205:85-88.

Both these publications of Beecher helped the medical community reach a more enlightened understanding of the ethical aspects of their work and of the need for public education about organ donation.

In 1968, during a symposium of the American Academy of Arts and Sciences on clinical experimentation, I spoke about the ethical problems of doing new things for the first time in the treatment of the sick. To innovate is essential for advance. How best can it be done? With what safeguards?

Moore, F.D. 1969. Therapeutic innovation: ethical boundaries in the initial clinical trials of new drugs and surgical procedures. *Daedalus* 98:502-522.

Other articles of mine on ethics and safeguards:

Moore, F.D. 1960. Symposium on the study of drugs in man. II. Biological and medical studies in human volunteer subjects; ethics and safeguards. *Clin. Pharmacol. Ther.* 1:149-155.

Moore, F.D. 1965. Ethics in new medicine. Tissue transplants. *Nation* 200:358-362.

Those who would stop the use of animals for research profess that they are motivated by ethical considerations. While the antivivisectionists are critical of scientists who use animals for experiments, they themselves daily violate the fundamental biblical ethic, "Do unto thy neighbor...." They refuse to engage in the discourse so essential to human relationships and the evolution of more lasting ethical values. On one occasion an executive of one of the antivivisection societies ssaid to me, "Dr. Moore, we don't want to win. But we don't want to lose either. All we want to do is keep the fight going because that's the way we raise our money." Since the antivivisectionists avoid public discourse with their opponents, preferring instead a blanket condemnation of those with other views, we do not have a chance to ask them what they would think of doing a new and hazardous operation to help a child without first testing it in laboratory animals.

Antivivisectionists and creationists are part of the anti-intellectual fringe of our society. They are not going to go away. In one form or another they—or other zealots of the fringe—have always been out there and always will be. Our most important function is to educate the public about the ways in which such people recruit the young and impede the growth of biological science in the care of the sick.

Marcia Angell, executive editor of *The New England Journal of Medicine*, has taken a firm stand on the need for physicians to confront and embrace the deeply felt emotions of patients who find life a burden because of pain and hopelessness. She has written a statement on this:

Angell, M. 1993. The right to die. *Bull. Am. Acad. Arts Sci.* 46:12-30.

Two recent statements further clarify the problem of physician-assisted death:

Cohen, J.S., S.D. Fihn, E.J. Boyko, A.R. Jonsen, and R.W. Wood. 1994. Attitudes toward assisted suicide and euthanasia among physicians in Washington State. *N. Engl. J. Med.* 331:89-94.

Miller, F.G, T.E. Quill, H. Brody, J.C. Fletcher, L.O. Gostin, and D.E. Meier. 1994. Regulating physician-assisted death. *N. Engl. J. Med.* 331:119-123.

The stories of patients in this chapter and this reference to Dr. Angell's work is a fitting way to close the scientific narrative of this book. New views of ethics and new scientific understanding are needed to move ahead in solving this problem of today in such a way that the solution will still be acceptable tomorrow. Breaking this barrier and enabling doctors to help with merciful death will be an ethical advance of which any generation can be proud. Maybe it will be the next generation. It certainly was not ours.

Termination of both pregnancy (at the start of life) and hopeless suffering (at the end of life) polarizes public opinion in similar ways, as mentioned in the text: free choice for self versus stubborn protection of all life. The two have another interesting common ground: they will be done whether we like it or not, whether or not the church opposes them, with or without legislative approval. This makes clear our job as physicians: we must help make these sad terminations, either of pregnancy or of suffering, clean, safe, and sure.

CHAPTER 34—Laura's Death; A New Life with Katharyn

Before Laura's death, she and I spent several years gathering the histories of the four grandparental families that together made up our genealogy:

Moore, F.D., and L.B. Moore. 1986. *Bartlett-Daniels-Huston-Moore; A Family Journey (Book I, Moderns; Book II, Ancestors; Book III, Potpourri; Book IV, Sources).* Boston, private printing.

Katharyn Watson Saltonstall's book about her years in Africa is based on her service there with her husband, William Gurdon Saltonstall, who in 1963 was asked by President Kennedy and Sargent Shriver (head of the Peace Corps) to be the Peace Corps representative in Nigeria. This was one of the largest of the Peace Corps efforts, with 750 volunteers under their supervision. Her book tells not only of the challenges and achievements of the Peace Corps, but also of some of the crises, illnesses, and even deaths in this service:

Saltonstall, K.W. 1986. *Small Bridges to One World.* Portsmouth, NH: Peter Randall.

Prior to their African adventure, William Saltonstall had been on the faculty of Phillips Exeter Academy for 32 years, the last 16 as Principal, succeeding Lewis Perry in that post. The biography of Perry was a collaborative project of Bill and Katharyn, just as were their Exeter years:

Saltonstall, W.G. 1980. *Lewis Perry of Exeter: A Gentle Memoir.* (Foreword by David McCord.) New York: Atheneum Books.

CHAPTER 36—Cool Streams, High Mountains, White Faces: Looking Back

With poetic nostalgia, Joseph Conrad wrote about Youth:

Conrad, J. 1923. *Youth.* Garden City, NY: Doubleday, Page & Co.

This book is sometimes referred to as "Conrad in quest of his youth"—a phrase that became a metaphor for nostalgic revisitations of any sort, such as ours to Wyoming in recent years.

Conrad wrote: *Only a moment; a moment of strength, of romance, of glamour—of youth!... A flick of sunshine upon a strange shore, the time to remember, the time for a sigh, and—Goodbye!—Night—Goodbye—!*

Photo Credits

Plate numbers appear in parentheses.

Class of 1931 (Pl. 3)	Courtesy of North Shore Country Day School
Harvard Lampoon cover (Pl. 4)	Courtesy of David B. Little
Return of the bulldog (Pl. 4)	AP/Wide World Photos; *The New York Times*, March 26, 1934
Certificate of Attendance (Pl. 6)	Courtesy of Francis A. Countway Library of Medicine
Warren's bill for services (Pl. 6)	Courtesy of Thomas Jansen
Portrait of W. Cannon (Pl. 7)	Courtesy of Harvard Medical School (Artist: Page)
Dean C.S. Burwell (Pl. 7)	Courtesy of Francis A. Countway Library of Medicine
C.E. Welch (Pl. 8)	*Modern Medicine*, with permission
R. Warren (Pl. 8)	Courtesy of Mrs. Richard Warren
A.B. Hastings (Pl. 8)	Courtesy of Francis A. Countway Library of Medicine
L.S. McKittrick (Pl. 9)	Courtesy of Francis A. Countway Library of Medicine
MGH White Building (Pl. 9)	Courtesy of 1939 *Aesculapiad*

F. Albright (Pl. 9)	Courtesy of Francis A. Countway Library of Medicine
E.D. Churchill (Pl. 9)	Courtesy of Dr. J. Gordon Scannell; with permission from the Francis A. Countway Library of Medicine
Cocoanut Grove (Pl. 10)	AP/Wide World Photos, with permission
Rabbit (Pl. 10)	*Journal of Clinical Investigation,* 1942, Vol XXI, p. 474, copyright 1942, The Society for Clinical Investigation
Moore Pavilion (Pl. 11)	Photo by Brad Herzog
J.H. Harrison (Pl. 11)	Courtesy of Francis A. Countway Library of Medicine
F.S. Deland (Pl. 12)	Courtesy of Mrs. F.S. Deland
J.E. Dunphy (Pl. 13)	Courtesy of Francis A. Countway Library of Medicine
G.J. Dammin (Pl. 13)	Courtesy of Francis A. Countway Library of Medicine
1934 PBBH aerial view (Pl. 14)	Courtesy of Brigham and Women's Hospital Archives
1994 BWH aerial view (Pl. 15)	Photo by Joseph Melanson
Moore, Mannick, and Tilney (Pl. 17)	Photo by John Nordell
Adolph Watzka (Pl. 17)	Courtesy of Francis A. Countway Library of Medicine; photo by Arthur Griffin
J.R. Brooks (Pl. 17)	Photo by Richard Sobol
Nobel ceremony (Pl. 18)	Courtesy of Dr. Joseph P. Murray
D.M. Hume (Pl. 18)	Courtesy of Mrs. Marshall K. Bartlett
Herrick operation (Pl. 18)	Courtesy of Dr. Joseph P. Murray
Twin leaving hospital (Pl. 19)	Courtesy of Dr. Joseph P. Murray
Calne and Starzl (Pl. 19)	Courtesy of *Cambridge Evening News*
Urine attribution (Pl. 19)	Courtesy of Dr. Joseph P. Murray
Transplanted dogs (Pl. 19)	Courtesy of Dr. Joseph P. Murray
Moore and Tosteson (Pl. 20)	Photo by John Nordell

Dean G.P. Berry (Pl. 20)   Courtesy of Francis A. Countway
                               Library of Medicine
Merrill and Murray (Pl. 20)   Courtesy of Dr. Joseph P. Murray
R.H. Ebert (Pl. 20)   Courtesy of Francis A. Countway
                               Library of Medicine
Edinburgh degree (Pl. 21)   Courtesy of University of Edinburgh,
                               with permission from The Scotsman
                               Publications, Ltd.
Korea, helicopter (Pl. 21)   Courtesy of Dr. John M. Howard
Korea, admitting (Pl. 21)   Courtesy of Dr. John M. Howard
Cover of *Time* (Pl. 21)   © 1963 Time Inc. Reprinted by
                               permission.
Moore and Vandam (Pl. 22)   Courtesy of *Focus*, published by
                               Harvard Medical School Office of
                               Public Affairs, June 5, 1980
1990 Wedding (Pl. 24)   Photo by Jane MacDonald

Also by
Francis D. Moore

Moore, F.D., and M.R. Ball. 1952.
The Metabolic Response to Surgery.
Springfield, IL: Charles C Thomas.

Jessiman, A.G., and F.D. Moore. 1956.
Carcinoma of the Breast: The Study and Treatment of the Patient.
Boston: Little, Brown.

Moore, F.D. 1959.
Metabolic Care of the Surgical Patient.
Philadelphia: W.B. Saunders Co.

Moore, F.D., K.H. Olesen, J.D. McMurrey, H.V. Parker,
M.R. Ball, and C.M. Boyden. 1963.
*The Body Cell Mass and Its Supporting Environment:
Body Composition in Health and Disease.*
Philadelphia: W.B. Saunders Co.

Moore, F.D. 1964.
Give and Take. The Development of Tissue Transplantation.
Philadelphia: W.B. Saunders Co.

Moore, F.D., S.I. Woodrow, M.A. Aliapoulios, and R.E. Wilson. 1967.
Carcinoma of the Breast.
(A monograph based on a Medical Progress Report
in the *New England Journal of Medicine.*)
London: J. & A. Churchill Ltd., Distributed by Little, Brown.

Moore, F.D., J.H. Lyons, Jr., E.C. Pierce, Jr., A.P. Morgan, Jr.,
P.A. Drinker, J.D. MacArthur, and G.J. Dammin.
*Post-Traumatic Pulmonary Insufficiency: Pathophysiology of Respiratory
Failure and Principles of Respiratory Care After Surgical Operations,
Trauma, Hemorrhage, Burns, and Shock.*
Philadelphia: W.B. Saunders Co.

Moore, F.D. 1972.
Transplant: The Give and Take of Tissue Transplantation (Revised Edition).
New York: Simon and Schuster.

Index